T0183194

Emerging Drugs in Sport

Olivier Rabin • Ornella Corazza

Editors

Emerging Drugs in Sport

Forewords by Witold Banka and Claude Guillou

With contributions by Elisabeth Prevete

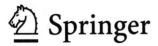 Springer

Editors
Olivier Rabin
Science and Medicine Department
World Anti-Doping Agency (WADA)
Montreal, QC, Canada

Ornella Corazza
Department of Clinical, Pharmaceutical and
Biological Sciences, School of Life and
Medical Sciences
University of Hertfordshire
Hatfield, Hertfordshire, UK

ISBN 978-3-030-79295-4   ISBN 978-3-030-79293-0   (eBook)
https://doi.org/10.1007/978-3-030-79293-0

This Springer imprint is published by the registered company Springer Nature Switzerland AG
The registered company address is: Gewerbestrasse 11, 6330 Cham, Switzerland

"Doping remains one of the greatest threats to the integrity of sport. We must never be tempted to turn our back on the problem and hope it will disappear.

At this moment in particular, the benefits of clean sport and the values it can bring to the world have never been more important. That is why this book with such a wide-ranging approach with experts from so many different fields is so valuable."

Thomas Bach, President, International Olympic Committee

"Physical activity is a vital part of healthy living, which is why doping in sport is not just an assault on fair competition, it's an assault on health. I strongly commend the impressive set of authors of this book for compiling the most advanced knowledge on emerging performance-enhancing drugs and for promoting health through sport."

Tedros Adhanom Ghebreyesus, Director-General, World Health Organization

In Memoriam of Auguste RABIN
(1933–2020) who always nurtured my
interest in science by showing me the
intrinsic beauty and the practical side of it.
O. RABIN

Foreword by Witold Banka

When tackling the issue of doping in sport, there is no single solution. One individual or interested body cannot make an impact without collaborating with all others within the anti-doping community to ensure equity and fairness. "Play true" represents more than a tag line for the World Anti-Doping Agency (WADA) as it encapsulates our core values of integrity, openness, and excellence, intended as guiding principle for all athletes at every level of competition. In that collaborative spirit, this important book explores the rapidly evolving doping landscape by examining emerging substances from various angles. It looks at how performance-enhancing drugs have been used in the past and in the present day, how anti-doping organizations, such as the WADA, have brought consistency to the regulatory framework within clean sport, but also the broader societal trends towards drug use, the prevalence of the win-at-all-cost mentality among many elite athletes and coaches, and an exploration of the challenges faced by the authorities in detecting and successfully prosecuting those who would take drugs to cheat the system. As a former sports minister of Poland and athlete at the international level, it was a great privilege for me to assume the presidency of WADA on 1 January 2020 and to become part of its mission to lead a collaborative worldwide movement for doping-free sport. In 2019, WADA celebrated its 20th anniversary. It has been two decades of progress, improvement and, of course, plenty of complex challenges. It is remarkable to think of how far WADA and, by extension, global anti-doping efforts have come in that short time. Back in the 1990s, there was no single approach to tackling doping in sport. Every sport had different rules. Countries had diverging laws. An athlete could be, for example, banned in one nation or sport but able to compete in others. Following a number of major doping scandals in sport, WADA was founded in 1999 as a unique 50-50 partnership between the Sports Movement and Governments of the world to promote, coordinate, and monitor activities towards the prevention, deterrence, and detection of doping. WADA's key activities include development of regulations, monitoring of compliance, and enforcement including through investigations. We also play a critical role facilitating scientific research, education, and capacity-building for athletes and anti-doping stakeholders. The backbone of our work is the World Anti-Doping Programme that is comprised of the

World Anti-Doping Code (the Code), International Standards and Guidelines, which together aim to ensure harmonization and best practice by almost 700 Code Signatories around the world. In parallel, the UNESCO Convention Against Doping in Sport that was adopted in 2005 provides public authorities with a legal framework to recognize the Code. Through the Convention, Governments can address specific areas of doping that are outside the domain of the Sports Movement. The Convention is now ratified by 191 countries, covering more than 99% of the world's population. Since the early days, the Code and International Standards have been revised three times following exhaustive consultation with all WADA stakeholders. The new versions, which were approved by WADA's Foundation Board and Executive Committee, respectively, in November 2019, came into force on 1 January 2021 and are further strengthening the World Anti-Doping Programme. WADA is leading the way, taking steps to tackle the issues with agility and innovation across all facets of anti-doping, not least in the area of emerging drugs. Through the consistent implementation of key initiatives, WADA is moving towards its vision of a future where all athletes can participate in a doping-free sporting environment. To do this, we continuously monitor trends, annually review the list of prohibited substances and methods, embrace innovation, and develop partnerships with leaders in various fields. Athletes and sports organizations now benefit from internationally harmonized rules, compliance and enforcement processes, and a network of partners to ensure that they are implemented in every corner of the world. There are not many aspects of modern life that have achieved the level of international cooperation of anti-doping. The end result is that we have a system that works well, despite numerous challenges. And that is the key—cooperation. In order to effectively lead an ambitious mission like the protection of clean sport, WADA knows that it needs to collaborate and work with a disparate group of experts, whether they are athletes, Government officials, sports administrators, regulators, scientists, educators, lawyers, law enforcement officers, those within the pharmaceutical industry, and many others. That is why this important book related to emerging drugs in sport resonates with me. The challenge of drugs in sport is not one posed exclusively to sport itself. It is clearly and inextricably tied up with the wider problem of drug abuse and misuse in society as a whole. The solutions, therefore, cannot be proposed and implemented by one group but will require the will, dedication, and investment of all those aforementioned groups as they join forces to protect sport, society, and the health of athletes. This excellent book brings together high-profile authors from various fields, united in the common goal of learning more about these substances and how they can threaten individuals, families, sports, and society, and what we can do about it, working together. Through cooperation, collaboration, and a global perspective, I believe we can overcome the scourge of drugs in society and, in the process, protect our values and the integrity of the sports we love.

Witold Banka
President, World Anti-Doping Agency
Montreal, QC, Canada

Foreword by Claude Guillou

I welcome the publication of this book and its multi-faceted approach to the phenomenon of doping and emerging drugs in sport.

The natural conclusion in Part VI is "The Next Challenge", which discusses what can be expected for the future. The size of that challenge can already be gauged from the various contributions gathered in the previous sections which provide an overview of the current complexity of the situation of drugs and doping in sports.

From untested or contaminated sports supplements to gene manipulations, the enhancement of performance in sports can involve a wide range of practices enabled by existing scientific knowledge and techniques.

As a consequence, the legal frame for controls and the international regulatory environment need to keep pace with the swift evolution of science and technology. For instance, the increase in the number of novel psychoactive substances (NPS) requires a continuous update of data by the international bodies in charge of monitoring these compounds. The testing laboratories also need to remain well-equipped and at the forefront of the detection technology.

The athlete remains the central actor in this environment. At the start of their career, as with many young adults, they may be easily influenced and persuaded to make choices without fully understanding the long-term consequences. When fully informed, they can take the right decisions for themselves, and also behave as examples for others.

All these aspects are well-presented and discussed by the eminent contributions and testimonies of the authors of this book.

Sophisticated doping practices are likely to remain within the sphere of world-class athletes and professional sport. In addition, the broad range and availability of a number of substances easily purchased through the internet is a growing concern also for amateur sport and beyond that also constitutes a threat to public health in general.

However, the voices of the athletes and their resonance in our society of mass communication and social media can play a central role in the fight against this threat if the right messages are disseminated.

Therefore, "Emerging Drugs in Sport", considered by some to be the problem of only a few, is not only relevant to specialists and professionals in sport, but it also speaks to each and every one of us. It may also help us to reflect on our own choices for our society regarding education of our younger generations, our public health, and our way of life in general.

I congratulate the editors, Ornella Corazza and Olivier Rabin, and all the authors who accepted to share their invaluable experience in the fields of anti-doping and new drugs. The book *Emerging Drugs in Sport* will make us better prepared for the next challenges to be faced in that very dynamic area.

Claude Guillou
European Commission, Directorate General Joint Research Centre,
Directorate F – Health, Consumers and Reference Materials
Ispra, Italy

Preface

We live in a world where an increase in the use of drugs has been recorded among those engaged with physical activities, mainly to alter bodily functions, boost their stamina, enhance muscle growth, or reduce body fat and weight. How many times have we read or heard this in magazines, reports, or discussed this phenomenon in expert conferences or symposia? Our contemporary societies are pushing individuals to constantly optimize or improve their performances and achievements in all sectors of life. However, the constant quest for optimal mental and physical well-being often contradicts the reality of professional lives, where performance maximization is the norm and the line between work and personal life has never been so blurred.

Caught by frenetic and digitalized lifestyles, technological advances, and cultural pressures on physical appearance, individuals are more inclined to use drugs to achieve their professional or personal goals, at a time when access to these pharmacological aids has never been so easy. Over the past decade, there has been a dramatic increase in the number of novel psychoactive substances (NPS) being discovered and synthetized across the world, with over 850 illicit compounds now identified globally by the United Nations Office on Drugs and Crime (UNODC). According to UNODC, NPS can be defined as substances of abuse, either in a pure form or a preparation, that are not controlled by international conventions, but which may pose a public health threat. However, the scope of this book encompasses a more global range of emerging drugs, which extend beyond the NPS categories listed above and includes any newly identified substances not approved by the public health authorities and being distributed as a single or combined active principle in one or more products via the Internet or elsewhere. Sometimes, consumers can be exposed to these by incidence, in particular when found in accessible preparations or fitness supplements. A wide range of sport foods (e.g., gels, bars, drinks, protein powders), ergogenic, herbal and botanical supplements, vitamins, minerals, amino acids, among other substances are often advertised with misleading marketing strategies as "natural" and "safer" alternatives to pharmaceutical products to improve performance (boost your energy, endurance, or muscle strength), physical appearance (lose fat or increase muscle mass) and well-being (sleep or recovery), making this a highly profitable business. Despite constant warnings from public or regulatory authorities, it appears that the dietary supplement industry benefits from lenient regulations in some countries exposing consumers to potentially dangerous substances, leading to unwanted side effects. Overall, applying the principle that the supply of emerging drugs exists because it meets an existing demand, we can safely conclude that a growing proportion of individuals in our societies is constituted by avid occasional or regular consumers of such illegal substances. The world of sport, which in essence represents only a microcosm of our larger society, is not immune to this general increasing drug trend. Even if athletes traditionally represent role models for a healthy lifestyle, and this remains valid for the vast majority of them, their exposure to a new wide range of fitness-enhancing drugs is a logical consequence of such new trends in society. The high pressure to constantly perform at elite level from training to major sport events, including often in their personal life, may negatively influence a fringe of the vulnerable athletic population and encourage them to use drugs outside or in the field of play. Sport authorities are acutely aware of the situation and consider doping in sport as the most serious threat to contemporary sport. The World Anti-Doping Agency (WADA) was established in 1999 to tackle doping in sport at the international level under all its forms. It was acknowledged both by the international sport movement and the public authorities that the issue of doping in sport was too complex to be tackled by one side alone, and a joint and coordinated effort in the form of an independent and dedicated agency was required to efficiently address this major issue. From the onset, WADA took the strong position of proactively banning all substances, known or unknown at present, falling under well-identified categories of performance-enhancing drugs, including but not limited to steroids, stimulants, and cannabinoids. This proactive approach was a strategy to position anti-doping rules ahead of the doping scheme and logically brought WADA into interactions and collaborations with other international organizations involved in the field of drugs of abuse. Beyond the aspects of performance enhancement and the risk to the essential value of fairness in sport, the protection of the health of the athletes is part of the World Anti-Doping Code, one of the founding documents applied by all organizations actively fighting against doping in sport.

While the global threat posed by emerging drugs is growing, the role played by the inter-sector collaboration between several international, public, law enforcement authorities, and academia has become of paramount importance in assessing the global risk and tackling such a complex phenomenon. So far joint efforts and resources have been mobilized to better understand, monitor, and prevent the deleterious health impact of emerging drugs on human beings, leading to the establishment of the International Society for the Study of Emerging Drugs (ISSED) among other initiatives.

In an age of global insecurity, it would be an illusion to believe that one organization alone could efficiently defy the tentacular criminal organizations, or the individual illegal initiatives, that are implanted around the world and support the development, manufacturing, and distribution of emerging drugs. More concrete operations in the field have taken place in recent years across different organizations to dismantle illegal networks. Notable is the multi-sector cooperation between WADA, the US Drug Enforcement Agency (DEA), and Interpol with significant achievements in promoting a deeper understanding of the dynamics supporting the detection and the seizure of illegal substances, which remain today the most promising way to efficiently protect the health of individuals voluntarily or unknowingly exposed to such substances.

In this context, our book aims to explore and advance knowledge on emerging drugs and NPS in sport and their impact on society. It offers a timely perspective on the rapidly changing doping scenario and the latest research advances and regulatory approaches, immersing the reader in the multi-faceted reality of tackling drug abuse.

It represents a useful resource designed for those working in sport, anti-doping, forensics, law—including legislative personnel drafting laws and regulating NPS, health care, policy making, and police forces as well as for athletes at any level and the professionals working with them. It has been written in a way that anyone with an interest in "clean sport" will be able to appreciate.

Not only leading experts in the field were solicited to contribute to this manuscript, but also high-level athletes who made the choice to use or reject such drugs. We found it important to hear from them about how they reflect today, sometimes years after the facts, on the situation they faced and the risk they accepted to take at the time they were taking substances, and included them as co-authors.

For clarity reasons, chapters have been presented in six interconnected parts.

Part I, "The Evolving Doping Scenario", introduces the evolution of emerging drugs used in sport and the challenges faced over time. It argues how in recent years there has been a significant increase in the number of doping cases with illegal stimulants related to amphetamines and cathinones as well as new synthetic cannabinoids.

Part II, "Navigating in a Difficult Regulatory Environment", explores regulatory approaches for doping agents and the role played by WADA and the UNODC to ensure "clean sport" and bring consistency to anti-doping policies and regulations within sport organizations and governments across the world. It highlights the specific rules presented by the list of prohibited substances and methods within and out of competition classification of restricted use.

Part III, "Towards a Doping Society?", examines how the wide availability of such fitness-enhancing products, along with the sponsored endorsements by popular elite sportsmen, have made ergo nutritional aids an essential part of the training of elite athletes, amateur athletes, or just recreationally active individuals and explores the health risks associated with such a trend.

Part IV, "Winning at Any Cost: Doping Experiences of World-Class Athletes", focuses on athletes and their journeys with doping. It presents the personal motivations behind their behaviours and explores their attitudes to win at any cost, sometimes scarifying their own health. We also highlight the personal story of an athlete who rejected doping and his motivations.

Part V, "Truth in the Test Tubes?", explores the challenges faced in the detection of doping agents among athletes and profiles the latest approaches and techniques to tackle the rise of NPS. It encourages the development of intelligence-based approach, aiming at identifying and purchasing such drugs to identify their chemical structures and assess their quality and purity with the objective to facilitate their identification and detection sometimes even before they appear on the market.

Finally, Part VI, "The Next Challenge", covers the key priorities in ongoing and future research and anticipates what the future challenges might be, while helping the development of a new direction.

We strongly believe this book is another example of effective collaboration among different actors to federate all the existing activities and competencies to address such a complex and multi-faceted risk faced by individuals and societies.

We hope you will enjoy it and find it a useful and informative resource. It is not meant to be left on a bookshelf. Clean sport deeply matters to us and although we do not necessarily know what the next challenge will be, by working together we are more prepared to face the future.

Olivier Rabin
Ornella Corazza

Acknowledgements

This book was written during a very challenging time for humanity due to the outbreak of the COVID-19 pandemic. While recognizing the suffering, the losses of dear ones, the increased workloads, and the necessity to stay all physically apart, we would like to express our deep gratitude to the 36 co-authors of this book, who felt the need to come together to share their knowledge and experience in support of clean sport. These include some world-class athletes who agreed to share their personal stories and opinions on doping, which have made our book even more valuable.

We also must thank Elisabeth Prevete who, with the support of Valentina Giorgetti and Riccardo Paci, led the editing of this book and the correspondence with the authors. We wish you all every success with your promising career as researchers in the field of emerging drugs. Highly capable and committed clinicians and scholars such as yourselves are greatly needed in our society.

We also own a debt of gratitude to the team at Springer for their restless interest, attention, and advice on our manuscript. It has been a long but enriching journey.

Olivier Rabin
Ornella Corazza

Contents

About the Editors

Olivier Rabin, PhD is the Senior Director in charge of Science and Medicine at the World Anti-Doping Agency (WADA). Over the years, he has established an international reputation as an expert in pharmaceutical research and development. With a background in fundamental and applied toxicology, he is the author of numerous scientific publications.

Ornella Corazza, PhD is Professor of Addiction Science at the University of Hertfordshire in the UK and leading scholar in the field of novel psychoactive substances. Her work has been presented in numerous peer-reviewed publications, books, and invited lectures and recognized internationally with various prizes and awards. She is the President of the International Society for the Study of Emerging Drugs (ISSED).

About the Contributors

Patricia Anielski, PhD Institute of Doping Analysis Dresden, Kreischa, Germany

Toby Atkins London, UK

Witold Banka, MA Poli Sci, President, World Anti-Doping Agency (WADA), Montreal, QC, Canada

Francesco Saverio Bersani, MD Department of Human Neurosciences, Sapienza University of Rome, Rome, Italy

Quentin Bigot Gandrange, France

Odile Cohen-Haguenauer, MD, PhD Unité d'Oncogénétique Clinique AP-HP, Nord-Université de Paris, DMU Icare, UFR de Médecine de l'Université de Paris, Unité de recherche INSERM UMR-S 976, Hôpital Saint-Louis, Paris, France

Ornella Corazza, LLM, MA, PhD Department of Clinical, Pharmaceutical and Biological Sciences, School of Life and Medical Science, University of Hertfordshire, Hatfield, Hertfordshire, UK

Conor Crean, BA (mod) Chem, PhD Laboratory and Scientific Section, Division of Policy Analysis, United Nations Office on Drugs and Crime (UNODC), Vienna, Austria

Asma Fakhri, BA (Hons) Laboratory and Scientific Section, Division of Policy Analysis, United Nations Office on Drugs and Crime (UNODC), Vienna, Austria

Renzo Ferrante, LLM Carabinieri, Comando Carabinieri Tutela Salute, Nucleo Antisofisticazioni (NAS), Florence, Italy

Sebastien Gaillard, LLM Interpol, Lyon, France

Claude Guillou, PhD Senior Expert, European Commission, Directorate General Joint Research Centre, Directorate F – Health, Consumers and Reference Materials, Ispra, Italy

Tyler Hamilton Missoula, US

Barrie Houlihan, BA, MSc, PhD, FAcSS Loughborough University, Loughborough, UK

Audrey Kinahan, PhD, BSc Pharm, DipFM, MPSI Eirpharm, Ennis, Co. Clare, Ireland

Prohibited List Expert Advisory Group, World Anti-Doping Agency (WADA), Montreal, QC, Canada

Tiia Kuuranne, PhD Swiss Laboratory for Doping Analyses, University Center of Legal Medicine, Genève and Lausanne, Centre Hospitalier Universitaire Vaudois and University of Lausanne, Epalinges, Switzerland

Emily D. Lockhart, MFS Drug Enforcement Administration (DEA), Special Testing and Research Laboratory, Dulles, VA, USA

Sigmund Loland, PhD Institute for Sport and Social Sciences, Norwegian School of Sport Sciences, Oslo, Norway

Swedish School of Sport and Health Sciences, Stockholm, Sweden

Irene E. Mazzoni, PhD Science and Medicine Department, World Anti-Doping Agency (WADA) Montreal, QC, Canada

Mike McNamee, BA, MA, MA, PhD Faculty of Movement and Rehabilitation Sciences, KU Leuven, Leuven, Belgium

School of Sport and Exercise Sciences, Swansea University, Swansea, Wales, UK

Jean-Pierre Morand, LLM Kellerhals-Carrard Law Firm, Lausanne, Switzerland

Attilio Negri, MD Department of Clinical, Pharmaceutical and Biological Sciences, School of Life and Medical Science, University of Hertfordshire, Hatfield, Hertfordshire, UK

Olivier Rabin, PhD Science and Medicine Department, World Anti-Doping Agency (WADA), Montreal, QC, Canada

Clare Jones de Rocco, BA (Hons) Laboratory and Scientific Section, Division of Policy Analysis, United Nations Office on Drugs and Crime (UNODC), Vienna, Austria

Silvia Rossato, PsyD Dual Diagnosis Unit, Clinica Parco dei Tigli, Padua, Italy

Angela Scoppettone, PsyD Dual Diagnosis Unit, Clinica Parco dei Tigli, Padua, Italy

Julien Sieveking, LLM Director, Legal Affairs World Anti-Doping Agency (WADA), Montreal, QC, Canada

Pierluigi Simonato, MD, PhD Department of Clinical, Pharmaceutical and Biological Sciences, School of Life and Medical Science, University of Hertfordshire, Hatfield, Hertfordshire, UK

Dual Diagnosis Unit, Clinica Parco dei Tigli, Padua, Italy

Yuliya Stepanova (née Rusanova) World Anti-Doping Agency (WADA), Montreal, QC, Canada

Mark Stuart, BPharm Centre for Metabolism and Inflammation, Division of Medicine, University College London, London, UK

International Testing Agency, Lausanne, Switzerland

Justice N. A. Tettey, BPharm (Hons), MSc, PhD, Hon LLD Laboratory and Scientific Section, Division of Policy Analysis, United Nations Office on Drugs and Crime (UNODC), Vienna, Austria

Mario Thevis, PhD Center for Preventive Doping Research – Institute of Biochemistry, German Sport University Cologne, Cologne, Germany

European Monitoring Center for Emerging Doping Agents, Cologne, Germany

Detlef Thieme, PhD Institute of Doping Analysis Dresden, Kreischa, Germany

Honor D. Townshend, BA, MSc, PhD (candidate) Department of Criminology, School of Law, University of Hertfordshire, Hatfield, Hertfordshire, UK

Ross Wenzel, MA (Oxon) Kellerhals-Carrard Law Firm, Lausanne, Switzerland

Gunter Younger Intelligence and Investigations Department, World Anti-Doping Agency (WADA), Montreal, QC, Canada

Meike Younger, BSc International Investigations Expert, Auckland, New Zealand

Nicolas Zbinden, MLaw, LLM Kellerhals-Carrard Law Firm, Lausanne, Switzerland

Part I
The Evolving Doping Scenario

The Evolution of Performance-Enhancing Drug Use in Sport

Barrie Houlihan

Introduction

Although the use of drugs in sport can be traced back to ancient Greece, the modern history of the use of performance-enhancing drugs (PEDs) begins in the late nineteenth century in connection with emerging professional endurance sports such as 5- and 6-day cycling events, long-distance swimming and horse and dog racing. Commonly used drugs at that time were caffeine, cocaine, alcohol and strychnine, which were used either individually or in combination. By the 1920s, there was growing awareness and concern among sport organisations with regard to drug use, and between 1910 and 1920, scientists were beginning to develop detection methods for some drugs, initially those involved in horse racing [1]. International federations (IFs) were also beginning to amend their rules to address the emerging problem of doping. One of the first IFs to amend their rules was the international federation for track and field (International Amateur Athletic Federation, IAAF) who in 1928 prohibited the use of stimulants. However, as there was no reliable test for stimulants, the prohibition was largely ineffective. Between the 1920s and the 1960s, an increasing number of IFs and major event organisers amended their rules to prohibit doping, but just as simply amending rules had little effect unless there were reliable tests available, it was also true that the availability of reliable tests also had little impact unless there was a process and funding for conducting the tests and for the laboratory analysis.

B. Houlihan (✉)
Loughborough University, Loughborough, UK
e-mail: B.M.J.Houlihan@lboro.ac.uk

© The Author(s), under exclusive license to Springer Nature Switzerland AG 2022
O. Rabin, O. Corazza (eds.), *Emerging Drugs in Sport*,
https://doi.org/10.1007/978-3-030-79293-0_1

The 1950s and 1960s: The Spread of PEDs Use in Sport

The two groups of substances that were to become the main PEDs used by doping athletes were stimulants and steroids. The stimulant amphetamine was first synthesised in the late nineteenth century, and testosterone (the base compound for the development of synthetic steroids) was first isolated in the mid 1930s [2]. However, it was not until the 1950s and 1960s that evidence of the extent of their use in sport began to emerge. Three factors were particularly important in stimulating PED use in sport in the 1950s: first, scientific experimentation during the Second World War with drugs designed to keep soldiers alert and increase their aggression; second, the increasing success in the synthesis of drugs; and third, the deepening of the Cold War. The use of amphetamines by soldiers during the Second World War not only stimulated scientific research into stimulants but perhaps more importantly made the performance-enhancing properties of the drugs widely known among athletes and the general public. Evidence of extensive use of stimulants first appeared in cycling. According to Müller (2010), "In a cycling competition in 1955, five samples out of 25 tested positive for amphetamine ... During several high-level cycling competitions (e.g., World Amateur Championship, Professional Cycling World Championship Zürich, Austria Tour) numerous cyclists (e.g., from Austria, the Netherlands and Poland) tested positive ..." [2]. Also in the 1950s, evidence of the increasing use of anabolic agents across a range of sports was emerging although there were significant challenges in distinguishing exogenous consumption of anabolic androgenic steroids from normal endogenous production. The entry of the Soviet Union to the Olympic Games in 1952 intensified the ideological rivalry with the USA and provided a powerful legitimation for increased experimentation and use of PEDs in both countries. However, it is clear that experimentation and use of PEDs in the 1950s and early 1960s was not confined to the two major powers but was evident across a wide range of countries including England, Italy, France and Belgium and was also evident in a wide range of sports including cycling and rowing [3], football [4] and swimming [5]. Also of considerable significance was the early evidence that the doping practices of elite level athletes were moving into wider society affecting, for example, the behaviour of young athletes well below the elite level. According to Novak (1964), "Since the high school athlete and coach are influenced by the professional and intercollegiate athletes, the amphetamines became popular even in interscholastic athletics" [6]. The factors that accelerated the use of PEDs in the 1950s and early 1960s, nationalism and Cold War rivalry, were intensified in the two subsequent decades but were also augmented by two further powerful factors, government investment in, and the rapid commercialisation of high performance sport. Although some governments, most notably the former German Democratic Republic (GDR) and the former USSR, had for some time treated elite sport as a diplomatic resource, most governments were reluctant to invest public money in sport. However, the willingness of an increasing number of governments from the 1980s to invest public funds in sport, especially elite sport, was due to the combination of (a) USA-USSR rivalry and the recognition of the diplomatic potential of sporting success, especially at the Olympic Games; (b) the rapid increase in sports broadcasting following the introduction of live satellite transmission of major sports events; and (c) the growing interest in sport as a solution (or at least a palliative) for a number of social ills, such as juvenile delinquency and poor public health. Government interest was also reinforced by the rising commercial value of the sports industry (especially broadcasting, events, leagues and clubs) as a source of employment and profit. In 1912, there were only 20 major international sports events. By 1970, the figure had increased to 350 and by 2005 to 900 [7]. The sports events market was valued at 21,274M USD in 2019 and, despite a severe drop in 2020, was forecast to rise to 31,029m USD by 2024 [8]. Government investment in elite sport has grown in parallel to commercial investment and has been driven by a variety of motives including diplomatic, tourism promotion and nation (re)branding [9]. As the following section will illustrate, the growth in the political and commercial (both corporate and personal) benefits of elite level success has been paralleled by consistent innovation and experimentation in PED use and by the concern of sport organisations and governments to reduce if not eliminate doping in sport. The first list of prohibited substances, compiled by the IOC for use at the 1968 Olympic Games, contained just two classes of substances – stimulants and narcotics [10]. The list has steadily expanded and is now the responsibility of the World Anti-Doping Agency (WADA) and is updated on an annual basis. The list now contains nine groups of PEDs, five that are prohibited at all times (anabolic agents; peptide hormones, growth factors and related substances; beta-2 agonists; hormone and metabolic modulators; and diuretics and masking agents) and four that are prohibited in-competition (stimulants; narcotics cannabinoids; and glucocorticoids). In addition, there are beta-blockers that are prohibited in selected sports, and three doping methods are also prohibited (manipulation of blood and blood compounds; chemical and physical manipulation; and gene and cell doping).

Evolution of PEDs Use

Table 1 provides a summary of some of the major PEDs and methods used in sport and an indication of their current scale of use. What is particularly striking is the relatively short time lag between the development of a particular class of substances and their use in sport.

Stimulants

Stimulants have a long history of exploitation in sport initially based on the use of natural products, but since the middle of the last century based on synthetic stimulants such as amphetamine. Unlike some of the other categories on the WADA Prohibited List, stimulant use developed first outside sport mainly in a military

Table 1 Summary of the most common PEDs and current scale of use

Drug	Approximate date of discovery	First use in sport	Extent of use	Major sports affected	Peak of use	Assessment of current level of use
Stimulants: Amphetamines	1880s (commercial development 1930s)	1940s	Heavy use between the mid-1950s and the late 1980s. Evidence of substantial use by cyclists as an ingredient in the "pot belge"	Cycling, American football, soccer (and many other endurance sports)	Late 1960s to late 1980s	Moderate, due to ease of identification and availability of alternatives
Cocaine	Pre-seventeenth century	Late nineteenth century	Heavy in the late 1960s, particularly among horse racing jockeys and tennis players and then moderate to present day	Many endurance sports and major team sports	Unclear	Moderate
Ephedrine	c1940s	1970s	Heavy use from the mid-1970s to the present	Most endurance sports and many major team sports	Consistent since the 1970s	Heavy
Blood manipulation (methods designed to increase red blood cell count)	Blood doping 1970s	1970s	Moderate	Endurance sports such as long-distance cycling, running, swimming and cross-country skiing	1980s	Moderate, but resurgence in the 2000s as the detection of EPO became easier
Narcotics	Pre-seventeenth century	Late nineteenth century	Heavy between the late 1960s and the present day, but often as recreational drugs as performance-enhancing effect is not clear. However, heroin was used as part of the "pot belge"	Some evidence of use in endurance sports to control pain	Not known	Generally light in elite sport, but still high in some sports/countries, e.g., tramadol abuse

Drug	Approximate date of discovery	First use in sport	Extent of use	Major sports affected	Peak of use	Assessment of current level of use
Anabolic steroids and anabolic agents	1930s	1950s	Heavy between the late 1960s and the late 1980s	Most Olympic sports and many major team sports	Consistent since the 1980s	Heavy
Peptide hormones: For example, EPO	rEPO 1987	Late 1980s	Light in late 1980s but heavily used from the 1990s	Endurance sports	Perhaps 2010s	Heavy to moderate
Human growth hormone	Mid-1980s	Late 1980s	Moderate	Body-building and a similar range of sports that attract anabolic steroid users	Yet to be reached	Moderate, but rising
Diuretics and other masking agents	Synthetic diuretics 1960s	1970s?	Moderate to heavy in the early 1970s	Weight-related sports, but all sports when used as a masking agent	Mid-1970s	Moderate use in weight-related sports or as a part of a dietary supplement, despite the relative ease of identification
Beta-blockers	1960s	1970s	Moderate use in small number of sports	Shooting, archery and snooker	Late 1980s	Light
Genetic manipulation	1970s	No confirmed cases	Rumours and speculation, but no evidence of use	Potential to affect all sports		None to negligible
Novel psychoactive substances	A fragmented history, but came to the notice of drug agencies in the late 1990s	1990s	Moderate, but difficult to determine accurately	Potential use in all sports	Probably not yet reached	Moderate to heavy

context and, in the 1960s and 1970s, as a recreational drug among adolescents. As mentioned previously the use of amphetamines and related stimulants was first identified in endurance events especially road cycling but also in long-distance running and swimming as well as some team sports such as football in the 1950s and 1960s. Since then a large number of stimulants that mimic the effects of amphetamine have been developed for therapeutic use and have subsequently been used by athletes. One of the most notable is ephedrine, a substance that was, at one time, common in over-the-counter cold remedies. The use of the drug in sport came to public attention in 1972 when the American swimmer Rick DeMont tested positive for ephedrine at the Munich Olympic Games. Since then ephedrine has been regularly detected in doping controls although other stimulants such as methylphenidate, cocaine, and heptaminol have been identified more frequently in anti-doping controls [11]. Stimulants remain a major concern for anti-doping organisations. Between 2014 and 2017, stimulant use was identified by WADA as a regular occurrence in most major sports including cycling, athletics, aquatics, weightlifting and boxing [12] and in WADA's 2018 anti-doping report stimulants was the second most commonly identified class of drugs [11].

Anabolic Agents

One of the first clinical uses of this class of drugs was to aid the recovery of patients suffering from starvation in the 1930s. Later during the Second World War, anabolic steroids were used in the German army to increase the aggressiveness and strength of soldiers. Reports of the use of anabolic steroids in sport began to emerge in the early 1950s. At the 1952 Helsinki Olympic Games, rumours circulated that members of the Soviet Union team had used anabolic steroids as part of their training preparations and that this partly explained the success of the team in winning 71 medals just five short of the USA total. Rather than these rumours leading to attempts to prevent further use, they fuelled the rivalry between the USA and the Soviet Union. The spread of anabolic steroid use in the USA was facilitated by the willingness of some doctors to supply PEDs to US athletes. As Goldman and Klatz noted, "When steroids first came on the scene there were many physicians, including the father of anabolic steroids, Dr. John Ziegler, who cautiously embraced them, and willingly prescribed them to athletes for whom they were responsible ... Patriotism was a factor as well. The feeling of these doctors was that if they could in any way help an American athlete bring home the gold, they had somehow struck a blow for freedom" [13]. Further evidence of the use of anabolic steroids by Soviet athletes emerged at the 1956 Olympic Games where the use of the drug was so great that, according to Voy (1991), some Soviet athletes had to be catheterised in order to pass urine due to the enlargement of the prostate gland [14]. Ziegler began to experiment with synthetic testosterone to test their performance-enhancing potential at about the same time that the Ciba pharmaceutical company was developing steroids for clinical use with burn victims. The outcome of the development was the steroid trade-named Dianabol. Ziegler persuaded three American weightlifters to experiment with Dianabol with the result that "all three experienced significant improvements in both strength and muscle mass. Following this success, the use of Dianabol spread rapidly among U.S. lifters and, from there, to other sports" [15].

The use of steroids was initially confined to the power sports such as weightlifting and throwing events but soon spread to other sports such as swimming. The increase in the use of this class of drugs was partly the result of the recognition that not only could the drugs be effective in adding muscle mass but that they were also effective in enabling athletes to train longer and recover faster from intensive periods of training. By the 1970s, the use of anabolic steroids was widespread, and it was not until a reliable test had been developed to detect the drugs that use began to slow. Tests were conducted at the Montreal Olympic Games in 1976, and eight athletes were disqualified for the use of anabolic steroids. However, rather than the development of a reliable test marking a decline in steroid use, it merely marked the first phase in an ongoing competition between steroid users and anti-doping organisations. Doping rule violations involving steroids continued into the 1980s. At the 1983 Pan-American Games many athletes withdrew when they were made aware of the likelihood of being tested for steroids, and 19 athletes tested positive for PEDs, some of which were steroids. However, it was later in the decade that the scale of steroid use began to become apparent. In 1987, 34 people, including the British Olympian David Jenkins, were indicted by the US Drug Enforcement Administration for smuggling steroids worth around $100m from Mexico to the USA. The following year Ben Johnson tested positive for steroids after winning the 100 m final at the Seoul Olympics. Evidence of the widespread use of steroids in high performance sport and increasingly among non-elite athletes and indeed non-athletes continued to emerge during the 1980s and 1990s. The enquiry into doping in sport in Australia [16] reported that around 70% of all positive doping controls in IOC-accredited laboratories were for steroids. The popularity of steroids among PED users continued into the twenty-first century with the WADA report [17] for PED use in 2010 noting that just under 81% of all reported findings were for steroids. Although the 2018 WADA testing figures reported that steroid use had dropped to 44% of all reported findings, this class of PEDs was still by far the most commonly found [11]. While the continued popularity of steroids among elite athletes is a substantial challenge for anti-doping authorities, the spread of steroid use beyond the confines of elite sport has emerged as a significant contemporary public health concern. Two developments in the spread of steroids are of particular concern: the spread among school-age young people and among gym users. According to Dandoy and Gereige (2012), the US National Youth Risk Behavior System which surveys over 16,000 9th to 12th grade students reported that the incidence of steroid use had risen from 2.7% in 1991 to 6.1% in 2003 before declining to 3.3% in 2009 [18]. The rise in steroid use was accompanied by a "sharp decline" in the perception of risk associated with steroid use. Further evidence came from the National Institute on Drug Abuse which estimated that over 500,000 8th and 10th grade students, predominantly those involved in sports including American football, baseball and basketball, were using steroids (NIDA 2004). In a later study, NIDA reported that steroid use among 8th and 10th grade high school students had peaked around 2000 and had "generally declined" although use among 12th grade students "increased from 2011 to 2015" before declining from 2015 to 2016 and then stabilising [19]. There are relatively few studies of adolescent steroid use outside the USA, but those that exist present a broadly similar picture. Nilsson et al. (2001) found that 3.6% of 16-year-old males in a survey of 5827 16- and 17-year-olds in Sweden admitted to using steroids (2.8% for 17-year-olds) [20]. A study in Poland reported that in their survey of 1175 male and female students, 9.38% of males and 2.08% of females reported having used steroids. The authors reported that the main motives for steroid use "were connected with shaping their bodies in a manner allowing realisation of cultural ideals of bodyshape" [21]. Broadly similar results were reported from a range of studies across Europe indicating a significant public health problem among adolescent males especially among those involved in youth sport (e.g., [22, 23]). Overlapping with the prevalence of steroid use among adolescents is the increasing use among gym users. Numerous studies have indicated that steroid use is evident among gym users although precise figures regarding usage are difficult to obtain. Stubbe et al. (2014) reported usage of steroids by 1% of gym users (with 0.8% reporting using prohormone and 1.1% using growth hormone or insulin) although the most frequently used PEDs were stimulants (4.8%) to help reduce weight [24]. McVeigh and Begley (2017) reported a substantial increase in steroid users (not all of whom were necessarily gym users) accessing local needle and syringe programmes in two counties in north-west England (553 clients in 1995 and 2446 in 2015) [25]. Christiansen (2015) summarised a number of studies from Nordic countries indicating a prevalence rate for steroid use of 3.8% (Sweden) and 5% (Denmark) [26]. He also noted that "for users in the gym environment most evidence suggests that use ... is restricted to a limited period of the individual's life ... from late teens to early thirties" [26]. Unlike the pattern of use of stimulants where use appeared to develop in elite sport and broader society in parallel, the spread of steroid use to junior athletes and to gyms appeared to have followed the demonstration effect of use by elite athletes.

Peptide Hormones: Human Growth Hormone

Human growth hormone (hGH) is one of the newer PEDs in sport and was developed in the mid-1970s as a replacement for natural endogenous growth hormone. By the late 1980s, there were reports of athletes using human growth hormone often at many times the recommended therapeutic levels even though there had been no peer-reviewed papers providing evidence of its performance-enhancing effect. Despite the lack of evidence, Sonksen et al. (2016) noted that "so great was the demand for GH that stocks of GH in pharmacies and warehouses and even trucks on the road were targeted" [27]. One of the earliest verified cases of use of human growth hormone was in evidence given to the Dubin Inquiry following the Ben Johnson scandal in 1988. The sprinter Angella Issajenko admitted using hGH along with other drugs. The report of the Inquiry noted that "Notwithstanding the strict control of growth hormone there was evidence of increased use by other sprinters, bodybuilders, weightlifters and intercollegiate football players whose sole source of supply has been the black market" [28]. Human growth hormones tend to be used by athletes seeking similar advantages as expected from steroids, but they are more attractive to those seeking to improve musculature rather than simply enhance muscle strength. However, the discovery of 13 vials of hGH in the luggage of a member of the China swimming team in Perth in 1998 suggests that the drug is also valued by those athletes in explosive and endurance events. The IOC identified GH use as a concern in the early 1990s, but it was not until the London 2012 Olympic Games that testing for GH took place. As Sonksen et al. (2016) note, "Knowledge about the misuse of GH is unreliable as our intelligence is largely based on hearsay and anecdotes as testing for GH has been limited but it appears to be particularly popular in sprint and power sports usually in combination with anabolic steroids" [27]. The latest WADA testing figures [11] indicate the continuing use of peptide hormones, growth factors, and related substances with them accounting for 3% of adverse analytical findings and 31% of atypical findings. WADA's report on 2018 testing figures expressed concern about the use of GH and encouraged an 18% increase in the number of tests between 2017 and 2018 [11].

Diuretics

Diuretics are drugs that are used to increase the rate of urine formation [29]. The modern suite of diuretics dates from the mid-1950s and has been used in sport for three main purposes: (a) to achieve rapid weight loss in weight-graded sports such as boxing and wrestling; (b) to flush other drugs out of the system; and (c) to counteract the fluid-retention properties of steroids. The last purpose is attractive to bodybuilders who use diuretics to achieve a more sharply defined musculature. While it can be assumed that the use of diuretics by elite athletes took place in the 1960s and 1970s, it was not until the 1980s that evidence of use by athletes began to accumulate. One of the earliest examples of the use of diuretics involved a Canadian athlete at the 1983 Caracas Pan-American Games, but as diuretics were not on the IOC list of prohibited substances, no anti-doping rule had been broken. Diuretics were added to the IOC list in 1985, and since then there have been regular reports of violations involving this class of drugs each year. Examples of anti-doping violations involving diuretics include the British judo athlete who tested positive for the diuretic furosemide in 1988, the cyclist Pedro Delgado who tested positive in the same year and Veronica Campbell-Brown (winner of three Olympic gold medals) who tested positive in 2013. Data from WADA indicates a steady rise in the proportion of adverse analytical findings that involve diuretics: in 2003, there were 142 occurrences (5.2% of all positives); in 2008, 436 occurrences (7.9%); and in 2018, 589 occurrences (14%). Outside of Olympic sports, use of diuretics is also evident among bodybuilders although use is far behind that of steroids (e.g., [24, 30, 31]).

Beta-Blockers

Beta-blockers are used to treat a range of medical conditions such as migraine and angina. In sport they are used to reduce anxiety levels, steady breathing and reduce heart beat frequency and muscle tremor. While they are of little value in most sports, they can be beneficial in those that require a steady hand such as shooting, archery, darts and snooker. Beta-blockers came to the notice of sports federations in the 1980s. Evidence of the use of beta-blockers was found among competitors in shooting events and modern pentathlon in the 1984 Olympic Games, and later in the 1980s, a number of snooker players were reported to have been using this class of drugs. Beta-blockers were not prohibited at the time of the Los Angeles Olympic Games although team doctors were obliged to notify the IOC of any team members taking the drug. The number of notifications, sometimes whole teams, alarmed the IOC who added beta-blockers to the prohibited list in 1985. Current usage of beta-blockers appears to be low [11] although there are occasional high-profile cases at Olympic Games such as the positive test for propranolol in the sample of the North Korean shooter Kim Jong-Su at the 2008 Games in Beijing.

Genetic Manipulation

The history of doping in sport provides ample evidence of the willingness of athletes to use drugs before clinical trials have been completed, to use drugs specifically designed for use in a veterinary context and to use drugs in amounts that far exceed therapeutic limits. It is, therefore, highly likely that this propensity for risk-taking will manifest itself in relation to genetic manipulation. An early warning of the interest from athletes in advances in gene therapies came when an email from the coach Thomas Springstein was read out in court in 2006 in which he enquired about the drug Repoxygen, a virus-based drug carrying the human EPO gene which would have similar blood-boosting properties to rEPO. WADA had added gene doping to its prohibited list in 2003, and research continues to identify detection methods. At present there are no verified cases of gene doping, but experimentation by athletes is inevitable. Lopez et al. (2020) summarise the potential candidate genes associated with sport performance and note that many of the current gene therapy trials are addressing clinical problems that have a clear cross over to doping in sport and include those associated with oxygen delivery, pain tolerance and muscle growth/repair [32]. The threat to clean sport from gene doping is substantial and is a major challenge for anti-doping authorities.

Novel Psychoactive Substances

Novel psychoactive substances (NPS) may be "novel" in a variety of ways. NPS may refer to "something newly created, an old drug that has come back into fashion, or a known NPS molecule being used in an innovative or unusual way" [33]. From 2004 to 2017, between 700 and 800 examples of NPS were identified by European and international drug agencies with the most common examples being "synthetic cannabimimetics, synthetic opioids, phenethylamines, designer benzodiazepines, and prescribed drugs" [33]. As Mazzoni et al. (2017) observed, "Among the doping substances, the most preoccupying is the increased supply of counterfeit and designer drugs, including NPS. NPS have a long history of abuse in sport" [34]. Most NPS fall within the categories of stimulants, narcotics and cannabinoids on the WADA list of prohibited substances and practices. The growth in the availability of NPS is proving to be a particularly daunting challenge for WADA. First, as Mazzoni et al. (2017) note, "the identification of prohibited substances… requires the previous knowledge of the chemical structure of the substance and its mass spectrum none of which are known for NPS recently introduced in the market" [34]. The acquisition of knowledge of the chemical structure of NPS relies on NPS being sent to WADA or its network of laboratories or the direct purchase of NPS from the Internet. Second, "the risk of inadvertent doping with supplements is high because it is common that NPS are not named on the labels or sometimes they are referred to with a fictional name … or by a purposely wrong chemical name" [34]. Third, detection of some NPS, particularly synthetic cannabinoids, is made more difficult as they appear to be unrelated to their natural counterparts. In addition to the problems of detection, there are serious challenges in limiting supply. It is estimated that 80% of the raw materials for the clandestine manufacture of counterfeit and illegal drugs abused in sport come from China. WADA is working closely with the Chinese authorities to reduce supply, but it remains to be seen how effective the Chinese efforts will prove to be.

Conclusion

Prior to the establishment of WADA, the fragmented and under-funded nature of anti-doping action meant that anti-doping authorities were always some way behind drug users both scientifically and organisationally. There was often a long delay between a PED being identified in sport and its incorporation into the IOC prohibited list and the development of a reliable test that would withstand legal challenge. The establishment of WADA has harmonised anti-doping regulations and provided valuable coordination of anti-doping research. Equally importantly the Agency has built links with the pharmaceutical industry, customs and excise departments and law enforcement agencies and established a secure whistleblowing procedure and an internal investigations capacity. These positive developments notwithstanding the Agency and sport organisations still face considerable challenges as innovation in the development, modification and administration of PEDs continues. In addition, the lack of consistent support for anti-doping from some governments and the ambivalent attitude of some international federations continue to pose problems for the implementation of an effective global response to the problem.

References

1. Prokop L (1970) The struggle against doping and its history. J Sports Med Phys Fitness 10:45
2. Müller RK (2010) History of doping and doping control. In: Thieme D, Hammersbach P (eds) Doping in sports: handbook of experimental pharmacology 195. Springer-Verlag, Berlin, pp 1–23
3. Dimeo P (2007) A history of drug use in sport 1876–1976: beyond good and evil. Routledge, London
4. Malcolm D, Smith A (2015) Drug use in professional football. In: Møller V, Waddington I, Hoberman JH (eds) Routledge handbook of drugs and sport. Routledge, London, pp 103–114
5. Koh B (2015) Drug use in swimming. In: Møller V, Waddington I, Hoberman JH (eds) Routledge handbook of drugs and sport. Routledge, London, pp 128–144
6. Novak (1964) In Dimeo P (2007) a history of drug use in sport 1876–1976: beyond good and evil. Routledge, London, p 272
7. Dejonghe T (2007) Sport in de wereld. Academia Press, Gent, Belgium
8. Statista (2020) Sport events worldwide. Available at: https://www.statista.com/outlook/272/100/sport-events/worldwide Accessed 19 Oct 2020
9. Houlihan B, Zheng J (2013) The Olympics and elite sport policy: where will it all end? Int J Hist Sport 30:338–355
10. Mazzoni I, Barroso O, Rabin O (2011) The list of prohibited substances and methods in sport: structure and review process by the World Anti-Doping Agency. J Anal Toxicol 35:608–612
11. WADA (2019) 2018 anti-doping testing figures. Montreal, WADA
12. Aguilar-Navarro M, Salinero JJ, Muñoz-Guerra J, del Mar PM, del Coso J (2020) Sport-specific use of doping substances: analysis of World Anti-Doping Agency doping control tests between 2014 and 2017. Subst Use Misuse 55:1361–1369
13. Goldman B, Klatz R (1992) Death in the locker room. Elite Sports Medicine Publications, Chicago, p 47
14. Voy RO (1991) Drugs, sport, and politics, vol. 10. Human Kinetics Publishers, Champaign, IL
15. Hunt TM (2007). Drug games: The international politics of doping and the Olympic Movement, 1960–2007. Doctoral dissertation. University of Texas at Austin, p 6
16. Government of Australia (1989) Drugs in sport, interim report of the senate standing committee on the environment, recreation and the arts. Australian Government Publishing Service, Canberra
17. WADA (2011) 2010 Adverse analytical findings and atypical findings reported by accredited laboratories. Montreal, WADA
18. Dandoy and Gereige (2012) Performance and enhancing drugs. Pediatr Rev 33(6):265–272
19. NIDA. Who uses steroids. Available at: https://www.drugabuse.gov/publications/research-reports/steroids-other-appearance-performance-enhancing-drugs-apeds/who-uses-anabolic-steroids Accessed 10 Sept 2020
20. Nilsson S, Baigi A, Marklund B, Fridlund B (2001) The prevalence of the use of androgenic anabolic steroids by adolescents in a county of Sweden. Eur J Public Health 11:195–197
21. Sas-Nowosielski K (2006) The abuse of anabolic-androgenic steroids by polish school-aged adolescents. Biol Sport 23:225–232

22. Grace F, Baker J, Davies B (2001) Anabolic androgenic steroid use in recreational gym users: a regional sample of the mid-Glamorgan area. J Subst Abus 6:189–195
23. Kokkevi A, Fotiou A, Chileva A, Nociar A, Miller P (2008) Daily exercise and anabolic steroids use in adolescents: a cross-national European study. Subst Use Misuse 43:2053–2065
24. Stubbe JH, Chorus AM, Frank LE, de Hon O, van der Heijden PG (2014) Prevalence of use of performance enhancing drugs by fitness Centre members. Drug Test Anal 6:434–438
25. McVeigh J, Begley E (2017) Anabolic steroids in the UK: an increasing issue for public health. Drugs Edu Prev Policy 24:278–285
26. Christiansen AV (2015) Drug use in gyms. In: Møller V, Waddington I, Hoberman JH (eds) Routledge handbook of drugs and sport. Routledge, London, p 424
27. Sonksen PH, Cowan D, Holt R (2016) Use and misuse of hormones in sport. Lancet Diabetes Endocrinol 4:882–883
28. Inquiry D (1990) Commission of Inquiry into the use of drugs and banned practices intended to increase athletic performance, commissioner, C.L. Canadian Government Printing Centre, Dubin, Ottawa, p 120
29. Cadwallader AB, De La Torre X, Tieri A, Botrè F (2010) The abuse of diuretics as performance-enhancing drugs and masking agents in sport doping: pharmacology, toxicology and analysis. Br J Pharmacol 161(1–16):882–883
30. Sánchez-Oliver AJ, Grimaldi-Puyana M, Domínguez R (2019) Evaluation and behavior of Spanish bodybuilders: doping and sports supplements. Biomol Ther 9:122
31. Tavares ASR, Serpa S, Horta L, Carolino E, Rosado A (2020) Prevalence of performance-enhancing substance use and associated factors among Portuguese gym/fitness users. Subst Use Misuse 55:1059–1067
32. Lopez S et al (2020) Gene doping and genomic science in sports: where are we? Bioanalysis 12(11):801–811
33. Schifano F (2018) Recent changes in drug abuse scenarios: the new/novel psychoactive substances (NPS) phenomenon. Brain Sci 8:1–3
34. Mazzoni I, Barroso O, Rabin O (2017) Anti-doping challenges with novel psychoactive substances in sport. In: Corazza O, Roman-Urrestarazu A (eds) Novel psychoactive substances. Springer, Berlin, pp 43–56

Contamination of Sports Supplements with Novel Psychoactive Substances: An Old History with New Players

Irene E. Mazzoni

Historic Background: Traditional Medicines and Natural Products

Since ancient times, humans have relied on nature for their basic needs including medicines. Plants are considered a rich source of bioactive chemicals and have been the basis of traditional medicine systems for thousands of years [1]. In addition, many active compounds have been identified and isolated from these plants and are part of modern conventional therapeutic medications [2]. Fossil records date human use of medicinal plants from 60,000 years ago. Among the ancient civilizations, India is known to be the richest repository of medicinal plants. Ancient China developed systemic pharmacopeias as early as 3000 BC. Aboriginal people from America, Africa and Oceania have been using natural products as medicines for centuries [3–7]. Drugs acting on the nervous system, including psychoactive substances (PS), are present in many plants. One of the first used analeptic stimulants was strychnine, an alkaloid obtained from *Strychnos nux-vomica*. The poisonous and medicinal effects of strychnine have been well known since ancient times in China and India and more recently was also used worldwide in medicinal tonics until the early twentieth century, when it was abandoned due to its toxicity [8, 9]. Other analeptics found in plants include bicuculline, present mainly in *Dicentra cucullaria* [8, 10], and picrotoxin, obtained from the shrub *Anamirta cocculus* [2, 7]. In addition, xanthines like caffeine, theophylline and theobromine, naturally occurring in coffee and tea, are also considered mild analeptics [8, 11]. Cardiostimulants like scillaren A can be found in *Urginea (Scilla) maritima* and was known by the ancient Romans and Syrians, who used it for the treatment of oedematous states [12]. Plants of the

I. E. Mazzoni (✉)
Science and Medicine Department, World Anti-Doping Agency (WADA),
Montreal, QC, Canada
e-mail: Irene.Mazzoni@wada-ama.org

© The Author(s), under exclusive license to Springer Nature Switzerland AG 2022 17
O. Rabin, O. Corazza (eds.), *Emerging Drugs in Sport*,
https://doi.org/10.1007/978-3-030-79293-0_2

Digitalis family are rich sources of cardiotonics such as digitalin, digoxin, digitoxin, deslanoside and lanatosides and have been used for heart conditions since the thirteenth century [2, 14]. The stimulant properties of coca leaves, the source of cocaine, were known to indigenous people of the Andes since prehistory [13]. Coca was widely used to combat cold, fatigue, pain and hunger as well as in religious ceremonies. During the Inca Empire, coca was reserved for the elite classes, but after the Spanish conquest, it was made available to all the population, as it enabled peasants to work longer and harder and suppressed their appetite [14]. *Papaver somniferum* has been cultivated for several thousands of years in Mesopotamia for its poppy seeds, used for baking, and for the milky latex, opium. The dried latex contains numerous alkaloids including morphine, codeine, thebaine, noscapine, narceine and papaverine, which account for most of opium's narcotic and medicinal properties such as analgesia, antitussive and antidiarrheal effects [15]. Finally, several plants containing PS with hallucinogenic properties have been used in religious rituals throughout history. Known as entheogens, they include the peyote cactus, widely used in the Aztec Empire which contains mescaline as PS [16]; the ayahuasca drink prepared by Amazonian natives since pre-Columbian times, which contains MAO and serotonin inhibitors [17]; "magic mushrooms" containing psilocybin, used for centuries by Mexican aboriginal people [18]; and the iboga plant containing ibogaine, utilized by tribes of West Africa, at low doses as a stimulant to prevent fatigue and dull hunger and thirst and at high doses as hallucinogens during religious rituals [19].

Classical Doping Psychoactive Substances in Supplements

PS have long been used to enhance physical and mental performance. For example, Inca messengers used coca to help them run long distances at high altitudes [20]. Stimulants have also been extensively used in warfare to enhance stamina and alertness and to cope with traumas of the battlefield. A mixture of herbs containing stimulants, painkillers and hallucinogens was reported to be used by the Zulu tribes during their stand against British troops in 1879 [21]. While cocaine was the drug of choice during World War I, amphetamine and methamphetamine were used extensively during World War II [21–23]. Carphedon (phenylpiracetam) was developed in 1983 as a medication for Soviet cosmonauts to increase physical, mental and cognitive activities in space [24]. Amphetamines are also used by the working class to extend their working hours or facilitate hard labour [25], while prescription drugs like methylphenidate or dexamphetamine are often used by students in an attempt to enhance their learning skills [26]. The pharmacologic properties of many PS make them very attractive and valuable doping substances in sport. Some even claim that the word doping is originally derived from the use by some African tribes of a stimulant liquor called "dop" [27]. Precursors of modern-day supplements containing PS include the mixture of brandy and the stimulant strychnine that almost kills Thomas Hicks, the winner of the 1904 Olympic marathon in St Louis [28].

Strychnine and mixtures of heroin, cocaine and caffeine were commonly used by high-level athletes until the 1920s [29]. The use of stimulants in-competition was first banned by the International Association of Athletics Federations (IAAF) in 1928. However, this did not deter their use which continued to increase, in parallel with a more liberal view of society on drugs. The phenethylamine derivative amphetamine has played a prominent role in doping. The Dane Kurt Jensen was the first recorded death at the modern Olympics, collapsing from an amphetamine overdose at the 1960 Rome games, while the British cyclist Tommy Simpson died during the 1967 Tour de France after consuming amphetamines and brandy to combat the effects fatigue [30]. As a response to the growing doping problem, the International Olympic Committee (IOC) issued the first list of prohibited substances for the 1968 Olympic Games. This list included PS encompassed under the categories "Sympathomimetic Amines (e.g., amphetamine), ephedrine and similar substances", "Stimulants of the central nervous system (strychnine) and analeptics" and "Narcotics and analgesics (e.g., morphine), similar substances" [31]. The World Anti-Doping Agency (WADA), who in 2001 took over the regulation of the use of substances and methods in sports, continued with the ban of PS under three different categories: stimulants, narcotics and cannabinoids [32, 33]. Nevertheless, amphetamine and cocaine are still at the top of positive doping control tests in the class of stimulants [34]. Ephedrine alkaloids also belong to the group of traditional PS found in supplements. The ephedra plant (Ma Huang), which apart from ephedrine also contains pseudoephedrine and minor components, has been used in China for medicinal purposes for thousands of years [35]. Ephedrine became the standard medication for treatment of asthma in the first half of the twentieth century until the arrival of more efficacious medicines like beta-2-agonists and glucocorticoids [36, 37]. Its decline in use as a prescribed medicine in the 1960s was followed by an increase as a prominent component of nutritional supplements marketed as "natural stimulants", targeting weight loss and sports performance enhancement [35, 37–40]. A number of deaths and hundreds of adverse reactions associated with the use of ephedra-containing supplements in the USA prompted their complete ban in 2004 [41–47]. Fatal cases included those of professional athletes such as Korey Stringer in 2001 and Steve Bechler in 2003 [48]. Nevertheless, ephedra supplements are still widely available on the Internet. Other appetite suppressants such as fenfluramine, phentermine, phenmetrazine, fencamfamine, mephentermine and benfluorex are also commonly found as supplements claiming anorexigenic effects [49]. One of the minor alkaloids present in Ma Huang plant is cathine (norpseudoephedrine), and as expected, it is also found in dietary supplements containing this plant and its extracts [35, 38, 45]. However, the main natural source of cathine is the evergreen shrub *Catha edulis* (khat), grown mostly in East Africa, Yemen and other Middle Eastern countries. Khat contains, in addition to cathine, other amphetamine-like alkaloids such as cathinine and norephedrine [50]. Khat is traditionally used for its stimulant properties, sought to increase work capacity, improve sports and mental performance and improve alertness [50]. Although consumption of khat is mainly restricted to the native growing areas, cathine and cathinone are also found as part of manufactured dietary supplements, not only as natural component of the ephedra-derived supplements as noted before but as adulterants or main component of the supplement as well [40, 51]. A number of discontinued medications with psychoactive properties are also part of the arsenal used in supplements targeting athletes. As examples, we find methylhexaneamine (also known as, e.g., methylhex-amine, 1,3-dimethylamylamine, 1,3-DMAA, dimethylamylamine), an indirect sympathomimetic marketed as an inhaled nasal decongestant from 1948 until the 1970s under the trade name Forthane [52]. It reappeared in dietary supplements in 2006 under the trademarked name Geranamine. In order to disguise its synthetic origin, the supplements listed "geranium oil" or "geranium extract" as source. However, currently there is no evidence that methylhexanamine is present naturally in plants [53–56]. Similarly, methylsynephrine is claimed to be a component of bit-ter orange (*C. aurantium*), but efforts to identify it as naturally present in plants have failed [57–59]. In fact, methylsynephrine is the approved drug oxilofrine which is used to treat hypotension in a handful of countries [60]. Finally, the stimulant and appetite suppressant sibutramine was withdrawn from the market in many countries due to the risk of cardiovascular adverse events. Nevertheless, sibutramine and derivatives such as desmethylsibutramine and didesmethylsibutramine are found as components of many diet pills and anorexigenic supplements [49, 61–63]. This is another example of how the dietary supplement industry surreptitiously re-introduces discontinued medications into their products.

Novel Psychoactive Substances (NPS) in Dietary Supplements and Doping

NPS in the Prohibited List

Novel psychoactive substances (NPS) are unregulated substances with no legitimate medical use and are made to copy the effects of controlled substances and evade detection [64]. They are introduced in and withdrawn from the market in quick suc-cession to escape or hamper law enforcement efforts to contain their manufacture and sale. Despite being advertised as "legal highs" with the pretention that they are safer than commonly used drugs of abuse, these synthetic designer versions are in many cases stronger than the natural product. As the dietary supplement market rapidly expands, the probability of introducing NPS into these products increases. The athletic population is commonly targeted for products marketed to enhance performance, power, focus and energy, and NPS that specifically address these needs are designed to bypass the testing menu of anti-doping laboratories. In addi-tion, athletes may follow societal trends and may consume NPS for recreational purposes.

Based on their pharmacological properties, NPS can be divided into six groups [65]:

- Stimulants
- Opioids
- Synthetic cannabinoid receptor agonists
- Dissociatives
- Classic hallucinogens
- Sedatives/hypnotics

The World-Anti Doping Code defines the criteria to include a substance or method in the Prohibited List (the List): (1) evidence that it has the potential to enhance or enhances sport performance; (2) represents an actual or potential health risk to the athlete; and (3) violates the spirit of sport, reflecting the values found in and through sport. The three criteria have the same weight, and two out of three need to be fulfilled in order to consider whether the substance or a method should be prohibited [66]. From the aforementioned NPS groups, only three of them have a place in the List: stimulants, opioids and synthetic cannabinoid receptor agonists [33]. Dissociatives (e.g. phencyclidine (PCP) and ketamine), classic hallucinogens (e.g., LSD, psilocybin) and sedatives/hypnotics (e.g. benzodiazepines, barbiturates) are not prohibited in sport because they do not fulfil two of the three criteria established by the Anti-Doping Code. In this regard, these groups of substances are physically and mentally performance detrimental, and therefore their use is incompatible with sport practice and competition. While they certainly represent a risk for the health of the athlete, they would not be considered a violation of the spirit of sport since their abuse is linked to recreational purposes or addiction rather than sport practice. As a consequence, they are outside WADA's responsibilities. In addition, serotonin reuptake inhibitors and modulators and pure nootropics affecting memory are not prohibited, as there is no evidence that they provide an unfair advantage in sport. All PS are prohibited in-competition only, since it is considered that their effects are short-lived. Although it can be argued that these substances may be advantageous out-of-competition during the training period as well, and should be prohibited at all times, this possibility has not been considered for the moment. As of 2021, the Code defines that the in-competition period starts at 11:59 pm of the day before the competition that the athlete is scheduled to participate and finishes at the end of the competition with the sample collection process [67]. The List also identifies prohibited substances and methods as specified on non-specified with regard to the application of sanctions, which range from a reprimand to a maximum of 4 years' ineligibility for a first offence [33, 66]. In the case of specified substances or methods, it is considered that there is a possibility they were used by an athlete for a purpose other than the enhancement of sport performance. Examples of specified substances would be those generally available in over-the-counter medicinal products, present in foodstuff, used mainly for recreational purposes or because they are less likely to be successfully abused as doping agents. Among the three classes of PS in the List, only a number of stimulants are clearly identified as non-specified (Class S6.a). These are mainly classical PS widely and effectively abused for doping in sport. S6.a is closed, meaning that only the substances named belong to this subclass. All other stimulants (S6.b) as well as narcotics (S7) and cannabinoids (S8) are specified substances [33]. The class of narcotics is also closed except with regard to fentanyl derivatives [33]. Specified stimulants (S6.b) and cannabinoids (S8) are open classes, meaning that only a number of examples are given in the List. Other drugs within the same category that are not named will fall into these categories by virtue of phrases such as "included but not limited" and "substances with similar chemical structure and/or similar biologic effect" to the ones listed. The purpose is twofold: (a) it would be practically not possible to name all substances existing worldwide within these categories, and (b) if a new substance comes onto the market, it will be automatically considered belonging to the class by virtue of its chemical structure and known or perceived pharmacological activity. Point (b) is particularly important for NPS, as any new designer drug will be covered within those categories as soon as WADA becomes aware of it and the chemical structure is verified, or the psychoactive effect inferred or reported. Any NP stimulant will automatically be classified as a specified stimulant. However, if WADA determines that the NPS has a profile that defines it as a non-specified stimulant (e.g., pharmacologically optimal for doping purposes, not available legally or over the counter), it will have to be included by name in the non-specified subclass. Since the List is updated every 1 January, the NP stimulant will temporarily be classified as specified during the course of the year and upgraded to non-specified by naming it in the S6.a section in the year that follows. All cannabinoids are specified substances, so all NPS in this class will be specified as well. Narcotics is a closed class, except for fentanyl and its derivatives, so any NPS that is derived from fentanyl will be automatically included. Any other type of narcotic NPS will need to be evaluated and included by name if it is deemed that it should be prohibited in sport. All drugs included in as narcotics are specified. The 2021 Code introduced the concept of "substances of abuse" [67], and the List will identify substances that are frequently abused in society outside of the context of sport. The 2021 List includes cocaine, diamorphine (heroin), methylenedioxymethamphetamine (MDMA/"ecstasy") and tetrahydrocannabinol (THC) [68]. This means that if an athlete can demonstrate that the use of any of these four substances was out-of-competition and unrelated to sport performance, the suspension imposed will be 3 months, with the possibility of reducing it to 1 month if the athlete completes a rehabilitation programme. Other drugs may be identified as "substances of abuse" in the future, but it is not expected that any NPS will be part of this group because there will be little data on the prevalence of use, the advantages offered in sports or their addiction potential. Evaluating the status of NPS is complex because very little is known about their effects. Not all PS are prohibited in sport as they must fulfil the criteria established in the Code. All NPS are potentially a risk for health (second criteria), as they are chemical products never tested for their safety profiles, produced in clandestine laboratories using unsophisticated techniques of synthesis and purification and prone to cross-contamination with other substances manufactured simultaneously. To define the potential performance-enhancing effect (first criteria) of an NPS, a first step is to determine the chemical structure to see if it fits any of the prohibited classes. For example, NP phenethylamines will mostly act as stimulants and be prohibited, but those containing methoxy groups on the two and five positions of the benzene ring are most likely hallucinogenic and, if so, will not be considered prohibited substances in sport [69]. Therefore, a lot can be inferred from the chemical structure. The biologic effects, however, will be more difficult to ascertain. Unlike experimental drugs in preclinical or clinical studies, it is not possible to test the psychoactive effects in controlled human studies, and the rapidity by which these NPS appear and disappear from the market does not make them attractive candidates for study in animals or in vitro. It is possible to gather some information on their effects by browsing Internet forums, where users/athletes exchange information about enhanced sport performance, and from forensic or emergency ward reports. Nevertheless, as written in the List, it is necessary to show chemical similarity or biologic effect, and in the vast majority of cases, it is relatively straightforward to establish one or the other. This task was further facilitated in the 2015 List, which identified the whole family of phenethylamine derivatives as prohibited, to address the growing number of NPS designer drugs derived from this chemical.

Trends

Traditional PS commonly used for doping purposes are easily detected by routine doping control analysis. However, it is more challenging to tackle that analysis and identification of NPS, which are steadily flooding the market. The ready access to raw materials, the simple chemical reactions involved in NPS synthesis, which facilitate mass production, and the growing influence of the underworld in doping activities favour the continuous supply of these drugs. In order to avoid detection, the product labels either do not list the NPS or do so under a fake name or a false chemical structure in an attempt to deceive the user and to delay or mislead the development of proper detection methods. As the structure of most NPS is unknown, the identification relies, mainly, on untargeted or retrospective screening analysis of doping control samples, analysis of material seized by law enforcement or the proactive purchase of supplements through Internet providers for its identification and validation of detection methods.

Three major groups can be identified as NPS in dietary supplements used for doping purposes.

i. *Stimulants*

The NPS included in dietary supplements are mainly derived from the "classic" doping stimulants described above. The most common can be divided into two groups:

- Phenethylamine (PEA) derivatives: this group includes derivatives of classical stimulants such as amphetamines, cathinones and ephedrines. The phenethylamine core can be slightly altered to produce a wide array of compounds that differ, for example, in the nitrogen terminus, the presence of alkyl chains at the α-carbon and a number of different phenyl ring substitutions. These structural minor changes can significantly impact the mechanism of action of designer phenethylamines, including monoamine release and/or reuptake inhibition, and the relative selectivity for the dopamine, norepinephrine and serotonin transporters [70–73]. The popularity of stimulants precedes the presence of this kind of NPS in supplements. They are routinely found in the analysis of products claiming to increase stamina as well as induce weight loss and are the source of numerous positive doping controls [34] as well as fatalities. Examples of these NPS include β-Methylphenethylamine (β-MePEA), α-Ethyl-phenethylamines (α-Ethyl-PEAs) and their derivatives [57, 74–79]. Synthetic cathinones such as mephedrone were first synthesised in the 1920s but remained largely unknown until they were rediscovered in the early twenty-first century. They were sold freely under names such as "bath salts", "plant food/fertilizers" or "research chemicals" and were at the time legal compounds. 3,4-Methylenedioxypyrovalerone (MDPV), a common synthetic cathinone, affects the brain in a manner similar to cocaine but is at least ten times more powerful [80]. Due to its link to several fatalities, MDPV and other synthetic cathinones have been recently classified as a controlled substance in some countries. However, synthetic cathinones are still readily available through the Internet in a wide array of replacement compounds with new chemical modifications in order to bypass law enforcement [81, 82].

- Aliphatic amines: the ban of 1,3-dimethylamylamine (methylhexaneamine) by sporting authorities led to an increase in the inclusion of similar aliphatic amines in supplements. Contrary to methylhexanamine, these new substances have never been approved as medications. These include 3-methylhexan-2-amine, 1,4-dimethylamylamine and 1,3-dimethylbutylamine [83–85]. Although octodrine (2-amino-6-methylheptane) cannot be technically considered an NPS, since it was commercialized in the past as a nasal decongestant, it has been recently reintroduced in the market of supplements, mainly targeting athletes [84].

ii. *Narcotics*

Despite the opioid and specifically the fentanyl crisis that has affected the world in recent years, it is not expected that these types of NPS will be purposely incorporated in dietary supplements targeting athletes. Fentanyl-derived NPS are 100 times more potent than morphine, so very low concentrations are needed to lethally overdose. This fact, combined with their addictive potential and side effects such as sedation, drowsiness, dizziness and respiratory depression, makes them rather incompatible and unattractive as components of sports dietary supplements.

To illustrate this point, mitragynine, an alkaloid with stimulant and opioid characteristics present in the plant product kratom, was included in the WADA Monitoring Program from 2014 to 2017, in order to determine patterns of abuse in athletes. Although mitragynine cannot be considered an NPS since it has been traditionally used in Southeast Asia, it has gained popularity as a dietary supplement in the western world in recent years [86–88]. However, the monitoring programme barely showed any use of mitragynine among the athletic population, further supporting that opioids NPS may not be of great concern in sports.

iii. *Cannabinoids*

Synthetic cannabinoids, such as "Spice", "herbal incense" and "K2", are man-made compounds that bind to the cannabinoid receptors, albeit with higher affinities when compared to tetrahydrocannabinol (THC) [89, 90]. While THC is metabolized to only one active metabolite, many NP synthetic cannabinoids metabolize to generate pharmacologically active metabolites prolonging the psychotropic effects of the parent compound and contributing to its toxicity. Although first synthesized in the mid-1960s, they became popular in the mid-2000s, as legal replacements to cannabis. Following reports of intoxications and deaths, Spice was banned, only to be replaced by other NP synthetic cannabinoids. Even though these products are mainly sold to be smoked, they are occasionally found in dietary supplements in the form of tablets, candies, cookies or liquids, usually mixed with other substances [91–93]. Although there is no solid evidence that these supplements are manufactured to enhance sport performance, they can certainly cause unintended doping when consumed for recreational purposes.

Prevention Strategies

The use of dietary supplements containing NPS by athletes is a serious concern, as a significant number of anti-doping rule violations have been attributed to the misuse of supplements [51, 94, 95]. Blaming a positive doping control to a poorly labelled dietary supplement is not an adequate defence in a doping hearing. The problems raised by NPS in supplements are globally twofold: those originating from the NPS themselves and those linked to the manufacturing of dietary supplements. The supplement industry is unregulated, and although the manufacturers are required to label their products, it is well known that discrepancies exist between ingredients listed on labels and the actual ingredients the products contain. The presence of NPS in a supplement could be intentional or could be due to subpar quality control during production. In addition, the lack of good manufacturing practices can lead to cross-contamination with other products in the manufacturing facility. This lack of regulation opens the door for fraudulent production of dietary supplements [96–102]. One way to deal with this problem is to regulate the supplement industry. However, this is within the jurisdiction and the will of the governments around the world, who are widely aware of the problem. With regard to sporting authorities, the best strategy lies with prevention achieved through education. This includes information offered via Internet access through the sports authorities' websites, active campaigns, reaching out to athletes during sports events, publications or conferences, to name a few. Athletes should be made aware that the risks of taking supplements far outweigh the potential benefits. Another strategy to avoid contaminated supplements is the use of products that have been subjected to a quality assurance scheme. However, WADA is neither involved in the testing of dietary/nutritional supplements nor in any certification process and therefore does not certify or endorse any products. In addition, the International Standard for Laboratories establishes that WADA-accredited laboratories cannot engage in analysing dietary supplements unless as part of a doping case investigation. Some third-party testers of supplements exist, and this may reduce the risk of contamination but not eliminate it. For example, even if one batch of a product is free of prohibited substances, there is no assurance that another batch will not be contaminated if the source of material and manufacturing practices are not controlled [100, 102–104]. However, regulating the supplement industry will only address part of the problematic of NPS in supplements. Many of the products originate from clandestine laboratories that are part of criminal rings dedicated to the production, smuggling and distribution of these products. Law enforcement authorities play a key role in identifying and clamping down these activities either through intelligence and investigations, seizures during raids or at border controls. However, once the NPS-containing supplement reaches the market, it is necessary to identify their presence both in the supplements and in the doping controls. While the approach of targeted screening for prohibited compounds or their metabolites in blood or urine is an effective approach for doping control, it has its limitations. In this regard, NPS are designer drugs intended to bypass targeted drug or doping control analysis, so a more untargeted approach is needed. Detection and identification of these substances, be it from seized material, online purchases, doping controls or forensic samples, is a major challenge. Therefore, once an NPS is identified, it is fundamental that the information is shared. Among the most comprehensive databases on NPS, the United Nations Office of Drug Control has developed the Early Warning Advisory portal that provides open access to basic information on these substances and, to registered users, specific information on their chemical structures and laboratory analysis [64, 65]. Other examples of information gathering include the National Forensic Laboratory Information System (NFLIS) as part of the Drug Enforcement Administration (DEA) programme that collect results of forensic analyses, the European Monitoring Centre for Drugs and Drug Addiction (EMCDDA) and the Inter-American Drug Abuse Control Commission (CICAD) [105–107]. Rapid access to information allows taking immediate preventive measures for NPS that may pose an immediate health threat to consumers and developing the appropriate analytical methods for early detection, to prevent widespread undetected use of these compounds.

Conclusion

The alarming production of NPS combined with the unregulated manufacturing of nutritional supplements targeted for athletes is a serious combination that should be tackled from different angles. The rapid response by anti-doping authorities to the appearance of an NPS that is not covered by anti-doping regulations or by the laboratories testing menus results in the synthesis and production of another NPS to once more start the cycle. The maintenance of and access to databases storing information on NPS are important elements to address the problem of these drugs in supplements. In addition, a tight and fluid interaction and exchange of information between government agencies, anti-doping organizations, law enforcement, analytical laboratories and researchers in the field, through scientific meetings, publications, articles or working groups, will certainly make this challenging task more efficient. In addition, pressure should be put on the authorities to regulate the industry manufacturing dietary supplements. Finally, athletes, who are the end consumer of these supplements, should be constantly reminded of the high risks of using these products, as they not only take a chance of producing a positive doping control test but are jeopardizing their health administering products that have not been subjected to preclinical studies. Through education, the demand should decrease, and if combined with a better controlled supplement industry and an effective NPS tracking and identification system, the difficulty of controlling NPS in supplements should be reduced to a minimum.

Acknowledgements I would like to thank Elizabeth Adams for helpful suggestions and proofreading.

References

1. Karunamoorthi K, Jegajeevanram K, Vijayalakshmi J, Mengistie E (2013) Traditional medicinal plants: a source of Phytotherapeutic modality in resource-constrained health care settings. J Evid Based Compl Altern Med 18:67–74
2. Fabricant D, Fansworth NR (2001) The value of plants used in traditional medicine for drug discovery. Environ Heath Perspect 109(Suppl 1):69–75
3. Falzon C, Balabanova A (2017) Phytotherapy: an introduction to herbal medicine. Prim Care 44:217–227
4. Bamola N, Verma P, Negi C (2018) A review on some traditional medicinal plants. Int J Life Sci Scienti Res 4:1550–1556
5. Sen T, Samanta SK (2015) Medicinal plants, human health and biodiversity: a broad review. Adv Biochem Eng Biotechnol 147:59–110
6. Taylor JLS, Rabe T, McGaw LJ, Jäger AK, van Staden J (2001) Towards the scientific validation of traditional medicinal plants. Plant Growth Reg 34:23–47
7. Shorter W, Kathryn Segesser K (2013) Traditional Chinese medicine and Western psychopharmacology: building bridges. Phytother Res 27:1739–1744
8. Campbel R, Young SP (2014) Central nervous system stimulants: basic pharmacology and relevance to anaesthesia and critical care. Anaesth Intensive Care Med 16:21–25
9. Patocka J (2015) Strychnine. In: Gupta RC (ed) Handbook of toxicology of chemical warfare agents, 2nd edn. Elsevier Inc, Amsterdam, pp 215–222
10. Henry TA (1949) The plant alkaloids, 4th edn. J & A Churchill
11. Taylor DA (2003) Central nervous system stimulants. In: IV Drugs affecting the central nervous system
12. Norn S, Kruse PR (2004) Cardiac glycosides: from ancient history through Withering's foxglove to endogeneous cardiac glycosides. Dan Medicinhist Arbog:119–132

13. Stolberg VB (2011) The use of coca: prehistory, history, and ethnography. J Ethnicity Subs Abuse 10:126–146
14. Lyon PJ (2004) The more things change. Latin Am Anthropol Rev 6:29–32
15. Presley CC, Lindsley CW (2018) DARK classics in chemical neuroscience: opium, a historical. Perspective ACS Chem Neurosci 9:2503–2518
16. Cassels BK, Sáez-Briones P (2018) Dark classics in chemical neuroscience: mescaline. ACS Chem Neurosci 9:2448–2458
17. Blainey MG (2015) Forbidden therapies: Santo Daime, Ayahuasca, and the prohibition of entheogens in Western society. J Relig Health 54:287–302
18. Geiger HA, Wurst MG, Daniels RN (2018) DARK classics in chemical neuroscience: psilocybin. ACS Chem Neurosci 9:2438–2447
19. Wasko MJ, Witt-Enderby PA, Surratt CK (2018) DARK classics in chemical neuroscience: Ibogaine. ACS Chem Neurosci 9:2475–2483
20. Chowdhury AN (1995) Drug abuse and eco-stress adaptation. Addiction 90:19–20
21. Kamienski L (2016) Shooting up. A short history of drugs and war. Oxford University Press, pp 31–304
22. Rasmussen N (2011) Medical science and the military: the Allies' use of amphetamine during world war II. J Interdiscip Hist 42:205–233
23. Defalque RJ, Wright AJ (2011) Methamphetamine for Hitler's Germany: 1937 to 1945. Bull Anesth Hist 29:21–24
24. Zvejniece L, Svalbe B, Veinberg G, Grinberga S, Vorona M, Kalvinsh I, Dambrova M (2011) Investigation into stereoselective pharmacological activity of phenotropil. Basic Clin Pharmacol Toxicol 109:407–412
25. Pedersen W, Sandberg S, Copes H (2015) High speed: amphetamine use in the context of conventional culture. Deviant Behav 36:146–165
26. Lakhan SE, Kirchgessner A (2012) Prescription stimulants in individuals with and without attention deficit hyperactivity disorder: misuse, cognitive impact, and adverse effects. Brain Behav 2:661–677
27. Yesalis CE, Bahrke MS (2002) History of doping in sport. In: Bahrke MS, Yesalis CE (eds) Performance-enhancing substances in sport and exercise. Human Kinetics, Champaign, IL, pp 1–20
28. Abbott K (2012) The 1904 Olympic Marathon may have been the strangest ever. Smithsonian Magazine, August 7 2012 https://wwwsmithsonianmagcom/history/the-1904-olympic-marathon-may-have-been-the-strangest-ever-14910747 Accessed 13 Oct 2020
29. Baron DA, Reardon CL, Baron SH (2013) Doping in sport. In: Baron DA, Reardon CL, Baron SH (eds) Clinical sports psychiatry: an international perspective. Wiley, Oxford, UK, pp 18–32
30. Verroken M (2000) Drug use and abuse in sport. Bailliere's Clin Endocrinol Met 14:1–23
31. Annex VIII (1968) Doping, report of the medical commission, minutes of the 66th session of the International Olympic Committee. New Town Hall, Grenoble, February 1–5
32. World Anti-Doping Agency. List of prohibited substances and methods (2004). https://www.wada-ama.org/sites/default/files/resources/files/WADA_Prohibited_List_2004_EN.pdf. Accessed 13 Oct 2020
33. World Anti-Doping Agency. List of prohibited substances and methods. (2020). https://www.wada-ama.org/sites/default/files/wada_2020_english_prohibited_list_0.pdf. Accessed 13 Oct 2020
34. World Anti-Doping Agency. Anti-Doping Testing Figures Report 2006–2018. https://www.wada-ama.org/en/resources/laboratories/anti-doping-testing-figures-report. Accessed 13 Oct 2020
35. Gurley BJ, Gardner SF, White LM, Wang PL (1998) Ephedrine pharmacokinetics after the ingestion of nutritional supplements containing Ephedra sinica (Ma Huang). Ther Drug Monit 20:439–445
36. Lee MR (2011) The history of ephedra (ma-huang) J Roy Coll Phys Edinburgh 41:78–84

37. Morton SC (2005) Ephedra. Stat Sci 20:242–248
38. Roman MC (2004) Determination of ephedrine alkaloids in botanicals and dietary supplements by HPLC-UV: collaborative study. J AOAC Int 87:1–14
39. Chang CW, Hsu SY, Huang GQ, Hsu MC (2018) Ephedra alkaloid contents of Chinese herbal formulae sold in Taiwan. Drug Test Anal 10:350–356
40. Miller SC (2004) Safety concerns regarding ephedrine-type alkaloid-containing dietary supplements. Military Med 169:87–93
41. Josefson D (1996) Herbal stimulant causes US deaths. Br Med J 312:1378–1379
42. Doyle H, Kargin M (1996) Herbal stimulant containing ephedrine has also caused psychosis. Br Med J 313:756
43. Ault A (1997) FDA proposes limits on ephedrine supplements. Lancet 349:1753
44. Nightingale SL (1996) Warning issued about the street drugs containing botanical sources of ephedrine. JAMA 275:1534
45. Haller C, Benowitz N (2000) Adverse cardiovascular and central nervous system events associated with dietary supplements containing ephedra alkaloids. N Engl J Med 343:1833–1838
46. Onakpoya IJ, Heneghan CJ, Aronson JK (2016) Post-marketing withdrawal of anti-obesity medicinal products because of adverse drug reactions: a systematic review. BMC Med 14:191–202
47. Lee MK, Cheng BWH, Che CT, Hsieh DPH (2000) Cytotoxicity assessment of Ma-huang (*Ephedra*) under different conditions of preparation. Toxicol Sci 56:424–430
48. Knight J (2004) Safety concerns prompt US ban on dietary supplement. Nature 427:90
49. Rocha T, Amaral JS, Oliveira MBPP (2016) Adulteration of dietary supplements by the illegal addition of synthetic drugs: a review. Comprehensive Rev Food Sci Food Safety 15:43–62
50. Wabe NT (2011) Chemistry, pharmacology, and toxicology of Khat (Catha Edulis Forsk): a review. Addict Health 3:137–149
51. Ros JJ, Pelders MG, De Smet PA (1999) A case of positive doping associated with a botanical food supplement. Pharm World Sci 21:44–46
52. (1950) New and nonofficial remedies: methylhexamine; Forthane. JAMA 143:1156
53. Lisi A, Hasick N, Kazlauskas R, Goebel C (2011) Studies of methylhexaneamine in supplements and geranium oil. Drug Test Anal 3:873–876
54. Elsohly MA, Gul W, Elsohly KM, Murphy TP, Weerasooriya A, Chittiboyina AG, Avula B, Khan I, Eichner A, Bowers LD (2012) Pelargonium oil and methyl hexaneamine (MHA): analytical approaches supporting the absence of MHA in authenticated *Pelargonium graveolens* plant material and oil. J Anal Toxicol 36:457–471
55. ElSohly MA, Gul W, Tolbert C, ElSohly KM, Murphy TP, Avula B, Chittiboyina AG, Wang M, Khan IA, Yang M, Guo D, Zhang WD, Su J (2015) Methylhexanamine is not detectable in Pelargonium or Geranium species and their essential oils: a multi-Centre investigation. Drug Test Anal 7:645–654
56. Austin KG, Travis J, Pace G, Lieberman HR (2014) Analysis of 1,3 dimethylamylamine concentrations in Geraniaceae, geranium oil and dietary supplements. Drug Test Anal 6:797–804
57. Pawar RS, Grundel E (2017) Overview of regulation of dietary supplements in the USA and issues of adulteration with phenethylamines (PEAs). Drug Test Anal 9:500–517
58. Venhuis B, Keizers P, van Riel A, de Kaste D (2014) A cocktail of synthetic stimulants found in a dietary supplement associated with serious adverse events. Drug Test Anal 6:578–581
59. Pawar RS, Sagi S, Leontyev D (2020) Analysis of bitter orange dietary supplements for natural and synthetic phenethylamines by LC-MS/MS. Drug Test Anal. https://doi.org/10.1002/dta.2871
60. Pohl K, Kriech W (1991) Therapy of orthostatic disorders of cardiovascular regulation. Placebo controlled double-blind study with oxilofrine. Fortschr Med 109:685–688
61. Yuen YP, Lai CK, Poon WT, Ng SW, Chan AY, Mak TW (2007) Adulteration of over-the-counter slimming products with pharmaceutical analogue-an emerging threat. Hong Kong Med J 13:216–220

62. De Carvalho LM, Cohen PA, Silva CV, Moreira APL, Falcao TM, Dal Molin TR, Zemolin G, Martini M (2012) A new approach to determining pharmacologic adulteration of herbal weight loss products. Food Addit Contam A 29:1661–1667

63. Park S, Lee JG, Roh SH, Kim G, Kwon CH, Park HR, Kwon KS, Kim D, Kwon SW (2012) Determination of PDE-5 inhibitors and appetite suppressants in adulterated dietary supplements using LC/PDA and LC/MS. Food Addit Contam B 5:29–32

64. UNODC Early warning advisory on new psychoactive substances. What are NPS? https://www.unodc.org/LSS/Page/NPS#:~:text=UNODC%20uses%20the%20term%20 %E2%80%9Cnew,pose%20a%20public%20health%20threat%E2%80%9D. Accessed 13 Oct 2020

65. UNODC Early warning advisory on new psychoactive substances. pharmacology. https://www.unodc.org/LSS/Page/NPS/pharmacology Accessed 13 Oct 2020

66. World Anti-Doping Agency. World Anti-Doping Code 2015. https://www.wada-ama.org/sites/default/files/resources/files/wada_anti-doping_code_2019_english_final_revised_v1_linked.pdf Accessed 13 Oct 2020

67. World Anti-Doping Agency. World Anti-Doping Code 2021 https://www.wada-ama.org/sites/default/files/resources/files/2021_wada_code.pdf Accessed 13 Oct 2020

68. World Anti-Doping Agency. List of prohibited substances and methods. (2021). https://www.wada-ama.org/sites/default/files/resources/files/2021list_en.pdf Accessed 13 Oct 2020

69. Fantegrossia WE, Murnanea AC, Reissigb CJ (2008) The behavioral pharmacology of hallucinogens. Biochem Pharmacol 75:17–33

70. Zamberlan F, Sanz C, Martínez Vivot R, Pallavicini C, Erowid F, Erowid E, Tagliazucchi E (2018) The varieties of the psychedelic experience: a preliminary study of the association between the reported subjective effects and the binding affinity profiles of substituted phenethylamines and tryptamines. Front Integrative Neurosci 12:1–22

71. Calinski DM, Kisor DF, Sprague JE (2019) A review of the influence of functional group modifications to the core scaffold of synthetic cathinones on drug pharmacokinetics. Psychopharmacol (Berl) 236:881–890

72. Peters FT, Martinez-Ramirez JA (2010) Analytical toxicology of emerging drugs of abuse. Ther Drug Monit 32:532–539

73. King LA (2014) New phenethylamines in Europe. Drug Test Anal 6:808–818

74. El Sohly MA, Gul W (2014) LC–MS-MS analysis of dietary supplements for N-ethyl-a-ethyl-phenethylamine (ETH), N, N-diethylphenethylamine and phenethylamine. J Anal Toxicol 38:63–72

75. Kwiatkowska D, Wójtowicz M, Jarek A, Goebel C, Chajewska K, Turek-Lepa E, Pokrywka A, Kazlauskas R (2015) N,N-dimethyl-2-phenylpropan-1-amine – new designer agent found in athlete urine and nutritional supplement. Drug Test Anal 7:331–335

76. Wójtowicz M, Jarek A, Chajewska K, Turek-Lepa E, Kwiatkowska D (2015) Determination of designer doping agent--2-ethylamino-1-phenylbutane--in dietary supplements and excretion study following single oral supplement dose. J Pharm Biomed Anal 115:523–533

77. Wójtowicz M, Jarek A, Chajewska K, Kwiatkowska D (2016) N,N-dimethyl-2-phenylpropan-1-amine quantification in urine: application to excretion study following single oral dietary supplement dose. Anal Bioanal Chem 408:5041–5047

78. Uralets V, App M, Rana S, Morgan S, Ross W (2014) Designer phenethylamines routinely found in human urine: 2-ethylamino-1-phenylbutane and 2-amino-1-phenylbutane. J Anal Toxicol 38:106–109

79. Cohen PA, Travis JC, Venhuis BJ (2014) A methamphetamine analog (N,-diethyl-phenylethylamine) identified in a mainstream dietary supplement. Drug Test Anal 6:805–807

80. Baumann MH, Walters HM, Niello M, Sitte HH (2018) Neuropharmacology of synthetic cathinones. Handb Exp Pharmacol 252:113–142

81. Riley AL, Nelson KH, To P, López-Arnau R, Xu P, Wang D, Wang Y, Shen HW, Kuhn DM, Angoa-Perez M, Anneken JH, Muskiewicz D, Hall FS (2020) Abuse potential and toxicity of the synthetic cathinones (i.e., "Bath salts"). Neurosci Biobehav Rev 110:150–173

82. Majchrzak M, Celiński R, Kuś P, Kowalska T, Sajewicz M (2018) The newest cathinone derivatives as designer drugs: an analytical and toxicological review. Forensic Toxicol 36:33–50

83. Cohen PA, Travis JC, Venhuis BJ (2015) A synthetic stimulant never tested in humans, 1,3-dimethylbutylamine (DMBA), is identified in multiple dietary supplements. Drug Test Anal 7:83–87

84. Cohen PA, Travis JC, Keizers PJH, Deuster P, Venhuis BJ (2018) Four experimental stimulants found in sports and weight loss supplements: 2-amino-6-methylheptane (octodrine), 1,4-dimethylamylamine (1,4-DMAA), 1,3-dimethylamylamine (1,3-DMAA) and 1,3-dimethylbutylamine (1,3-DMBA). Clin Toxicol (Phila) 56:421–426

85. Riley PA (2012) DMAA as a dietary supplement ingredient. Arch Intern Med 172:1038–1039

86. Han C, Schmitt J, Gilliland KM (2020) DARK classics in chemical neuroscience: Kratom. ACS Chem Neurosci. doi: https://doi.org/10.1021/acschemneuro.9b00535

87. Mudge EM, Brown PN (2018) Determination of alkaloids in *Mitragyna speciosa* (Kratom) raw materials and dietary supplements by HPLC-UV: single-laboratory validation, first action 2017.14. J AOAC Int 101:964–965

88. Chien GCC, Odonkor C, Amorapanth P (2017) Is Kratom the new 'legal high' on the block?: the case of an emerging opioid receptor agonist with substance abuse potential. Pain Phys 20:E195–E198

89. Alipour A, Patel PB, Shabbir Z, Gabrielson S (2019) Review of the many faces of synthetic cannabinoid toxicities. Ment Health Clin 9:93–99

90. Walsh KB, Andersen HK (2020) Molecular pharmacology of synthetic cannabinoids: delineating CB1 receptor-mediated cell signaling. Int J Mol Sci. https://doi.org/10.3390/ijms21176115

91. Heo S, Yoo GJ, Choi JY, Park HJ, Do JA, Cho S, Baek SY, Park SK (2016) Simultaneous analysis of cannabinoid and synthetic cannabinoids in dietary supplements using UPLC with UV and UPLC–MS-MS. J Ana Toxicol 40:350–359

92. Choi H, Heo S, Choe S, Yang W, Park Y, Kim E, Chung H, Lee J (2013) Simultaneous analysis of synthetic cannabinoids in the materials seized during drug trafficking using GC-MS. Anal Bioanal Chem 405:3937–3944

93. Rianprakaisang T, Gerona R, Hendrickson RG (2020) Commercial cannabidiol oil contaminated with the synthetic cannabinoid AB-FUBINACA given to a pediatric patient. Clin Toxicol (Phila) 58:215–216

94. Parr MK, Pokrywka A, Kwiatkowska D, Schänzer W (2011) Ingestion of designer supplements produced positive doping cases unexpected by the athletes. Biol Sport 28:153–157

95. US Anti-Doping Agency. Case studies and arbitration decisions. https://www.usada.org/athletes/substances/supplement-411/realize-safety-issues-exist/case-studies-arbitration-decisions/ Accessed 14 Oct 2020

96. Walpurgis K, Thomas A, Geyer H, Mareck U, Thevis M (2020) Dietary supplement and food contaminations and their implications for doping controls. Foods. https://doi.org/10.3390/foods9081012

97. Martínez-Sanz JM, Sospedra I, Ortiz CM, Baladía E, Gil-Izquierdo A, Ortiz-Moncada R (2017) Intended or unintended doping? A review of the presence of doping substances in dietary supplements used in sports. Nutrients 9:1093. https://doi.org/10.3390/nu9101093

98. Geyer H, Parr MK, Koehler K, Mareck U, Schänzer W, Thevis M (2008) Nutritional supplements cross-contaminated and faked with doping substances. J Mass Spectrom 43:892–902

99. Kohler M, Thomas A, Geyer H, Petrou M, Schänzer W, Thevis M (2010) Confiscated black market products and nutritional supplements with non-approved ingredients analyzed in the Cologne doping control laboratory 2009. Drug Test Anal 2:533–537

100. Attipoe S, Cohen PA, Eichner A, Deuster PA (2016) Variability of stimulant levels in nine sports supplements over a 9-month period. Int J Sport Nutr Exerc Metab 26:413–420

101. Uchiyama N, Matsuda S, Kawamura M, Kikura-Hanajiri R, Goda Y (2014) Identification of two new-type designer drugs, piperazine derivative MT-45 (I-C6) and synthetic peptide

Noopept (GVS-111), with synthetic cannabinoid A-834735, cathinone derivative 4-methoxy-α-PVP, and phenethylamine derivative 4-methylbuphedrine from illegal products. Forensic Toxicol 32:9–18

102. Australian Sports Anti-Doping Authority Supplements in sport. https://www.asada.gov.au/substances/supplements-sport Accessed 14 Oct 2020

103. UK Anti-Doping Managing supplements risks. https://www.ukad.org.uk/athletes/managing-supplement-risks Accessed 14 Oct 2020

104. de Hon O, Coumans B (2007) The continuing story of nutritional supplements and doping infractions. Br J Sports Med 41:800–805

105. Drug Enforcement Administration. National Forensic Laboratory Information System. https://www.nflis.deadiversion.usdoj.gov/ Accessed 14 Oct 2020

106. European Monitoring Centre for Drugs and Drug Addiction. https://www.emcdda.europa.eu/ Accessed 14 Oct 2020

107. Inter-American Drug Abuse Control Commission. http://www.cicad.oas.org/main/default_eng.asp Accessed 14 Oct 2020

Untested Supplement Use Among Athletes: An Overlooked Phenomenon?

Attilio Negri, Honor D. Townshend, and Ornella Corazza

Untested Sport Supplements: A Growing Public Health Concern

Dietary and sports supplement is an umbrella term that includes products containing vitamins, minerals, herbals and botanicals or enzymes, which are available in various forms (bars, powders, gels, liquids, tablets or capsules) and are used to add further nutritional value to a usual diet [1, 2, 3]. A great number of these products are marketed and promoted as compounds able to correct or prevent nutritional deficiencies, improve overall health status, enhance physical performance, lose weight or reduce pain, and they are often considered a safer and more natural alternative to prescription medicines. However, whilst prescription drugs are subject to stringent manufacturing processes by national and international medicine regulatory agencies, including premarketing clinical trials and post-marketing assessments, supplements are not subject to the same scrutiny, and guidelines vary broadly from country to country. This therefore may allow manufacturers to sell products that have had no official control or testing as to their purity, safety and efficacy. This allows these producers to increase their revenues and profits whilst potentially exposing consumers to adverse effects and health risks, due to the presence of contaminants and impurities generated by the superficial production processes [4]. The International Olympic Committee (IOC) has recently intervened on this matter stating that "it takes considerable effort and expert knowledge to identify which

A. Negri (✉) · O. Corazza
Department of Clinical, Pharmaceutical and Biological Sciences, School of Life and Medical Science, University of Hertfordshire, Hatfield, Hertfordshire, UK
e-mail: attilio.negri@unimi.it

H. D. Townshend
Department of Criminology, School of Law, University of Hertfordshire, Hatfield, Hertfordshire, UK

products are appropriate, how to integrate them into the athlete's sports nutrition plan, and how to ensure that any benefits outweigh the possible negative side effects, including the potential for an adverse drug reaction" [5]. Despite this growing concern, the global sales of supplements have skyrocketed in recent years, especially in the USA and China, recording revenues of over $120 billion in 2017 with the prediction to reach more than $180 billion in the next 5 years, at the unprecedented annual growth rate of almost 9% [6]. However, despite this increasing concern, there is also evidence that generally speaking, supplements are good for overall health. Seventy-five percent of US adults take dietary supplements such as multivitamins, multiminerals and proteins, with no significant differences according to age, gender, income or education level. An increase in the use of herbals and botanicals products has also been recorded among consumers, totalling a 13% increase in the past 5 years. The most common reasons cited for this use of supplementations are as follows: to improve health, to benefit general wellness, to gain energy and/or to fill nutritional gaps [6].

Patterns of Supplement Use

The wide availability of supplements, sometimes endorsed by popular elite athletes, has made ergonutritional aids an essential part of the training for the majority of those engaging in physical activities. This population includes elite as well as amateur athletes and even generally recreationally active individuals seeking to boost or optimize their physical performance. Although the use of dietary supplements and ergogenic aids in sport competitions has been evidenced dating back as far as the first Olympic Games [7], their consumption has seen a notable increase, particularly in certain population groups (e.g., high-performance athletes) where the prevalence of use is estimated to range between 60% and 90% [8–11]. This evidence has also been confirmed by a recent meta-analysis on more than a hundred studies showing how elite athletes are more likely to use dietary supplements than their amateur counterparts [12]. Lun and colleagues also identified a positive association between sport supplement intake, total weekly training hours and participation in endurance-based sport events [13]. Furthermore, a recent cross-sectional study on Dutch elite and sub-elite athletes showed that almost the totality of the respondents (97.2%) used supplements. Interestingly, those receiving dietary counselling by a professional nutritionist were also more likely to use dietetic supplements, such as vitamin D, recovery drinks, energy bars, protein bars, isotonic drinks, dextrose, beta-alanine and sodium bicarbonate [12]. The trends of this consumption would suggest that this use appears to increase with age and is more frequent in men than in women [7]. It also usually involves the use of multiple compounds, correlating with the phase of the workout (e.g., "stacking") or in cycles of different lengths. In a survey of 800 high-performing athletes, 82.6% of the sample declared using more than one supplement and 11.5% reported regularly using more than five [14]. Although the use of supplements in sport is well documented across relevant literature, the existing evidence is often quite fragmented and collected with different methodologies across heterogeneous populations. It can thus be argued that patterns of use of sports supplements still represent a major knowledge gap, which needs to be addressed, particularly due to the exponential growth of this market in recent years. Researchers have referred to the intake of supplements as a positive reinforcement towards doping practices in athletes as a "grey zone" [7]. This conceptual framework, also known as the "gateway hypothesis" [15], is best modelled with Kandel's theory on psychoactive drugs which showed that the use of nicotine, alcohol and cannabis in adolescents may escalate to the consumption of more addictive illicit drugs later in adulthood [16]. Similarly, the gateway concept suggests that supplement use may precede, or facilitate, the intake of other prohibited substances at a later stage. In other terms, using a compound to improve performances, lose/gain weight or increase energy may be the first step to the consumption of other substances, including hormones, stimulants and other substances prohibited by the World Anti-Doping Agency (WADA). This model further argues that supplement use and doping share a common intent of performance enhancement: a prolonged goal-oriented behaviour, in order to increase physical strength or endurance, and thus they may ultimately lead to the use of doping substances. Although no direct causality has been established between sports supplement use and doping, it has been reported that doping is more prevalent in athletes that take supplementation products than in those who do not [16, 17]. Further to this point, a recent study among athletes by Hurst and colleagues found an association between ergonutritional aids, doping attitudes and doping likelihood, leading them to state that "if athletes perceive sport supplements as beneficial for performance, they may subsequently be more likely to consider doping" [18]. It has additionally been argued that athletes may follow a "more is better" philosophy, consuming increasing doses of multiple supplements encouraged by the belief that rivals are taking even higher doses [6]. Supporting evidence also emerged from our recent "Keep Fit" study, conducted among almost 2000 exercisers across the EU [19]. A large percentage (39.8%) of study participants declared using a variety of different fitness products, including supplements, unprescribed medical products (e.g., anabolic steroids; diuretics; growth hormones) and illicit drugs (e.g., amphetamine). These products were predominantly bought online and were taken with no medical supervision. The sample also highlighted a previously unexplored association between the use of supplements and various psychopathologies, such as exercise addiction (EA) and body dysmorphic disorders (BDD), including muscle dysmorphia (MD) [19].

Health Risks and Contamination Issues

Whilst the hypotheses that supplement use can reinforce a "doping attitude" requires further evidence to be confirmed, it is known that a growing number of athletes have tested positive for prohibited substances due to the intake of supplements. Cases have ranged from Olympic sprinters to swimmers, basketball players, martial arts fighters, professional drivers and even professional bridge players who have blamed an adulterated sport supplement for their failed doping test. Among the unlabelled contaminants allegedly within these supplements were stimulants, anabolic steroids, estrogen receptor modulators, diuretics and other pharmaceuticals. However, there are a number of factors to consider regarding these claims of unintentional doping. Primarily, from the perspective of the athlete, the intake of a prohibited substance has often become a key legal strategy to appeal against doping suspensions [20–22]. Another consideration is that the mislabelling or contamination might also be unintentional on the part of the producers. In fact, cross-contamination of an otherwise legal supplement may happen for those manufacturers who produce a variety of compounds, such as prohormones. In addition, the counterfeit products do not follow any type of quality control, and in most cases, inorganic compounds like lead, arsenic, zinc, mercury and chromium were found as well as residual bacterial products from the production of recombinant proteins, indicating poor purification processing processes [23]. However, where this is the case, the concentration of contaminants is usually low. As such, when the concentrations of prohormones or stimulants are high, it is plausible to consider that they might have been added intentionally by the manufacturers in the attempt to boost the effects of the products with pharmacological doses of active adulterants. Although the consumers of these contaminated supplements may be unaware of the actual content of such products, if a doping control proves positive due to this use, it is still considered the responsibility of the athlete. Therefore, it is the athlete, not the manufacturer or the distributor, who will face sanctions if tested positive, potentially damaging their career, credibility and possibly their own health, depending on the dose and type of contaminant. This adulteration of supplements might be more common than once assumed. A recent analysis of FDA's *Tainted Products Marketed as Dietary Supplements* database identified 776 adulterated products between 2007 and 2016, with 443 of these (57.1%) being reported from 2012 to 2016 [4]. These were mainly sold as fat burners, weight-loss aids or muscle-building compounds but contained variable quantities of unlabelled prohibited compounds, from testosterone to growth hormone (GH). Studies involving the analysis of sports supplements with gas or liquid chromatography-mass spectrometry in order to detect undisclosed substances also always reported relatively high percentages of positive results [20, 21, 24, 25]. As it will be better examined in the athletes' testimonies presented in this book, when the goal is to succeed in such a high-performance culture, athletes may be more inclined to use supplements following the aforementioned "more is better" philosophy, therefore consuming high doses of multiple supplements, encouraged by the belief that rivals are taking more [7]. Such hazardous behaviours can have serious and long-lasting health consequences and, with the prevalence of potential contaminants, can be considered high risk. An analysis by Geller et al. reported 23,000 accesses to US emergency rooms between 2004 and 2013 due to side effects from dietary supplements, of which almost one out of ten resulted in prolonged hospitalisations [26]. The primary issue is that athletes at various levels of their career may have limited knowledge of the potential risks associated with supplement use, such as these adverse events or contamination [27, 28], and as such may not take harm-reductive actions that may be beneficial. Evidencing this misinformation is a survey on 164 teenager elite athletes, only one third was informed of the risk of contamination, and among those unaware, only a small percentage expressed the need for a better information on the topic [8].

Need for a Shared Global Regulatory Framework

Laws and regulations regarding dietary and sports supplements are not uniform across countries and have been a matter of concern for national and international agencies in recent years. In the USA, the Dietary Supplement Health and Education Act (DSHEA) regulates supplements as foods, which thus requires producers to be responsible for their own products' safety and appropriate labelling of ingredients [29]. Therefore, it is only down to the Food and Drug Administration (FDA) to remove any product from the market if an adulteration, misbranding, risk of illness or adverse event is reported. In 2006, the Dietary Supplement and Non-prescription Drug Consumer Protection Act updated these regulations. Subsequently it was required that the producers of sports and dietary supplements, as well as manufacturers and distributors of other over-the-counter drugs, report any adverse event which may have been caused by one of their products. However, a high percentage of them initially failed to accomplish this requirement [27]. In Europe, the European Food Safety Authority (EFSA) provides similar guidelines, as well as a list of specific substances or compounds that may be intended as sports or dietary supplements [30]. However, member states lack a harmonized regulation and classification, and consequently quality controls of manufacturing may significantly vary across European countries. In Australia, supplements may be regulated as either food or medicine, dependant on whether they meet the requirements outlined in the Food Standards Code, or the Therapeutic Goods Act (TGA) [31]. Due to this guideline which means supplementation products may be regulated as either therapeutic goods or food, consumers in Australia may also use a "food-medicine interface guidance tool" which aids them in determining which standards these products are regulated by [31]. In Asia, China recently updated the national regulation of dietary supplements with the new Food Safety Law of 2015. These new parameters require companies to apply and obtain a health food registration certificate, as well as a full testing report generated from analysis of three samples before placing health food into the Chinese market [32]. However, the law establishes that certain supplements (e.g., minerals and vitamins) may bypass the China Food and Drug Administration's (CFDA) registration process due to a notification-based system. In the absence of a shared global regulatory framework, the market of dietary and sports supplements remains largely unregimented and unexplored, in particular considering the virtually unlimited possibilities provided by the Internet, both in terms of online sales and information sharing among users.

An Alarming Netnographic Snapshot
of the Supplement Market

More and more athletes have found online communities reliable virtual spaces to exchange information on sport routines, equipment or products, including dietary supplements. Whilst previously dietary advice was predominantly obtained from coaches, medical professionals and other trusted and accountable persons, such reputable formats have progressively been replaced by the Internet and social media [7, 33, 34]. A major issue with this shift is that members of these online communities often exchange information, or provide unsolicited advice [35], without any professional medical surveillance on adverse effects and risks, including those of intentional or involuntary doping [36]. A higher proportion of athletes are also more inclined to buy products directly from Internet websites than before, trusting claims and advertisements rather than verifying brands certification of controls and safety [1]. In a globalised society, which relies on Internet communication and content sharing, such risks are no longer confined to competing athletes but now permeate to lower-level athletes as well as amateur gym-goers of all ages, making this a potential public health issue [23]. Such a drastic evolution in the sport and health sector emphasises the need to pay more attention to online, or as we prefer to call it, "netnographic" content regarding supplement use. Since social networks and online forums have become an essential part of the online world, new techniques of investigation such as netnography (i.e. ethnography on the Internet) have been developed. Netnography is defined as the utilization of social science research methods to carry out ethnographic research, which encompasses both online and archival communication networks. This type of research allows the researcher to select and collect online data by the regular observation of these online networks, in order to collect and analyse data from these digital networks quantitatively and qualitatively [37]. Netnographic studies can therefore be described as research into "the nature of online social experience and interaction" [38]. We have successfully piloted such methodologies to conduct an analysis of posts on sport and fitness forums, in order to identify personal factors linked to supplement use. This included considerations such as motivations of use, perceived risks of use, self-reported side effects and attitudes towards doping and sport values, among other features [1]. We summarise in this section some of the key highlights of our study. An initial systematic monitoring of the Internet was carried out. Generic keywords such as "sport supplement", "fitness supplement", "dietary supplement", "workout supplement", "ergogenic aid" and "nutraceutic" were searched through an automated online tool (Brand24®) for a total period of 30 days. The tool provides a real-time analysis of the web across multiple channels (consisting of news sites, social media, blogs, forums and advertisement sites, among others), analysing mentions for different keywords and collecting references, discussion volumes and sentiment analysis for the content. This tool uses natural language processing, text analysis, computational linguistics and biometrics to systematically identify, extract, quantify and study affective states and subjective information. This allowed us to identify the most

Table 1 Top five supplements discussed online

Keyword	Number of mentions	Positive (%)	Negative (%)	Number of interactions	Number of shares	Number of mentions related to doping or contamination (%)
Creatine	9375	2335 (75)	789 (25)	6108	779	30 (0.32)
Branded chain amino acid/ BCAA	8290	3377 (87)	485 (13)	10,598	638	14 (0.16)
Whey protein	17,438	5532 (82)	1255 (18)	44,954	1206	35 (0.20)
Nitric oxide/ nitric oxide booster	10,392	580 (69)	259 (31)	1502	316	15 (0.14)
Multivitamin	9063	2750 (81)	649 (19)	27,912	3302	24 (0.26)

discussed fitness products, as well as the most relevant online forums, for further manual qualitative analysis. Overall, we were able to identify 19,835 references related to sport supplements with a social media reach of around 4 million individuals. Social networks (19.2%), blogs (35.3%) and Internet fora (3.9%) were the most common online resources identified. The most popular hashtags associated with supplements online were "#fitness", "#workout", "#gym" and "#health", and an automated sentiment analysis on the mentions revealed that 86% of them were classified as "positive" content. Only 218 (1.17%) of the collected mentions were related to adulteration, contamination or doping issues. The most cited substances or type of supplements in our sample were creatine, branded chain amino acid (BCAA), whey protein, nitric oxide boosters and multivitamin supplements. "Whey protein" was the most discussed fitness supplement, appearing in 17,438 references of our sample with 44,954 interactions and 1,206 shares among Internet users. This was followed by multivitamins and BCAA, reference, interaction and rates for which can be viewed in Table 1.

The most positively rated compounds as per this analysis were "branded chain amino acids" (87%) and "whey protein" (81%): related hashtags were linked to wellness, healthy nutrition and lifestyle. A limited number of references for each of the five most popular products were collected when filtered to select doping-related mentions, consisting of 30 (0.32%) for creatine, 14 (0.16%) for BCAA, 35 (0.20%) for whey protein, 15 (0.14%) for nitric oxide supplements and 24 (0.26%) for multivitamin supplements. Within the subsequent manual qualitative analysis, a wide range of motivations for use of sport and dietary supplements emerged from our analysis. Muscle mass gain was by far the highest mentioned reason for supplement usage, with 39 out of 123 (23%) fora threads referring to this as a significant or the sole reason for the use of supplements. Muscle mass gain was cited in the context of body image, as opposed to strength, which was only mentioned only eight times (4% of mentions in fora threads). This evident correlation between supplementation is significant, due to previous research finding connections between mental health and problematic health routines, particularly in men, whom made up 76% of posts on the assessed fora threads. The second most common self-reported motivation for use of all supplements was to aid in increasing energy, with 23 (17%) fora threads mentioning the positive effects on energy levels that supplements can have. This was particularly relevant with regard to BCAAs, creatine and multivitamins. The aspiration for increased energy was directly linked to the individual wanting to continue their sporting activities, as opposed to the want for energy in other elements of life. Other motivations cited were weight loss/gain, the negating of the side effects of other substances or to contribute to their effects, fat loss, injury recovery and muscle maintenance. The second theme of our qualitative analysis regarded the availability of information on supplement intake. Users in our sample consulted a number of sources to gain advice about nutrition supplement compounds: surprisingly, the highest referenced point of information collection was academic studies and papers, with 30% of posts referring to academic literature as a citation for their information. However, very few comments were made on posts of these nature, and of those comments that did exist, many stated that the language was too difficult to be understood by non-academic readers. Therefore, a few key fora users would act as interpreters and disseminators of the information. This validates the importance of continued academic development and research in the field in order to ensure the maintenance of relevant literature available for the fora users. It also shows the interest of users in evidence-based information to mitigate any potential concerns. However, this is also problematic for several reasons. Despite academic materials being the most cited source, it was still only mentioned in 30% of posts, meaning that key harm-reducing information is potentially being missed by individuals to whom it would be beneficial. Another issue is that the requirement of a fora user to act as the interpreter requires this individual to be construing the information correctly. As such, there is a recommendation that academic findings ought to be disseminated in a number of alternative formats to the traditional papers, such as posters, presentations, leaflets and other forms utilising new media formats, as well as posts on fora to ensure a wider reach of reputable information. The second most cited reference for finding information was generically termed in our research as "online", which included supplement-dedicated websites and social media, with 21% of fora users referring to these sources. This was followed by so-called fitness influencers, with 17% of assessed posts referring to these sources. Fitness influencers refer in this context to individuals, who may be professional athletes or otherwise, with high social media presence and reach, who post about their gym activity and supplement use. This is particularly worthy of note due to the lack of current regulation of these types of posts, either legally or site-specifically, meaning that the information is uncertified and potentially inaccurate. Other sources of information were cited as supplement manufacturers (13%), worth noting due to the potential bias of this information, magazines (8%), blogs (2%), nutritionists (2%), doctors (2%), and brand ambassadors (2%). Various side effects were mentioned in fora posts, with 14% of all posts discussing this topic. The most common side effects forming the basis of entire discussion threads were acne (9%) and water retention

(9%). The former was predominantly linked to discussions of whey protein, though did also come up in relation to the use of multivitamins. Specifically, nitric oxide supplements were mentioned with one fora user stating "Since I started using my new supplements from NO, I have been having some rather bad acne. This is the first time it is happening to me—never thought that just supplements can cause these problems". With regard to water retention, this was mentioned solely in relation to the use of creatine. Though the water retention was not explicitly stated to be causing harm to anyone in the assessed posts, it was an undesirable side effect noted by many. Following these in most-mentioned side effects were rashes, erectile issues and stomach pain, all with 7% of posts referring to these side effects. The rashes discussed varied in bodily location and were mentioned only in relation to whey protein. Erectile issues refer to either additional erections or difficulties in obtaining erection and were predominantly discussed in relation to nitric oxide and its perceived positive impact on this function. Stomach pain was mentioned in posts discussing BCAAs, whey protein and multivitamins and was actively linked by fora contributors as a direct causal effect from the supplements, with one post entitled "I think my new protein is giving me bad stomach pains". In terms of perceived health risks associated with supplement intake, the biggest concern for fora users was damage to the kidneys, with 15% of all posts discussing risks to health considering this as a significant risk. This was predominantly discussed in relation to creatine, though was also mentioned in a thread regarding multivitamins and their impact on the potential development of kidney stones according to one fora user. The use of creatine was regularly mentioned in the context of its use to alleviate some of the issues associated with the use of anabolic androgenic steroids (AAS), and one poster stated confusion regarding the negative association of creatine and these health issues, stating "I can't see any reason for why everybody says Creatine is a waste of time during Steroids and will hurt the kidney". Although being one of the motivations for supplement intake, another concern regularly discussed (in 10% of relevant posts) was weight gain. This was perceived as a significant concern to the population of fora users who, as mentioned earlier, often have a collective goal of weight loss and/or muscle gain. This was mentioned as a perceived risk from BCAAs, creatine and whey protein, with the latter being cited as a concern by one forum user regarding the development of gynecomastia (cited as "man boobs") if dosage was not properly regulated. This closely relates to the concerns regarding water retention, which has a frequency of 8% in this sub-section. The predominant concern about water retention was its impact on physical appearance, as opposed to any perceived direct risks to health, but it was still considered an important theme to be noted. Finally, a prominent theme was generic "health concerns" (10%), with users predominantly asking advice for any perceived health risks from other individuals who had previously used a supplement type, showing that users are indeed worried about the use of their supplements and the potential side effects. Posts containing concerns on supplement contamination (26%) and possible doping implications also emerged from our analysis. For instance, a consumer stated: "Oxandrolone isn't supposed to cause water retention so I doubt it's that. And no they aren't D-bol, the pills match the description" insinuating that supplements with different effects are being labelled and sold incorrectly. Concerns about specific brands/websites selling such products were also often shared with other users. For instance, a fora user stated that "most supplements out there have tons of fillers and a pathetic amount of ingredients/dosages. they are worthless. [Brand] actually puts in tons of ingredients in their stuff". Additional concerns included counterfeit products (10%) and the presence of illicit substances (10%), the latter encompassing the contamination of products specifically with illicit drugs (AAS). Regarding the use of illicit substances alongside supplements, a post discussed the links between the use of supplements and illegal drug dealing. Interestingly, though, despite the concerns of contamination with legal and illegal products, along with concerns about the legitimacy of purchased products, only 6% of the screened posts mentioned concerns around "cheating" or ethical/moral aspects around the intake of supplements in either a professional sporting or personal achievement sense. One fora poster stated: "Do you feel that creatine is cheating? I want to earn my muscles the hard way and don't want to cheat to get them", evidencing the latter interpretation of cheating. On a thread discussing a specific product, a profile posted to say, "I don't know if you guys remember or ever used this product, I was a faithful user until it was banned by FDA, I'm wondering if is there is out there a product similar to it?". The abstinence from a product due to its status as a banned product evidences conscientiousness regarding not appearing to be cheating. Additionally, 6% of assessed posts suggested a causal link between the use of supplements and the use of illicit substances, insinuating a "gateway" principle. One fora user stated that "Creatine and Bulgarian tribulus are also gateway drugs", with another post referencing an academic article that discussed the link between teenagers who use supplements going on to take AAS. A variety of other issues were covered by this subtopic, including fora posts regarding hidden ingredients, banned supplements, content scepticism, legal questions and quality concerns [1].

Conclusion

The explosion in the popularity of untested fitness supplements and the increase of their intake have the potential to cause adverse effects among users, due to the undeclared presence of illicit substances and other contaminants. In the absence of strict regulations, online distributors and physical retailers can easily sell counterfeit products to unaware customers, such as present/future amateur and professional athletes. This phenomenon might also be seen a "new gateway to doping". It has been hypothesized that if non-athletes perceive sport supplements as beneficial for their performance, and are encouraged to take them because of the positive online narrative and the captivating marketing strategies, they may also be subsequently more likely to consider doping when involved in a competitive activity, if not educated otherwise. Among the web content retrieved in our study, we found numerous health blogs reviewing supplements' brands, sports fora discussing specific workout programmes and social media threads providing counselling for beginners. This justifies the need for more targeted prevention strategies by regulatory agencies, health professionals and academic institutions: this should not be limited to elite athletes but more inclusive of this new at-risk cohort who are less likely to receive any medical advice or supervision regarding their supplementations. Furthermore, a wide range of side effects and perceived risks were posted online by supplement users, such as overuse of supplements, combining supplements, cramping, dehydration, hidden ingredients and quality concerns. Reported side effects were usually attributed by fora moderators and blog owners to subjective intolerances, who it is believed may also interfere in the discussions by deleting negative comments or promoting positive ones for their commercial interests. The risks of an uncontrolled supplement potentially concern not only the cited physical issues but also a variety of psychopathological features that can emerge, sustain or worsen underlying psychiatric symptoms, such as anxiety, low self-esteem, exercise addiction and low body satisfaction. Medical professionals, often unaware of such risks, might disregard such conditions in both the assessment and treatment of their patients. It is thus of paramount importance to raise awareness to trained medical doctors on such emerging issues, particularly when considering the high availability of such supplements in the market. And finally, more precise information on every advertised compound should be available online for each user to better be able to avoid risky supplementation and the associated possible adverse effects. In a globalised and rapidly changing society, novel approaches are overall required to complement laboratory analysis in verifying the presence of potential adulterants, including substances incorporated in the WADA List of Prohibited Substances and Methods. It is crucial to develop more sophisticated tools and methods for the rapid identification of new licit and illicit compounds available on the web and to be able to anticipate future trends. The large amount of data collected in our preliminary study suggests a wide scope for future netnographic investigations, which could be invaluable to the health and safety of athletes and other supplement users. The advent of new technologies such as "big data" and artificial intelligence (AI), which are currently specifically developed for and incorporated in general pharmacovigilance and toxicovigilance programmes, may further facilitate and expand the research process [39]. Novel approaches and technologies may contribute to the creation of online resources and accessible databases designed to address the issue of uncontrolled supplement use and their possible contamination. An even stronger collaboration between regulatory agencies and academic institutions would be needed at the global level to anticipate future trends: this should involve also public authorities, in order to strengthen and harmonize regulations worldwide, provide stricter pre-marketing requirements and enhance the control role by health agencies. We can no longer act in isolation.

References

1. Catalani V, Negri A, Townshend H, Simonato P, Prilutskaya M, Tippett A, Corazza O. (2021) The market of sport supplements in the digital era: A netnographic analysis of perceived risks, side-effects and other safety issues. Emerging Trends in Drugs, Addictions and Health 1, 100014. https://doi.org/10.1016/j.etdah.2021.100014

2. Mazzoni I, Barroso O, Rabin O, 2017. Anti-doping challenges with novel psychoactive substances in sport, in: Novel Psychoactive Substances: Policy, Economics and Drug Regulation. Springer International Publishing, pp. 43–56. https://doi.org/10.1007/978-3-319-60600-2_4

3. US Food and Drug Administration (FDA) (2020) Dietary supplement products & ingredients. Available at http://www.fda.gov/Food/DietarySupplements/ProductsIngredients/default.htm

4. Tucker J, Fischer T, Upjohn L, Mazzera D, Kumar M (2018) Unapproved Pharmaceutical Ingredients Included in Dietary Supplements Associated With US Food and Drug Administration Warnings. JAMA Network Open 1:e183337

5. Maughan RJ, Burke LM, Dvorak J, Larson-Meyer DE, Peeling P, Phillips SM, Rawson ES, Walsh NP, Garthe I, Geyer H, Meeusen R, Van Loon LJC, Shirreffs SM, Spriet LL, Stuart M, Vernec A, Currell K, Ali VM, Budgett RG, Engebretsen L (2018) IOC consensus statement: dietary supplements and the high-performance athlete. Br J Sports Med 52:439–455. https://doi.org/10.1136/bjsports-2018-099027

6. Council for Responsible Nutrition (CRN) (2018) Consumer Survey on Dietary Supplements. Available at www.crnusa.org/CRNConsumerSurvey

7. Garthe I, Maughan RJ (2018) Athletes and supplements: Prevalence and perspectives. Int J Sport Nutr Exerc Metab 28:126–138. https://doi.org/10.1123/ijsnem.2017-0429

8. Braun H, Koehler K, Geyer H, Kleiner J, Mester J, Schanzer W (2009) Dietary supplement use among elite young German athletes. Int J Sport Nutr Exerc Metab 19:97–109

9. Baylis A, Cameron-Smith D, Burke LM (2011) Inadvertent doping through supplement use by athletes: assessment and management of the risk in Australia. Int J Sport Nutr Exerc Metab 11:365–383

10. Froiland K, Koszewski W, Hingst J, Kopecky L (2004) Nutritional supplement use among college athletes and their sources of information. Int J Sport Nutr Exerc Metab 14:104–120

11. Wardenaar FC, Ceelen IJM, Van Dijk JW, Hangelbroek RWJ, Van Roy L, Van Der Pouw B, De Vries JHM, Mensink M, Witkamp RF (2017) Nutritional supplement use by Dutch elite and sub-elite athletes: Does receiving dietary counseling make a difference? Int J Sport Nutr Exerc Metab 27:32–42. https://doi.org/10.1123/ijsnem.2016-0157

12. Knapik JJ, Steelman RA, Hoedebecke SS, Austin KG, Farina EK, Lieberman HR (2016) Prevalence of dietary supplement use by athletes: systematic review and meta-analysis. Sports Med 46:103–123. https://doi.org/10.1007/s40279-015-0387-7

13. Lun V, Erdman KA, Fung TS, Reimer RA (2012) Dietary supplementation practices in Canadian high-performance athletes. Int J Sport Nutr Exerc Metab 22:31–37. https://doi.org/10.1123/ijsnem.22.1.31

14. Petroczi A, Naughton DP (2008) The age-gender-status profile of high performing athletes in the UK taking nutritional supplements: Lessons for the future. J Int Soc Sports Nutr 5:2. https://doi.org/10.1186/1550-2783-5-2

15. Backhouse SH, Whitaker L, Petroczi A (2013) Gateway to doping? Supplement use in the context of preferred competitive situations, doping attitude, beliefs, and norms. Scand J Med Sci Sports 23:244–252

16. Kandel D (1975) Stages in adolescent involvement in drug use. Science 190:912–914

17. Lazuras L, Barkoukis V, Mallia L, Lucidi F, Brand R (2017) More than a feeling: the role of anticipated regret in predicting doping intentions in adolescent athletes. Psychol Sport Exerc 30:196–204

18. Hurst P, Kavussanu M, Boardley I, Ring C (2019) Sport supplement use predicts doping attitudes and likelihood via sport supplement beliefs. J Sports Sci 37(15):1734–1740. https://doi.org/10.1080/02640414.2019.1589920

19. Corazza O, Simonato P, Demetrovics Z, Mooney R, van de Ven K, Roman-Urresterazu A, Rácmolnár L, De Luca I, Cinosi E, Santacroce R, Marini M, Wellsted D, Sullivan K, Bersani G, Martinotti G (2019) The emergence of exercise addiction, body dysmorphic disorder, and other image-related psychopathological correlates in fitness settings: a cross sectional study. PLoS ONE 14:e0213060. https://doi.org/10.1371/journal.pone.0213060

20. Geyer H, Parr MK, Koehler K, Mareck U, Schanzer W, Thevis M (2008) Nutritional supplements cross-contaminated and faked with doping substances. J Mass Spectrom 43:892–902

21. Martello S, Felli M, Chiarotti M (2007) Survey of nutritional supplements for selected illegal anabolic steroids and ephedrine using LC-MS/MS and GC-MS methods, respectively. Food Addit Contam 24:258–265
22. Ayotte C, Lévesque JF, Cléroux M, Lajeunesse A, Goudreault D, Fakirian A (2001) Sport nutritional supplements: quality and doping controls. Can J Appl Physiol Rev Can Physiol Appl 26:S120–S129
23. Mazzoni I, Barroso O, Rabin O (2017) Anti-doping challenges with novel psychoactive substances in sport. In: Novel psychoactive substances. Springer, Berlin, pp 43–56
24. Van Thuyne W, Van Eenoo P, Delbeke FT (2006) Nutritional supplements: Prevalence of use and contamination with doping agents. Nutr Res Rev 19:147–158
25. Judkins CMG, Teale P, Hall DJ (2010) The role of banned substance residue analysis in the control of dietary supplement contamination. Drug Test Anal 2:417–420
26. Geller AI, Shehab N, Weidle NJ, Lovegrove MC, Wolpert BJ, Timbo BB et al (2015) Emergency department visits for adverse events related to dietary supplements. N Engl J Med 373:1531–1540
27. Mathews NM (2018) Prohibited contaminants in dietary supplements. Sports Health 10:19–30. https://doi.org/10.1177/1941738117727736
28. Tian HH, Ong WS, Tan CL (2009) Nutritional supplement use among university athletes in Singapore. Singapore Med J 50:165–172
29. US Food and Drug Administration (FDA) (1994) Dietary Supplement Health and Education Act (DSHEA). Available at https://ods.od.nih.gov/About/DSHEA_Wording.aspx
30. European Food Safety Authority (EFSA) (2015) Food supplements. Available at: http://www.efsa.europa.eu/en/topics/topic/food-supplements
31. Therapeutic Goods Administration (TGA) (2019) Sport supplements in Australia. Available at https://www.tga.gov.au/media-release/sports-supplements-australia#:~:text=Supplements%20may%20be%20regulated%20as,medicine%20can%20sometimes%20be%20complex.
32. Deng H (2015) Chinese new regulation for health food products. Natural Products Insider Website. Available at: http://www.naturalproductsinsider.com/articles/2015/10/chinese-new-regulation-for-health-food-product.aspx. Updated 2015.
33. Denham BE (2017) Athlete information sources about dietary supplements: A review of extant research. Int J Sport Nutr Exerc Metab 27:325–334
34. Heikkinen A, Alaranta A, Helenius I, Vasankari T (2011) Dietary supplementation habits and perceptions of supplement use among elite Finnish athletes. Int J Sport Nutr Exerc Metab 21:271–279
35. Pilgrim K, Bohnet-Joschko S (2019) Selling health and happiness how influencers communicate on Instagram about dieting and exercise: mixed methods research. BMC Public Health 19:1–9. https://doi.org/10.1186/s12889-019-7387-8
36. Martínez-Sanz JM, Sospedra I, Ortiz CM, Baladía E, Gil-Izquierdo A, Ortiz-Moncada R (2017) Intended or unintended doping? A review of the presence of doping substances in dietary supplements used in sports. In Nutrients 9:10. https://doi.org/10.3390/nu9101093
37. Corazza O, Assi S, Simonato P, Corkery J, Bersani FS, Demetrovics Z, Stair J, Fergus S, Pezzolesi C, Pasinetti M, Deluca P, Drummond C, Davey Z, Blaszko U, Moskalewicz J, Mervo B, Furia LD, Farre M, Flesland L, Pisarska A, Shapiro H, Siemann H, Skutle A, Sferrazza E, Torrens M, Sambola F, van der Kreeft P, Scherbaum N, Schifano F. (2013) Promoting innovation and excellence to face the rapid diffusion of novel psychoactive substances in the EU: the outcomes of the ReDNet project. Hum Psychopharmacol 28(4):317–23. https://doi.org/10.1002/hup.2299
38. Kozinets RV (2015) Netnography: redefined. Sage, London
39. Negri A, Townshend H, McSweeney T, Angelopoulou O, Banayoti H, Prilutskaya M, Bowden-Jones O, Corazza O. (2021) Carfentanil on the darknet: potential scam or alarming public health threat? International Journal of Drug Policy, 91: 103118. https://doi.org/10.1016/j.drugpo.2021.103118

Challenges Posed by Gene Manipulations and Sport Performance

Odile Cohen-Haguenauer

Introduction

Doping is a threat to the fairness of sport competition and might also compromise athletes' health. Although there is no current proof of evidence that gene doping has been used, the recent clinical successes in gene-therapy endeavours, along with the progress of emerging techniques and the recent advertisement of do-it-yourself gene therapy, altogether increase the likelihood of abuse based on human gene transfer. In fact, the field of gene therapy is rapidly evolving [1]. New milestones are being achieved every year, such as the approval both in Europe and the United States of a gene therapy treatment for spinal muscular atrophy type I (Zolgensma) [2, 3] resulting in spectacular neuromuscular functional recovery in otherwise deeply affected young children. There are several other gene-based drugs that have received marketing authorization (MA) from the US Food and Drug Administration and the European Medicines Agency. Success has been met in treating children with near-fatal immune-deficiencies, improving the outlook and quality of life of patients with a variety of blood disorders such as Wiskott-Aldrich syndrome and restoring some vision to someone nearly blind from Leber's amaurosis [1]. There are also encouraging developments with respect to debilitating degenerative diseases, and glimmers of hope for major scourges like coronary artery disease, HIV infection and cancer with the CAR-T cell revolution [1, 4]. Important progresses have been made towards the treatment of diseases such as hemophilia A and B, Duchenne muscular dystrophy and several in vivo and ex vivo approaches for gene therapy of

O. Cohen-Haguenauer (✉)
Unité d'Oncogénétique Clinique AP-HP, Nord-Université de Paris, DMU Icare, UFR de Médecine de l'Université de Paris, Unité de recherche INSERM UMR-S 976, Hôpital Saint-Louis, Paris, France
e-mail: odile.cohen-haguenauer@aphp.fr

inherited and metabolic disorders [5, 6], which will continue to enrich the pipeline of market-approved treatments in the near future.

Advances in Gene Therapy and Their Potential Impact on Sport Performance

There basically are two main strategies to achieve gene therapy for genetic diseases: (i) either genetically modify autologous progenitor cells ex vivo, with integrating vectors and reinfuse them into the patient with the concurrent risk of insertional mutagenesis when integration occurs randomly in the genome; (ii) or deliver the vector and its transgene cargo directly in vivo, addressing long-lived post-mitotic cells or slowly dividing cells which do not require integration into the genome of the target cells. Enormous progress has been made since the first attempt at in vivo gene therapy and the death of an 18-year-old subject enrolled in a clinical trial using an adenovirus-derived vector for the treatment of ornithine transcarbamylase (OTC) deficiency. This tragic accident resulted in a major setback for the field as a whole and for the use of adenoviral vectors except for vaccines and cancer therapy [7]. Several investigational gene therapy drugs based on the safe and efficient adeno-associated virus (AAV) vector platform [8] currently are in clinical trials for a number of inherited metabolic disorders, including OTC deficiency, Crigler-Najjar syndrome mucopolysaccharidosis (MPS) type IIIA and IIIB, glycogen storage disease (GSD) type 1a and 2 (Pompe disease), phenylketonuria, methylmalonic acidemia (MMA), Fabry's disease, familial hypercholesterolemia and type 1 diabetes [9] among others. Clinical trials show extremely promising results. Yet, the presence of pre-treatment neutralizing antibodies directed against the virus poses a major limitation to AAV gene transfer, since they block the transfer into target tissues even at relatively low concentrations. This is even more problematic when considering the need of a second injection for therapeutic purpose [10]. In fact, currently ongoing technological optimization of AAV vectors is aiming at evading pre-existing immune reaction to the virus or making in vivo redosing possible [11], as well as viral vectors with enhanced ability to transduce a given target cell [12]. The field of ex vivo gene transfer also experienced parallel setbacks arising in the first clinical trials which shown the best at first and the worse to follow with the outbreak of viral vector-induced leukemias [7]. The occurrence of the malignancies was demonstrated to result from insertional mutagenesis of first-generation vectors driven by the integration of the vector and its cargo at the locus of a gene involved in the target cell proliferation (LMO2 specifically) [13]. At present, safer lentivirus-based vectors have been developed, yielding unprecedented results in the cure of diseases such as metachromatic leukodystrophy and adrenoleukodystrophy and Wiskott-Aldrich syndrome, among others [1, 14]. In addition, clinical trials are also ongoing for the treatment of metabolic disorders such as mucopolysaccharidosis I and

Fabry's disease, which are currently showing promising results in patients. Further optimization of integrative vectors for ex vivo [15] or in vivo [16] gene transfer is underway with the use of post-transcriptional regulatory elements within lentivectors or transposon-derived vectors. Novel therapeutic strategies are now showing besides the classical "gene addition" using integrating viral vectors, such as nonviral delivery of DNA. Among other emerging technologies, mRNA-based delivery is now being tested in patients [17]. This other nucleic-acid-based strategy has been initially developed towards RNA-based vaccines as recently demonstrated against the SARS-Cov-2 coronavirus at the origin of the COVID-19 pandemic. It is currently being used in a phase I/II clinical trial for methylmalonic acidemia (MMA). This technological approach is likely to fulfil important medical needs, such as severe metabolic liver diseases associated with early lethality, for instance. RNA-based technology has also been investigated in order to mediate gene silencing which can be achieved making use of antisense oligonucleotides which bind to its target mRNA and inhibit its association with ribosomes, preventing expression. Another approach involves small interfering RNAs (siRNA), which result in the degradation of its mRNA target, in order to abolish or diminish the synthesis of the corresponding protein and prevent its action. Adding to the panel of novel technologies, many approaches for genome editing are either in a development phase or in the clinic, mostly based at present on the cluster regularly interspaced short palindromic repeats (CRISPR)-Cas (CRISPR-associated) system [18]. With genome editing, like for any innovative therapy, current investigations will help define which parameters should be refined to prove both safe and efficient in order to achieve clinical success. More recently, Anzalone et al. [19] have described the unprecedented power and subtlety of the "Prime" system, which is more likely to fit the ex vivo gene therapy setting. When considering gene doping to enhance sport performance, direct in vivo administration of the gene vectors, or performance-modifying sequences, would present as the most probable option. As shown, gene therapy can treat a variety of human diseases through the systemic administration of AAV vectors with excellent safety records in clinical trials so far and long-term expression of the transgene of interest in a variety of post-mitotic tissues including the liver and skeletal muscle [8]. The current manufacturing scale is able to meet the demands for in vivo gene transfer to treat rare monogenic conditions, which fall into the definition of orphan drugs. Accordingly, the event of gene doping is unlikely to require very large vector doses to achieve a meaningful clinical result. Altogether, the same characteristics that make AAV-derived vectors a very good platform for clinical gene therapy may set the basis for its misuse to deliver genes for doping purposes in order to improve muscle performance or slow down ageing. There is thus a need to develop strategies able to detect gene doping, particularly resulting from illegal applications of gene transfer and AAV-based manipulations.

Gene and Cell Doping

Definition
According to the *World Anti-Doping Agency (WADA) List of Prohibited Substances and Methods*, the following, with the potential to enhance sport performance, are prohibited:

1. The use of nucleic acids or nucleic acid analogues that may alter genome sequences and/or alter gene expression by any mechanism. This includes but is not limited to gene editing, gene silencing and gene transfer technologies.
2. The use of normal or genetically modified cells.

Approaches to the Detection of Gene and Cell Doping
In view of the above-described progress in the field of gene transfer, one may recapitulate main characteristics which establish in vivo AAV-mediated gene transfer as the most probable candidate for gene doping, as follows:

- Direct in vivo injection: "a gene in a needle"
- Favourable risk/benefit profile
- Very good safety and efficacy records in clinical trials
- Muscle and liver tropism
- Relative ease for product manufacture
- Evidence for the absence of vector circulating in blood or urines after few days following administration

Detection programmes as applied in anti-doping have to adapt accordingly. In addition, given the highest level of performance challenge from the athletes' standpoint and in the interest of preserving their potential, preference should be given to non-invasive methods of athletes' sampling with view to detecting gene doping. As a priority, blood takes should be privileged for screening and biopsies reserved to confirmation procedures only. Interestingly, clinical trials aiming at therapeutic muscle gene transfer have shown that DNA sequences derived from AAV vectors can be detected in human blood months after intramuscular (IM) injection [20]. Similarly, the presence of AAV vector genomes in serum and human peripheral blood mononuclear cells (PBMCs) has been documented for a long period of time, following intravascular delivery of AAV vectors to transduce the liver [21]. In large animal models, the persistence of AAV vector genomes has been reported up to almost 2 years in PBMCs after IM administration of AAV1 and AAV8 vectors [22, 23] even when very low vector doses were used. Furthermore, there is robust evidence indicating that cell-free DNA increases in blood after exercise [24, 25], thus offering an opportunity to detect AAV vector genomes in serum/blood samples. Assays are directed for examples towards detection of EPO intended at increasing endurance or IGF-1 to increase strength or inhibition of a gene that suppresses muscle growth such as myostatin. Importantly, detection programmes under development are challenging methods and protocols in samples from clinical and pre-clinical studies that involve gene transfer. In addition, and in order to secure reproducibility, protocols need to be independently tested in accredited reference laboratories.

Direct Detection of Nucleic Acids: Vector and Transgene Sequences

Polymerase chain reaction (PCR) methods have been developed for the detection of transgenic sequences resulting from in vivo administration of gene transfer vectors, either systemically or locally, e.g., intramuscularly. Currently available platforms are based on the detection of transgenic sequences—either vector-related or which belong to the gene of interest—in nucleic acids extracted from peripheral blood mononuclear cells (PBMC): these samples are easy to store following small-sized blood collections and high-quality DNA easily extracted from them. Published methods for detection of gene doping initially make use of PCR-based assays or loop-mediated isothermal amplification (LAMP) which target specific sequences [26–34]. The detection potential can reach a high level of sensitivity and specificity. When it comes to being legally defensible, these strategies require particular attention as most procedures make use of nested PCR to increase sensitivity, with the collateral risk for carry-over of contaminations. Refined assays have been developed towards detection of EPO intended at increasing endurance. Gene transfer usually makes use of intron-less transgenes, namely cDNA sequences derived from the messenger RNA in order to reduce the size of the vector cargo instead of introns-containing genomic DNA. Therefore, exon-exon junctions can be targeted toward detection of transgene sequences because they are not present within the endogenous locus of the corresponding gene, in the genomic DNA of human cells. Baoutina (2020) [35] and her team have developed an analytical procedure aimed at detecting EPO gene doping, based on several complementary PCR assays, which have been designed to specifically target exon/exon junction sequences, in particular. With this combination of tests, the presence of a transgenic sequence can be accurately detected. Because the exon-exon sequence junctions of doping genes are known, short PCR primers annealing can be compromised by slight sequence modifications. The latter may allow evading detection through current PCR-based methods, which can be achieved by modifying the doping gene with synonymous mutations, resulting in false-negative PCR data. However, the multiple targets assay set up by Baoutina et al. make it unlikely to compromise transgene detection. While the modification of one transgene exon/exon junction may be possible, altering each transgene exon-exon junction may be extremely challenging with a risk to compromise mRNA stability in creating (e.g. cryptic splicing sites and/or the function of the transgenic protein). In addition, an EPO Reference Material (RM-EPO) is used to standardise the procedure, while its melting and size characteristics can be distinguished from the functional cDNA sequences. PCR analysis includes one assay as part of the "initial testing procedure" and a different assay as part of the "confirmation procedure" used in anti-doping testing.

Gene Doping Detection by Next-Generation Sequencing

Deep Sequencing-Based Detection in Nucleic Acids from Peripheral Blood Mononuclear Cells (PBMCs)

Because unknown sequences can be evidenced using next-generation sequencing (NGS), this approach stands as a unique methodology to address the detection of sequences which have been modified to avoid identification. It thus harbours a high detection power in the fight against gene doping. NGS is also able to cover the detection of small genes with intact introns (e.g., EPO or GH1). An issue that might also further complicate the detection of doping would be the simultaneous use of a combination of genes rather than a single one. Along this line, deep sequencing of expanded range of transgenes and sequences is currently being considered with a variety of target genes; regulatory sequences such as promoters, enhancers and miRNAs; as well as doping with multiple genes. Both increased performance and more accessible related costs of next-generation sequencing (NGS) have revolution-ized genetics-based diagnosis and translated into an immense interest of the medical community. Different approaches are currently being implemented, depending on the field of interest and the main focus, e.g., towards diagnosis or search for discov-ery: (i) whole exome sequencing (WES), with most functional mutations likely to be in or near exons; (ii) whole genome sequencing (WGS) which is more expensive than WES and more challenging to interpret—this approach could detect intronic, regulatory, intergenic as well as unknown variations; (iii) RNA-seq which could detect both relative gene expression and variants and could be integrated with DNA sequencing or miRNA-seq; (iv) utmost refined cutting-edge single cell-based meth-ods (WGS, RNA-seq, etc.) which could detect lower frequency mutations in hetero-geneous samples; and (v) targeted, capture-based DNA sequencing which is a cost-effective method intended to focus sequencing to a coding region or other regions of interest of the genome under study. The sample DNA is fragmented, and then regions of interest are captured by hybridization to synthetic biotinylated probes in solution, which are further isolated by magnetic pulldown, in order to enrich the test DNA in known target regions further submitted to sequence analysis. Target capture NGS is suited for clinical practice, because it is scalable and acces-sible in terms of cost and allows for greater sensitivity in the analysis of identified targets, when compared to whole exome (WES) or whole genome sequencing (WGS). Moreover, targeted gene sequencing also generates a smaller, more man-ageable data set compared to approaches with broader coverage. Subsequent analy-sis and interpretation of data are thus facilitated. Of note, the versatility of custom targeted sequencing is also being implemented in the screen for transposon or viral integration sites into the host genome following gene therapy [36]. De Boer et al. (2019) [28] have developed a targeted next-generation sequencing-based assay for the detection of all exon-exon junctions of potential doping genes, such as EPO, IGF1, IGF2, GH1 and GH2. Using this assay, all exon-exon junctions of cDNA of doping genes could be detected with a sensitivity of a few hundreds of cDNA copies per mg of genomic DNA. In addition, the design of the assay makes it resistant to tampering. Promoter regions and plasmid-derived sequences are readily detectable in sequencing data. The authors thus claim that expanding the panel in order to detect other sequences would be straightforward, such as genes with manipulated junctions, promoter regions as well as plasmid or virus-derived. Van der Grond et al. (2013) [37] have selected a list of candidates for doping which include erythropoietin, insulin-like growth factor, growth hormone, myostatin, vascular endothelial growth factor, fibroblast growth factor, endorphin and enkephalin, α-actinin 3, peroxisome proliferator-activated receptor-delta (PPARδ) and cytosolic phosphoenolpyruvate carboxykinase (PEPCK-C). The following genes which are currently being screened include *EPO, EPOR, VEGFA, MSTN, IGF1, FST, PPARD* and *AMPK,* but the list of genes which can be analysed can be further expanded. The next question to be addressed is the relative sensitivity of this approach compared to PCR-based assays.

CRISPR-Cas-Based Detection of Specific Sequences in Nucleic Acids from Blood: CARMEN

More recently, a scalable and multiplexed technology to quickly and inexpensively identify any circulating pathogen has been established and named after "CARMEN" [38]. The assay is sensitive, specific and statistically robust. A similar strategy could be applied to the detection of gene doping-based abuse. Fast, economically accessible detection methods, such as CRISPR-based approaches, antigen-based tests, PCR or loop-mediated isothermal amplification (LAMP), were identified to detect only one or a small number of pathogens in a given reaction. Combining the strengths of these approaches and in the pursuit of an ideal diagnostic, screening and surveillance technology, Ackerman et al. (2020) have developed CARMEN to enable both highly multiplexed nucleic acid detection and scale up to hundreds of samples at once. As described, the inputs to CARMEN-Cas13 are samples that have been amplified by PCR or recombinase polymerase amplification (RPA) and Cas13 detection mixes, which contain Cas13, a sequence-specific CRISPR RNA (crRNA) and a cleavage reporter. CARMEN-Cas13 benefits from the specificity of SHERLOCK: sequence-specific identification is achieved through Cas13-crRNA binding and recognition, mitigating concerns about off-target amplification that are common in other nucleic acid detection methods. The CARMEN assay has been designed to test dozens of samples in parallel for all 169 human-associated viruses (HVs) and shown to achieve high specificity. In the fight for fairness in sport and against doping, CARMEN-based assays could be developed based on known sequences likely to be used for doping purpose with a capacity to test many samples in parallel. Similar to PCR-based and NGS capture-based DNA sequencing assays, only already identified sequences would be detected. NGS-based assays will add to the system as both a confirmation and refinement of CARMEN-based findings, with each sample being analysed separately for precise identification. The relative specificity and sensitivity characteristics will further need to be compared and final assays established based both on accuracy and interlaboratory reproducibility and related costs.

Indirect Detection

Immune Response Following In Vivo Administration of Gene Transfer Vectors

There now is strong evidence in human subjects undergoing clinical trials that gene transfer with AAV vectors leaves an immunological footprint, which can clearly be distinguished from a naturally occurring AAV infection with a wild-type virus counterpart. This feature holds potential to translate into a robust biological marker, which also is long lasting and provides a prolonged window of detection for several months at least. Both humoral and cell-mediated immunity to wild-type AAV have been documented in healthy donors and, at least in the case of anti-AAV antibodies, have been shown to have an impact on the outcome of gene transfer. The high homology with the parental wild-type AAV virus, which often infects humans, thus brings limitations related to immune responses associated with this vector platform. Several factors can contribute to the overall immunogenicity of rAAV vectors; meanwhile, vector design and the total vector dose appear to be responsible for immune-mediated toxicities. In any event, this robust biological marker harbours a detection potential, reminiscent of vector passage into the body which is long lasting and provides a window of detection which might extend to several months. Based on this body of evidence, a main objective is to establish a detection method for AAV-mediated gene doping based on the quantitative analysis of anti-AAV humoral response, in comparing healthy control subjects with AAV-treated individuals. Importantly, while immunosuppression given at the time of AAV treatment could reduce the cytotoxic immune response, results in non-human primates suggest that anti-AAV antibodies raise to unprecedented levels even when placed under immunosuppression at the time of AAV vector administration [8, 39]. Assays are currently being developed that address a variety of AAV capsids; the latter define both the AAV serotype and their corresponding tropism following in vivo infusion [39].

Rationale for Other Indirect Biomarkers

In principle, there is space for considering additional indirect biomarkers, among which the detection of either (i) exogenous protein product, e.g. designer nucleases, including CRISPR-Cas related or antibodies raised by the recipient against the latter

[40]; (ii) longitudinal changes in biomarkers, similar to the principles of the Athlete Biological Passport, such as cells, proteins [41], metabolites or RNA levels (arrays, RT-PCR or RNA-seq), the latter may very well fit the situation where epigenetic modifications will have been intended that result in both qualitative and quantitative changes in the target gene expression profile; and (iii) altered posttranslational modification patterns which have been described with, e.g., the product of intramuscular EPO cDNA [23].

Strategies to Improve Detection

Cell-Free DNA (CfDNA) Analysis

In their study in human athletes, Atamaniuk et al. (2008) [24] investigated the effects of an ultra-marathon on cell-free plasma DNA in mononuclear blood cells (MNCs). Blood samples were drawn from 14 athletes before and immediately after 6-h run. In addition, blood samples were also collected and analysed 2 h and 24 h after the end of the run. The authors show that levels of plasma DNA were significantly increased immediately after the marathon and were still higher 2 h later (P < 0.005) but significantly lower than those immediately after the race (P < 0.05). Cell-free plasma DNA returned to pre-race levels 24 h after the run. In an interesting report, Tug et al. (2015) [25] investigated the cellular origin of cfDNA in sex-mismatched haematopoietic stem cell transplantation (HSCT) and liver transplantation (LT) human patients by determining the relative proportion of Y-chromosomal to total nuclear cfDNA. Total nuclear cfDNA and Y-chromosomal cfDNA concentrations were determined in blood plasma before and after an incremental exercise test via quantitative real-time PCR (qPCR). Their results strongly suggest that cells from the haematopoietic lineage are the main source of cfDNA released during acute bouts of exercise. These findings might open a window for the use of cfDNA as an easy substrate for detection of gene doping, with increased accuracy in particular in the context of athlete's intensive exercise during high-level competitions.

Challenges Posed by the Detection of Gene Editing

Another possible option for gene doping in sports in the future is gene editing making use of the CRISPR-Cas system [18]. For instance, CRISPR-Cas could be used to disrupt a negative regulator of muscle growth, such as myostatin [42]. A major risk of CRISPR-Cas in human cells relates to off-target effects. Therefore, it is unlikely to be used in vivo in the near future. Recent studies have evidenced the occurrence of genetic scars such as on-target indels causing unwanted dysfunctional protein and/or unexpected chromosomal truncations [43]. These authors further show that a single nickase is safer than the nuclease approach when considering clinical translation of CRISPR-Cas-mediated gene therapies. To obtain on-target scarless gene correction, Prat et al. [44] showed that a mutant allele-specific guide was free of on-target collateral damage, this design being likely to prevent genotoxicity. For this type of gene doping to be detected, modification of methods will be required by changing the input material to RNA (converting to complementary DNA) and adding probes targeting genes of interest and housekeeping genes. Also and as mentioned, it is most probable that gene editing will be performed ex vivo in progenitor cells later to be infused in recipient patients. If unlikely to be used directly in vivo, should this be nevertheless attempted, it will require a vector system to drive its journey before it reaches its target. Detection methods directed against vector administration in circulating blood cells would be easiest to detect and might come into play if needed, according to the aforementioned procedures. Such detection strategies will be much more relevant than invasive methods involving tissue biopsies aiming at detecting gene editing-based sequence modifications.

From Suspicion to Conviction

Each of the previously described approaches designed to detect gene doping harbours its own detection profile, sensitivity and specificity. Altogether, indirect methods may be insufficient proof of drug abuse or gene manipulations. But they might hold instrumental as a first screening step to raise suspicion and guide further steps. Conviction can be won through direct evidence that a substance, a product or a sequence is present for a fact. The strategy to be implemented from suspicion to conviction requires gathering evidence from a cascade of tests: starting upstream with the more simple, widely applicable yet sensitive assays and at the lowest possible costs to be followed by precise downstream identification which may require more sophisticated techniques with the most accurate specificity and at a higher cost. A similar rationale is described in the development of CARMEN, with a very high throughput and large-scale assay being used in order to detect a specific signal amidst a combination of many sequences from very many individuals, which is followed by downstream steps intended at identifying the unique sample which gave the said signal. In the fight against gene doping, with a panel of several accurate assays which are available at present and each able to contribute specific information, a combinatory strategy making use of these assets will result in a powerful and robust characterisation of abuse that cannot be disputed.

Ethical Considerations

With the use of deep sequencing technologies able to read a whole genome in no time comes the evidence that incidental findings may reveal. Capture-based NGS strategy target known sequences from which disease-related genes are likely to be excluded. Similarly, amplification of genomic endogenous DNA sequences should be prevented, considering that the targets for doping detections are focused to exon-exon junctions. De Boer et al. (2019) show that genomic sequences of doping genes were the only unsolicited findings after alignment to the specific gene doping reference genomes. Moreover, genomic fingerprinting of intragenic genomic areas can be used to prove that the result does belong to a specific person, thus excluding the event of either contamination or confusion of identity. Conversely, ethical tensions may arise from the use of broader NGS-based tests. In fact, expanding to WGS or WES might result in incidental findings, which could raise concerns about the disclosure of unsolicited genetic information and privacy. Incidental findings might raise ethical dilemmas. Relevant modalities to handle these situations are currently being covered in appropriate fora and advisory committees worldwide. WADA is actively addressing ethical considerations related to gene doping detection with its ethical experts in order to ensure full applicability of gene detection methods in the anti-doping context.

Conclusion

Since the first conference on gene doping convened by WADA in 2002 and the prohibition of gene doping in sport for the first time in 2003 to now the routine application of gene doping detection in the anti-doping context, a long and challenging path has been covered to expose this new form of doping. Even if only a few anecdotal and never proven references to gene doping are found in the recent sport history, the recent phenomenal progress of gene therapy combined with the access to such methodologies by the general public makes it a sufficiently significant threat to be taken seriously to develop the arsenal of detection methods in which anti-doping authorities have invested in the past 15 years. Today as gene therapy comes to a certain degree of maturity as recognized by the regulatory approval of some of these methods, so does gene doping detection with advanced anti-doping methods being implemented in anti-doping laboratories. With the detection of gene doping, anti-doping experts have long anticipated this new dimension and acted to prevent manipulation of the human genome for the sole purpose of enhancing athletic performance.

References

1. High KA, Roncarolo MG (2019) Gene therapy. N Engl J Med 381:455–464
2. Hoy SM (2019) Onasemnogene abeparvovec: first global approval. Drugs 2019(79):1255–1262
3. Mendell JR, Al-Zaidy S, Shell R et al (2017) Single-dose gene-replacement therapy for spinal muscular atrophy. N Engl J Med 377:1713–1722
4. Luzzatto L, Verma IM (2012) Foreword. The CliniBook: Clinical gene transfer Edited by Odile Cohen-Haguenauer – EDK, Paris

5. Zabaleta N, Hommel M, Salas D et al (2019) Genetic based approaches to inherited metabolic liver diseases. Hum Gene Ther 30:1190–1203
6. Poletti V, Biffi A (2019) Gene-based approaches to inherited neurometabolic diseases. Hum Gene Ther 30:1222–1235
7. Couzin J, Kaiser J (2005) Gene therapy. As Gelsinger case ends, gene therapy suffers another blow. Science 307:1028
8. Mingozzi F, High KA (2011) Therapeutic in vivo gene transfer for genetic disease using AAV: progress and challenges. Nat Rev Genet 12:341–355
9. Callejas D, Mann CJ, Ayuso E et al (2013) Treatment of diabetes and long-term survival after insulin and glucokinase gene therapy. Diabetes 62:1718–1729
10. Colella P, Ronzitti G, Mingozzi F (2018) Emerging issues in AAV-mediated in vivo gene therapy. Mol Ther Methods Clin Dev 8:87–104
11. Leborgne C, Barbon E, Alexander JM, Hanby H, Delignat S, Cohen DM, Collaud F, Muraleetharan S, Lupo D, Silverberg J, Huang K, van Wittengerghe L, Marolleau B, Miranda A, Fabiano A, Daventure V, Beck H, Anguela XM, Ronzitti G, Armour SM, Lacroix-Desmazes S, Mingozzi F (2020) IgG-cleaving endopeptidase enables in vivo gene therapy in the presence of anti-AAV neutralizing antibodies. Nat Med 26(7):1096–1101
12. Zhang L, Rossi A, Lange L et al (2019) Capsid engineering overcomes barriers toward adeno-associated viral (AAV) vector-mediated transduction of endothelial cells. Hum Gene Ther 30:1284–1296
13. Hacein-Bey-Abina S, Garrigue A, Wang GP et al (2008) Insertional oncogenesis in 4 patients after retrovirus-mediated gene therapy of SCID-X1. J Clin Invest 118:3132–3142
14. Naldini L (2015) Gene therapy returns to Centre stage. Nature 526:351–360
15. Sii-Felice K, Castillo Padilla J, Relouzat F et al (2019) Enhanced transduction of *Macaca fascicularis* hematopoietic cells with chimeric lentiviral vectors. Hum Gene Ther 30:1306–1323
16. Milani M, Annoni A, Moalli F et al (2019) Phagocytosis-shielded lentiviral vectors improve liver gene therapy in nonhuman primates. Sci Transl Med 11:eaav7325
17. Martini PGV, Guey LT (2019) A new era for rare genetic diseases: messenger RNA therapy. Hum Gene Ther 30:1180–1189
18. Anzalone AV, Koblan LW, Liu DR (2020) Genome editing with CRISPR-Cas nucleases, base editors, transposases and prime editors. Nat Biotechnol 38(7):824–844
19. Anzalone AV, Randolph PB, Davis JR, Sousa AA, Koblan LW, Levy JM, Chen PJ, Wilson C, Newby GA, Raguram A, Liu DR (2019) Search-and-replace genome editing without double-strand breaks or donor DNA. Nature 576(7785):149–157
20. Brantly ML, Chulay JD, Wang L, Mueller C, Humphries M, Spencer LT, Rouhani F, Conlon TJ, Calcedo R, Betts MR, Spencer C, Byrne BJ, Wilson JM, Flotte TR (2009) Sustained transgene expression despite T lymphocyte responses in a clinical trial of rAAV1-AAT gene therapy. Proc Natl Acad Sci U S A 106(38):16363–16368
21. Manno CS, Pierce GF, Arruda VR, Glader B, Ragni M, Rasko JJ, Ozelo MC, Hoots K, Blatt P, Konkle B, Dake M, Kaye R, Razavi M, Zajko A, Zehnder J, Rustagi PK, Nakai H, Chew A, Leonard D, Wright JF, Lessard RR, Sommer JM, Tigges M, Sabatino D, Luk A, Jiang H, Mingozzi F, Couto L, Ertl HC, High KA, Kay MA (2006) Successful transduction of liver in hemophilia by AAV-Factor IX and limitations imposed by the host immune response. Nat Med 12(3):342–347
22. Ni W, Le Guiner C, Gernoux G, Penaud-Budloo M, Moullier P, Snyder RO (2011) Longevity of rAAV vector and plasmid DNA in blood after intramuscular injection in nonhuman primates: implications for gene doping. Gene Ther 18(7):709–718
23. Toromanoff A, Chérel Y, Guilbaud M, Penaud-Budloo M, Snyder RO, Haskins ME, Deschamps JY, Guigand L, Podevin G, Arruda VR, High KA, Stedman HH, Rolling F, Anegon I, Moullier P, Le Guiner C (2008) Safety and efficacy of regional intravenous (r.i.) versus intramuscular (i.m.) delivery of rAAV1 and rAAV8 to nonhuman primate skeletal muscle. Mol Ther 16(7):1291–1299
24. Atamaniuk J, Stuhlmeier KM, Vidotto C, Tschan H, Dossenbach-Glaninger A, Mueller MM (2008) Effects of ultra-marathon on circulating DNA and mRNA expression of pro- and anti-apoptotic genes in mononuclear cells. Eur J Appl Physiol 104(4):711–717

25. Tug S, Helmig S, Deichmann ER, Schmeier-Jürchott A, Wagner E, Zimmermann T, Radsak M, Giacca M, Simon P (2015) Exercise-induced increases in cell free DNA in human plasma originate predominantly from cells of the haematopoietic lineage. Exerc Immunol Rev 21:164–173

26. Baoutina A, Coldham T, Fuller B, Emslie KR (2013) Improved detection of transgene and nonviral vectors in blood. Hum Gene Ther Methods 24:345–354

27. Baoutina A, Coldham T, Bains GS, Emslie KR (2010) Gene doping detection: evaluation of approach for direct detection of gene transfer using erythropoietin as a model system. Gene Ther 17:1022–1032

28. de Boer EN, van der Wouden PE, Johansson LF, von Diemen CC, Haisma HJ (2019) A next-generation sequencing method for gene doping detection that distinguishes low levels of plasmid DNA against a background of genomic DNA. Gene Ther 26:338–346

29. Moser DA, Braga L, Raso A, Zacchigna S, Giacca M, Simon P (2014) Transgene detection by digital droplet PCR. PLoS One 9:e111781

30. Neuberger EW, Perez I, Le Guiner C, Moser D, Ehlert T, Allais M et al (2016) Establishment of two quantitative nested qPCR assays targeting the human EPO transgene. Gene Ther 23:330–339

31. Ni W, Le Guiner C, Moullier P, Snyder RO (2012) Development and utility of an internal threshold control (ITC) real-time PCR assay for exogenous DNA detection. PLoS One 7:e36461

32. Perez IC, Le Guiner C, Ni W, Lyles J, Moullier P, Snyder RO (2013) PCR-based detection of gene transfer vectors: application to gene doping surveillance. Anal Bioanal Chem 405:9641–9653

33. Salamin O, Kuuranne T, Saugy M, Leuenberger N (2017) Loop mediated isothermal amplification (LAMP) as an alternative to PCR: a rapid on-site detection of gene doping. Drug Test Anal 9:1731–1737

34. Zhang JJ, Xu JF, Shen YW, Ma SJ, Zhang TT, Meng QL et al (2017) Detection of exogenous gene doping of IGF-1 by a real-time quantitative PCR assay. Biotechnol Appl Biochem 64:549–545

35. Baoutina A (2020) A brief history of the development of a gene doping test. Bioanalysis 12(11):723–727

36. Miyazato P, Katsuya H, Fukuda A, Uchiyama Y, Matsuo M, Tokunaga M, Hino S, Nakao M, Satou Y (2016) Application of targeted enrichment to next-generation sequencing of retroviruses integrated into the host human genome. Sci Rep 6:28324

37. van der Gronde T, de Hon O, Haisma HJ, Pieters T (2013) Gene doping: an overview and current implications for athletes. Br J Sports Med Jul 47(11):670–678

38. Ackerman CM, Myhrvold C, Thakku SG, Freije CA, Metsky HC, Yang DK, Ye SH, Boehm CK, Kosoko-Thoroddsen TF, Kehe J, Nguyen TG, Carter A, Kulesa A, Barnes JR, Dugan VG, Hung DT, Blainey PC, Sabeti PC (2020) Massively multiplexed nucleic acid detection with Cas13. Nature 582(7811):277–282

39. Ronzitti G, Gross DA, Mingozzi F (2020) Human immune responses to adeno-associated virus (AAV) vectors. Front Immunol 11:670

40. Chew WL, Tabebordbar M, Cheng JKW, Mali P, Wu EY, Ng AHM, et al. (2016) A multifunctional AAV–CRISPR–Cas9 and its host response. http://doi.org/f864xc

41. Macedo A, Moriggi M, Vasso M, De Palma S, Sturnega M, Friso G, et al. (2012) Enhanced athletic performance on multisite AAV-IGF1 gene transfer coincides with massive modification of the muscle proteome http://doi.org/chnqvg

42. Carnac G, Vernus B, Bonnieu A (2007) Myostatin in the pathophysiology of skeletal muscle. Curr Genomics 8:415–412

43. Cullot G, Boutin J, Toutain J, Prat F, Pennamen P, Rooryck C, Teichmann M, Rousseau E, Lamrissi-Garcia I, Guyonnet-Duperat V, Bibeyran A, Lalanne M, Prouzet-Mauléon V, Turcq B, Ged C, Blouin JM, Richard E, Dabernat S, Moreau-Gaudry F, Bedel A (2019) CRISPR-Cas9 genome editing induces megabase-scale chromosomal truncations. Nat Commun 10(1):1136

44. Prat F, Toutain J, Boutin J, Amintas S, Cullot G, Lalanne M, Lamrissi-Garcia I, Moranvillier I, Richard E, Blouin JM, Dabernat S, Moreau-Gaudry F, Bedel A (2020) Mutation-specific guide RNA for compound heterozygous porphyria on-target scarless correction by CRISPR/Cas9 in stem cells. Stem Cell Reports. 15(3):677–693

Part II
Navigating in a Difficult Regulatory Environment

The "Forced" Union of Science and Law

Julien Sieveking

Introduction

What has been achieved by the anti-doping community since the creation in 1999 of the World Anti-Doping Agency (WADA) is quite significant. WADA has been legitimately established to lead a collaborative worldwide movement for doping-free sport and has developed harmonized anti-doping rules and policies across all sports and countries.[1] Strong and harmonized rules and processes have been established, are in place, and are evolving over time. New tools and analytical methods have been developed[2] by scientists and validated by arbitration panels and courts, and the level of expertise and competences of all persons involved in the defence of clean sport, including the anti-doping laboratories, has dramatically increased over the past 20 years. The counterpart—and sometimes also the cause—of this positive evolution for clean sport is that in parallel, doping techniques and protocols have also evolved, logically. New substances appear and doping regimes have become more sophisticated. Every time anti-doping authorities added a substance to the Prohibited List or developed a new analytical method to their arsenal for the defence of clean athletes, the "other side" immediately started working on challenging its prohibition, its validity, or on developing alternate techniques aimed at providing the same performance enhancement benefits. Further, elaborate defensive scenarios have been presented in cases of trial, with the support of cunning physicians,

---

[1] More information is available from: https://www.wada-ama.org/en/governance

[2] For example, among other progresses, the development of the athlete biological passport, the long-term storage of samples for future re-analysis, and the development of new analytical methods

J. Sieveking (✉)
Director, Legal Affairs World Anti-Doping Agency (WADA), Montreal, QC, Canada
e-mail: julien.sieveking@wada-ama.org

© The Author(s), under exclusive license to Springer Nature Switzerland AG 2022
O. Rabin, O. Corazza (eds.), *Emerging Drugs in Sport*,
https://doi.org/10.1007/978-3-030-79293-0_5

self-proclaimed experts, and hard-biting lawyers. Pharmaceutical companies have been indirectly nurturing chemical performances by producing medications sometimes in quantities more than human-estimated medical needs. This is of importance given that most of the substances used by cheats are registered medications. This issue has fortunately been addressed, thanks to the long-lasting efforts made by WADA as nowadays most of the world-leading pharmaceutical companies understand that a cooperation with the anti-doping community could only be beneficial to their work and image. Last but not least, the sometimes-passive attitude of sport sponsors, burying their heads in the sand, intentionally or not, for what relates to how their protégés get their brands on headlines, and the attitude of some governments using sports achievements by their athletes to enhance the national pride are both counter-productive to an efficient fight against doping in sport.

Global Context

Sport competitions, whatever their level, and artificial enhancement of performance have been intertwined since humans existed.[3] Nowadays, the ever-growing professionalization of sport, the social statute of the athlete, and media coverage of sports generate huge business opportunities and potential financial profits. As an example, the very profitable sponsorship deals offered to the "winners",[4] as well as the incredible difference in prize moneys between a winner and a runner up,[5] are some of the factors that lead the ones who favour their personal interests over clean sport to resort to doping, to organize it, and/or to turn a complicit blind eye on it. This is only the tip of the iceberg as amateur sports are also affected by doping, in a society that cherishes only winners, leading often to underestimated public health issues and costs for the taxpayers. Even if it may look like a fish swimming against the current in this over-medicalized society where all kinds of doubtful treatments and nutritional supplements are available to allegedly boost all that can be boosted in human minds and bodies, the fight against doping remains essential and of public interest.[6] As presented in more details in other chapters, the availability of all these products

---

[3] Performance-enhancing practices already existed during the Greek era (see, e.g., https://www.nationalgeographic.com/history/article/olympics-scandal-doping-ancient-greece-lochte)

[4] The estimated global amount spent yearly by commercial companies in sports sponsorship is close to 50 billion USD (see, e.g., https://www.marketingdive.com/news/sports-sponsorship-spend-to-increase-the-most-in-a-decade-report-says/571295/)

[5] For example, in 2019, the Wimbledon winner's prize money amounted to 2,954,247 USD, while the runner-up's prize money was half of this amount (https://www.perfect-tennis.com/prize-money/wimbledon/)

[6] The European Court of Human Rights considered that the fight against doping in sport was of public interest and stated that "while action to combat doping is a public-health issue in professional sport, it concerns all athletes. The above-mentioned reports show that doping affects amateur sports to a worrying extent, in particular among young athletes". More information is available in: http://hudoc.echr.coe.int/eng?i=001-180442

is also boosted due to their accessibility on the Internet and the absence of strong international regulations.

The Anti-doping Regulatory Framework

WADA appeared in the game following a doping scandal which gripped cycling at the time[7] and made it clear that doping was causing damage way beyond the sports world. Many realized that athletes and their support personnel were not the only ones involved. Government participation was thus required where a sport organization could not act. In response, WADA was created as a hybrid and unique structure, being composed of and funded equally by the international sport movement and the governments of the world working together, in a complementary way. While the sport movement ensures that the most recent anti-doping rules and supportive programmes are adequately adopted and implemented, governments intervene in trafficking and distribution of banned substances to athletes and address performance-enhancing drug abuse beyond elite sport and within wider society.[8] However, as WADA is a private organization registered as a foundation under Swiss law, these anti-doping rules and policies only apply, once implemented, to the sports movement. Indeed, governments, despite comprising half of WADA, cannot be bound by the rules established by a private entity. On their end, the governments recognize the fundamental role of an anti-doping regulatory framework and its principles via the UNESCO International Convention against Doping in Sport adopted in 2005.[9]

A Three-Level Anti-doping Regulatory Framework

As indicated earlier, harmonization of the anti-doping rules was an absolute necessity as in pre-WADA time, the prohibited substances and potential sanctions varied from one sport to another and from one country to another. These unbalanced treatments among athletes could not favour an adequate defence of sports integrity on a global scale. To reach this objective, a common and unique regulatory framework was established. It is composed of three levels, a structure which has not changed over the time.

---

[7] See https://en.wikipedia.org/wiki/Festina_affair

[8] https://www.wada-ama.org/en/governance

[9] https://en.unesco.org/themes/sport-and-anti-doping/convention

The First Level

At the top of the pyramid is the World Anti-Doping Code ("the Code"). Emphasis must be placed on "world" as the Code is the fruit of a global consensus among the anti-doping community and is, as such, the fundamental and universal document upon which the World Anti-Doping Program is based. It sets out the key principles required for an efficient and harmonized fight against doping: from the definition of doping, the anti-doping rule violations, the adjudication process, the sanctions, as well as rules on testing and education, including science-related provisions, addressing questions such as prohibited substances and the analysis of samples or research. The Code is a living document that evolves to ensure it always remains fit-for-purpose. Since the first version of the Code, which was adopted in 2003, three revision processes[10] have taken place leading to enhanced versions of the Code which entered into force in 2009, 2015, and 2021. Each new version was the fruit of a vast consultation where all stakeholders could submit their comments. Each time, the main challenge is obviously to reach a consensus and create solutions on subjects on which stakeholders have divergent, and sometimes polarized, opinions. Further, before its adoption, each new version of the Code is reviewed by experts in different fields such as ethics or human rights. It is important to stress that the Code is not self-applicable. It becomes binding only upon its acceptance by organizations and, by doing so, becomes signatories and commits to implement its rules in their own set of anti-doping rules.[11] It is a contractual agreement.[12]

The Second Level

The second level comprises the international standards and the so-called technical documents. The international standards contain technical and operational rules for the implementation of the Code principles. They are mandatory for all signatories, but unlike the Code, they are directly applicable without the need to implement them in the signatories' rules. The international standards are regularly revised,

---

[10]These subsequent review processes were driven by small drafting teams, comprised of senior WADA staff and external experts. Their goal was to review and analyse stakeholders' feedback and incorporate it into successive working drafts of the Code at each phase of the consultation process, until the adoption of the final version by the WADA Foundation Board

[11]As set out in article 23.1 of the Code, the International Olympic Committee, International Federations, the International Paralympic Committee, National Olympic Committees, National Paralympic Committees, Major Event Organizations, National Anti-Doping Organizations, and other organizations having significant relevance in sport may become Code signatories

[12]For some of the signatories, it is somewhat a "forced agreement". Indeed, the International Federations included in the Olympic programme and other organizations that are part of the Olympic movement (e.g. national Olympic committees) must accept and implement the Code (see article 43 of the Olympic Charter)

when necessary, in consultation with the stakeholders, to ensure they always remain fit-for-purpose. There are currently eight international standards covering the following areas: compliance,[13] testing and investigations,[14] prohibited substances and methods,[15] laboratories,[16] therapeutic use exemptions,[17] data protection and privacy,[18] results management,[19] and education.[20] This second level also includes the technical documents, which contain mandatory technical requirements on specific anti-doping topics as set forth in an international standard. They allow WADA to respond promptly to certain emerging problems. These documents are key to ensure anti-doping remains at a state-of-the-art level, in particular in science.[21] The technical documents have been enumerated in the 2021 version of the Code as one of the main elements of the World Anti-Doping Program. They are mandatory and become effective immediately upon publication by WADA unless a later date is specified.

---

[13] The purpose of the International Standard for Code Compliance by Signatories (ISCCS) is to set out the relevant framework and procedures for ensuring Compliance by Signatories to the Code (www.wada-ama.org/sites/default/files/resources/files/worldconferencebackgrounder_0.pdf)

[14] The International Standard for Testing and Investigations (ISTI) establishes mandatory standards for all that relates to conducting anti-doping testing (from planning, sample collection, transport, etc.) and also establishes mandatory standards for an efficient and effective gathering, assessment, and use of anti-doping intelligence and for the efficient and effective conduct of investigations (www.wada-ama.org/sites/default/files/resources/files/worldconferencebackgrounder_0.pdf)

[15] The Prohibited List identifies the substances and methods prohibited in- and out-of-competition and in particular sports (www.wada-ama.org/en/what-we-do/international-standards# ProhibitedList)

[16] The purpose of the International Standard for Laboratories (ISL) is to ensure production of valid test results and evidentiary data and to achieve uniform and harmonized results and reporting from all accredited laboratories (www.wada-ama.org/en/what-we-do/international-standards# Laboratories)

[17] The purpose of the International Standard for Therapeutic Use Exemptions (ISTUE) is to ensure that the process of granting Therapeutic Use Exemptions (TUEs) is harmonized across sports and countries (www.wada-ama.org/sites/default/files/resources/files/worldconferenceback-grounder_0.pdf)

[18] The purpose of the International Standard for the Protection of Privacy and Personal Information (ISPPPI) is to ensure that organizations and persons involved in anti-doping in sport apply appropriate, sufficient, and effective privacy protection measures to the personal information they process (https://www.wada-ama.org/sites/default/files/resources/files/worldconferencebackgrounder_0.pdf)

[19] The purpose of the International Standard for Results Management (ISRM) establishes mandatory standards for minimal requirements that all anti-doping organizations (ADOs) must follow in respect to the results management and hearing processes of potential anti-doping rule violations (www.wada-ama.org/sites/default/files/resources/files/worldconferencebackgrounder_0.pdf)

[20] The International Standard for Education (ISE) establishes mandatory standards for the planning, implementation, monitoring and evaluation of effective education programmes (www.wada-ama.org/sites/default/files/resources/files/worldconferencebackgrounder_0.pdf)

[21] For an exhaustive list of all Technical Documents, see https://www.wada-ama.org/en/resources/science-medicine/technical-documents-index

The Third Level

The third level comprises non-binding documents such as guidelines and models of best practice which are intended to assist Code signatories in implementing the rules of the World Anti-Doping Program.

The Anti-doping Regulatory Framework and the Law

The anti-doping regulatory framework is not isolated from other sectors of law. First, it must comply with universally recognized legal principles, such as the principle of proportionality, and above all with human rights. The respect of these principles is necessary to ensure athletes' rights are protected. Any breach may be challenged before state courts. Specific anti-doping provisions or decisions rendered in their application have in fact already been challenged before state courts and before the European Court of Human Rights.[22] Any decision rendered in application of Code-compliant rules may be appealed as a last resort before the Court of Arbitration for Sport ("the CAS"), an independent arbitration tribunal, recognized by the Swiss judicial order. Under the applicable Swiss legislation, CAS decisions may be appealed to the Swiss Federal Tribunal. This tribunal will review the decision to ensure they are not in breach of the so-called public order.[23] Further, on some occasions, the application of provisions of the Code or international standard may breach a national law. For example, the Code requirement to publicly disclose the outcome of decisions by which an athlete is sanctioned following an anti-doping rule violation is restricted under some national legislations. In such case, the national law prevails.

The Interaction of Science and Law

Perspective

The parallel evolution and sophistication of both the fight against doping and the doping practices has shed light on a necessary union: the union of science and law. Science and law are very different disciplines that genuinely do not constantly

---

[22] See, for example: http://hudoc.echr.coe.int/eng?i=001-180442 and http://hudoc.echr.coe.int/eng?i=001-186828

[23] This review is limited to questions such as jurisdiction, the composition of the CAS hearing panel or the respect of key principles (right to be heard, equal treatment of parties, etc.). The Swiss Federal Tribunal does not conduct a review of the merits of a case and cannot amend a CAS decision. It can only refer the case back to the CAS if irregularities are established

interact, but whose unnatural alliance is the cornerstone of the fight against doping in the frame of which they constantly interact, guide, and almost emulate each other. From the inclusion of a substance on the Prohibited List to the detection of this substance in an athlete's sample, from establishing an anti-doping rule violation to determining the appropriate sanction, from the research and development of a new analytical method to its implementation in the anti-doping laboratory procedures, and from therapeutic exemptions to the contamination appearing in natural and unprocessed foodstuffs, law and science are inevitably intertwined. Science is asked to always remain fit-for-purpose in an environment that is in constant evolution and where research and development take time. It must be secure enough to resist any challenge in legal procedures. Indeed, law requires certainty, and science is asked to provide answers to determine if applicable legal standards are met. Without strong science flourishing in and nurturing a fit-for-purpose regulatory framework, few cheats could be estranged from sports competitions by anti-doping tribunals. The science must be transcribed into the rules. The rules must establish clear criteria and standards addressing the numerous questions of a scientific nature: How it is decided, when and by whom, and based on which criteria that a substance is to be prohibited? What standards must anti-doping laboratories comply with in their analytical process for their result to constitute evidence meeting the required standard of proof? How is an analytical method validated? The system needs to provide strong answers to ensure that the anti-doping rule violation was duly established. Some may even say that the anti-doping law is a law based on science, and it is mostly right. Only 2 out of the 11 anti-doping rule violations listed in the Code—the presence of a prohibited substance in an athlete's sample[24] and the use of a prohibited substance or method[25]— have an exclusive or dominant scientific component and the first one constituting the majority of the reported anti-doping rule violations.[26] In summary, anti-doping science and anti-doping law both support each other. Sometimes science supports law, and sometimes law supports science: an unnatural but necessary symbiosis.

Science in Support of Law

To highlight how science supports the law, we will present in a detailed fashion the questions surrounding the anti-doping rule violation of the presence of a prohibited substance in an athlete's sample, from its inclusion on the List to the determination

---

[24] See article 2.1 of the Code

[25] See article 2.2 of the Code. The use of a prohibited substance can be established by any reliable means (see article 3.2 of the Code). All cases brought forward as a result of the Athlete Biological Passport system are "use" case, as the substance is not directly detected in the athlete's sample but its use is established due to the effect its intake had on selected blood parameters

[26] For example, in 2015, a total of 1929 anti-doping rule violations were established, among which 1649 were the consequence of the presence of a prohibited substance in the athlete's sample; see https://www.wada-ama.org/sites/default/files/resources/files/2015_adrvs_report_overview_web.pdf

of the sanction by anti-doping hearing panels. We will also highlight this support with other practical examples such as the question of the so-called substances of abuse and the therapeutic use exemptions.

The Presence of a Prohibited Substance in an Athlete's Sample

Establishing the Violation

The most common anti-doping rule violation, the presence of a prohibited substance in an athlete's sample, is a good example of science supporting the law. First, let's go back in time: In 1963, the Council of Europe proposed the following definition: "The administration, by any means, to an individual in good health of a substance foreign to the body or of abnormal quantities of physiological substances, with the sole aim of artificially or unfairly enhancing individual performance in a competition".[27] No need to be a sound lawyer to understand that this legal definition of doping made it almost impossible to prosecute doping practices: the anti-doping prosecutor being obliged to establish, inter alia, that the athlete was in good health, that he was administered the doping agent to enhance his performance, and that it was the only reason for which the substance was administered. This legal definition needed to be changed and it happened with WADA. Since the first edition of the Code in 2004, doping is defined in the form of a list: *Doping is defined as the occurrence of one or more of the Anti-Doping rules violations set forth in article 2 of the Code.*[28] The presence of a prohibited substance in an athlete's sample is the first one on the list of doping violations. For the anti-doping organization, it now suffices to establish that a prohibited substance was detected in the athlete's sample. No need to establish that the athlete intentionally ingested the substance to enhance his or her sporting performance. Once the presence is established, and if the athlete has no therapeutic use exemption for the substance at stake, the burden of proof shifts to the athlete who will have to establish either failures in the doping control or analytical processes or other circumstances to avoid a sanction or that he/she is eligible for a reduced sanction.[29] This is called the strict liability principle. Athletes must exercise the so-called utmost caution as they are responsible for any prohibited substance detected in their bodily fluids. This new legal approach, with a reduced burden of proof for the anti-doping prosecutor, is exclusively science-based as science determines that (1) the substance is prohibited and that (2) it was detected in the athlete's sample. There is no subjective element here. Science is responsible to

---

[27] Accessed   from: assembly.coe.int/nw/xml/XRef/X2H-Xref-ViewHTML.asp?FileID-9025 &lang=eng

[28] Article 1 of the Code

[29] For example, an athlete can benefit from a reduced sanction if he/she is able to establish at the required standard of proof how the substance entered his/her body and that the his/her fault or negligence is not significant

support the law by establishing a list of prohibited substances and guaranteeing high-level analytical protocols. Science must be robust as the consequences of a positive finding may be potentially career-ending for an athlete.

The Prohibited Substances

The prohibited substances are set out in the List of Prohibited Substances and Methods[30] (Prohibited List), which is the sole of the eight international standards that is reviewed every year, due to the evolution of the science and the regular emergence of new substances or methods. The List Expert Group, which is composed of scientific and medical experts, is responsible to ensure the List remains fit-for-purpose year after year.[31]

As the presence of a prohibited substance in an athlete's sample is a constitutive element of an anti-doping rule violation, the Prohibited List—which sets out which substances or methods are prohibited—has a legal component that triggers two consequences:

1. It must be as stable as possible to offer an appropriate legal certainty. Any amendment shall be scientifically justified and necessary for the fight against doping. It must be also legally reviewed given the potential consequences any change can trigger.
2. Establishing the List must comply with several legal requirements as set out in the rules; for example:

(a) The Code sets out three criteria[32] to be considered for the inclusion of a substance on the List, out of which two must be met[33]: (1) the potential to enhance sport performance, (2) a potential risk for the athlete's health,[34] and (3) the violation of the spirit of sport.[35] The first two of these criteria set out in the rules are obviously science-based, and their assessment of the substance must be based on strong scientific evidence.

---

[30] Article 4.1 of the Code

[31] The amended List is always circulated for stakeholder comment and is then to be approved by WADA Executive Committee, where the proposed changes sometimes create some debate and political challenge, as the perception of and the resort to a particular substance may vary among countries and cultures. This was the case for the inclusion of meldonium, for example, which was only used in countries of the former Soviet Union. The consumption of coca leaves, which leads to cocaine-positive, is another example

[32] Article 4.3.1 of the Code

[33] A substance may also be included on the List if it has the potential to mask the use of another prohibited substance (see article 4.3.2 of the Code)

[34] In the 2021 Code, health has been moved to the top of the list of rationales and is specifically mentioned in a sentence preceding that list (see Fundamental Rationale for the World Anti-Doping Code, page 13 of the Code)

[35] See Fundamental Rationale of the 2021 World Anti-Doping Code

(b) The Code also requires that each substance (or methods in case of use) be either specified or non-specified.[36] This mandatory distinction made by the law, for legal purposes, is not of a science nature but must be addressed by science to be applied. Science is asked to support the law.

Specified substances are defined in the Code as being more likely to have been consumed by an athlete for a purpose other than the enhancement of the sport performance, for example, by taking a medication sold without prescription and which contains a prohibited substance.

This distinction was legally necessary to have more flexibility to address cases where the substance is more likely to have been consumed inadvertently. For questions of proportionality, an inadvertent intake, albeit still constituting a violation, should not lead to the same sanctions as, for instance, the deliberate use of an anabolic agent.

(c) Other questions are to be addressed by the List Expert Group for each substance, given that all determinations made must be solid and resist challenges:

- Whether the substance must be prohibited only "in-competition" or at all times (i.e., in-competition and out-of-competition)
- Whether a reporting threshold shall be established[37]

The Detection of the Prohibited Substance in the Athlete's Sample

The second constitutive element of the presence of a prohibited substance is the detection of this substance in the athlete's sample. The reporting of a positive finding must therefore be irreproachable, in particular taking into account the presumptions of validity set out in the Code:

(a) The anti-doping laboratories are presumed to have conducted the sample analysis and custodial procedure in compliance with the International Standard for Laboratories.[38]

To support this first presumption of validity established in the Code, the International Standard for Laboratories sets out very strict conditions that a laboratory must fulfil to obtain and maintain the WADA accreditation and establishes a strict monitoring process and disciplinary consequences in case a laboratory does not perform at the required level.[39]

(b) The analytical method used is presumed to be scientifically valid.

To legitimize this presumption of validity, the Code requires that any analytical method used must be approved by WADA, after consultation with the relevant

---

[36] Article 4.2.2 of the Code

[37] For example, when determined that below a certain level, the effect on performance is negligible

[38] Article 3.2.1 of the Code

[39] CAS 2018/A/599: "Doping is an offence which requires the application of strict rules. If an athlete is to be sanctioned solely on the basis of the provable presence of a prohibited substance in his body, it is his or her fundamental right to know that the Respondent, as the Testing Authority, including the WADA-accredited laboratory working with it, has strictly observed the mandatory safeguards"

scientific community or which has been the subject of peer review.[40] Science is again required to support the established rules.

Fixing the Sanction

The role of science, as reflected above, is essential in establishing the violation, but its close interaction with and support of the legal process does not end here. Once the presence of a prohibited substance in an athlete's sample is established, science's input is often required to ensure an appropriate outcome of the adjudication phase. The Code sets forth different possibilities for a reduction, or even an elimination, of the otherwise applicable sanction depending, for example, on whether the athlete's fault or negligence is significant or not, or even absent. The common requirement for the application of any of the clauses offering the possibility to reduce or eliminate the otherwise applicable sanction is for the athlete to show how the substance entered his or her system. The explanations provided by the athletes often lead to a scientific opinion, which is provided to a panel to determine whether the athlete's explanation is realistic from a scientific standpoint. The questions to be reviewed by scientists have often a pharmacokinetic nature as it is necessary to ensure that the alleged date and time of ingestion, the way the substance was taken, as well as the alleged quantity match with the estimated concentration of the prohibited substance detected in the athlete's sample. These questions may become complex, for example, for substances for which the List does not establish any reporting threshold and for which the concentration reported by the laboratory is qualitative and not quantitative. To support the law and an appropriate outcome to a case, scientists are asked to provide answers, precise answers, as lawyers are always looking for a yes or a no and do not like answers such as "it cannot be excluded" or "unlikely". Depending on the substance at stake, studies or available research may well be very limited, when the substance is emerging, illegal or not used in any medication licensed around the world. Besides, the scenarios brought forward by athletes are sometimes surprising and unique and may be complicated to evaluate due to the lack of related scientific research. For example, French kissing a cocaine addict, drinking diuretic-contaminated tap water, maintaining sexual intercourse with a person using a steroid, drinking from a glass cleaned in the same dishwasher as the shaker used by a brother who ingested a prohibited substance, and consumption of contaminated meat are some examples of alleged sources of intake where science input is required in support of the adjudication process.

---

[40] Article 3.2.1 of the Code

Other Situations Where Science Supports the Law

The Substances of Abuse

The fight against doping in sport aims at ensuring fair competitions where no results are obtained with the support of enhancing substances or other doping practices. Some of the prohibited substances, in particular cocaine which is a powerful doping agent due to its strong stimulating effect, are also widely used in a social context at a time when perhaps the athlete is not participating in any competition and where the consumption of the substance is not even prohibited under the anti-doping rules. Indeed, stimulants such as cocaine are prohibited in competition only, as their effect is immediate and not long lasting, unlike anabolic agents or some hormones. The increased use of this cocaine in society and the parallel improvement of the laboratories' capabilities to detect lower levels led to the reporting of an important number of cocaine cases; cocaine is a non-threshold substance, so its mere presence at any level in an athlete's sample constitutes an anti-doping rule violation.[41] One can sarcastically say that science created the very problem it then helped the law to solve. It became obvious that the situation had to be addressed. Sanctioning athletes who are "only" partying or even addicts who do not intend to cheat with similar sanctions as real cheats was considered by many as unjustified with regard to the objective of the fight against doping and was also resource-consuming for anti-doping organizations without producing any tangible benefit to clean sport. It is not the role of anti-doping to address social issues. The rules were therefore amended, first in 2015, but the minimum sanction was still 1 year.[42] This still was not satisfactory. The 2021 Code now sets out that if the substance detected is a so-called substance of abuse and that the athlete can establish that the intake occurred out-of-competition and was unrelated to sport, the applicable sanction is 3 months.[43] This is what the rule says; law has found a solution, but a solution whose applicability requires science support, on different aspects:

1. First, science must establish which substances are to be considered "of abuse": the Code sets out that substances of abuse are substances identified as such on the Prohibited List. In other words, the law makes it mandatory for science to address this specific point.[44]

---

[41] The CAS considered in a decision that "the circumstance that the concentration was lower than 50% of the MRPL for cocaine is irrelevant. In fact, cocaine is a non-threshold substance and the finding of any quantity in an athlete's sample constitutes an anti-doping rule violation, whatever the laboratory reporting obligations are" (CAS 2017/A/5078)

[42] This minimum 1-year ban could only be pronounced if the athlete was able to establish at the required standard of proof that the substance at stake was used out of competition in a context unrelated to sport performance (see article 10.23 of the 2015 Code)

[43] Article 10.2.4 of the Code

[44] As soon as this solution appeared to be supported by most stakeholders during the Code revision process and before going any further with it, the Code drafters liaised with the List Expert Group

2. Another key aspect where science input is necessary is again the validation, most of the time at a pharmacokinetics level, of the athlete's scenario, which is sometimes complex due to the absence of scientific studies. Science is required to confirm that the intake occurred out-of-competition and that the level detected in-competition is low enough to exclude any potential performance-enhancing effect.

The Therapeutic Use Exemptions

As aforementioned, most of the prohibited substances detected in athletes' samples are active ingredients of legitimate and authorized medications. Athletes have, as any human being, the right to proper medical care and therefore to take medications when medically required. Prohibiting athletes to use the same treatments as any other persons, when prescribed in the frame of a legitimate medical treatment, would have been not only philosophically unsustainable but also would have been disbanded by the first tribunal being called to address this question. The law, therefore, proposed a solution called Therapeutic Use Exemptions (TUE). Athletes can apply for an authorization to use a substance for legitimate medical reasons. No need to present that question in detail in this chapter, but several of the conditions to be met by the athlete to be granted this authorization also require science input. For example, the dosage prescribed shall not produce any enhancing effect other than restoring a normal health condition. Therefore, when an athlete benefiting from a TUE is tested in competition, the anti-doping organization must determine whether the level detected matches the prescribed and authorized dosage. Should it not be the case, the athlete faces the risk of being sanctioned. Again, science is asked to provide the answers for the law to be applied in a fair manner.

Law in Support of Science

The interaction of law and science is constant. We have provided some examples underlying the key role of science in the anti-doping legal process. However, this support goes both ways as the law also supports science. First, the law gives science a legal status, a recognition. Indeed, the law sets the rules of the game. It tells science what is expected from it and the conditions that science shall be able to meet to support the legal process and resist challenges.[45]

---

[45] For example, it gives a WADA-accredited Laboratory a presumption of compliance, which is a necessary support, but also clearly establishes the standards to be met to benefit from this presumption, and thus guides the science

Some Examples of the Legal Protection and Support of Science

The law protects the science by establishing the way and conditions it can be challenged and enhances the status of science when it resists a legal challenge and is validated in a decision rendered by an anti-doping panel. It also guides science by pointing out how it must evolve when a challenge is upheld by a hearing panel.

Challenges of Decision Limits or Analytical Methods in Legal Processes

Science is asked to be robust enough to meet the required standard of proof set out in the Code.[46] In the same way as the presumption of compliance of the analytical processes conducted by the WADA-accredited laboratory, the Code provides additional support for science by setting out the presumption that the analytical methods and decision limits approved by WADA are scientifically valid. This support also takes the form of what we can call a guidance as the steps to be followed by science to reach this presumption of validity are clearly indicated: a consultation with the relevant scientific community[47] or a peer review is required.[48] Another protection offered by the Code to science is through the setting of clear conditions under which an analytical method or a decision limit may be challenged. Indeed, as the validation process is led by WADA, the latter is best placed to defend the outcome. Therefore, the Code makes it mandatory that WADA is duly informed when any method or limit is challenged during an adjudication process. This does not give science a guarantee to resist any challenge but that any challenge is properly addressed to avoid declaring a method is unfit for purpose based on weak or wrong scientific allegations. This system has led to fruitful results. Indeed, where a method is challenged but validated by the Court of Arbitration for Sport, it is reinforced and less likely to fail any further challenge. This was the case, for example, of the erythropoietin analytical method, which was specifically developed for anti-doping purposes and challenged several times and always resisted these challenges, enhancing its presumption of scientific validity. In case a method is not validated by the Court of Arbitration for Sport, which can occur, for example, with a decision limit, science is given some homework that indirectly supports it as it guides the way to resist the next challenge.[49] This is exactly what happened with the human growth hormone decision limit as it resisted the following challenges and was reinforced.[50]

---

[46] See article 3.2.1 of the Code

[47] This is important as anti-doping science cannot be validated by scientists involved in anti-doping matters. By requiring such a recognition, the Code further protects the science as it makes it more difficult to be challenged

[48] It is also to be noted that this rule has evolved over time as in the 2015 Code: indeed, under the 2015 Code, the consultation and the peer review were required. The bar has been somewhat lowered

[49] In the decision CAS 2011/A/2566, the Panel considered that the appellant (WADA) failed to meet the required burden of proof that the decision limits were reliable

[50] In the decision CAS 2014/A/3488, the Panel considered that "the Joint Publication Paper has addressed the doubts expressed by the Panel in the case CAS 2011/A/2566 and that it has done so in a manner that appears to be convincing"

Retesting

The appearance of new doping protocols and doping agents is sometimes faster than what can be reasonably expected from science as the inclusion of a substance or method on the List, as well as the development, validation and implementation of a new robust analytical method, takes time and resources. By setting a statute of limitation of 10 years to prosecute a potential anti-doping rule violation[51] and by permitting the storage of a sample for further analysis at a later stage,[52] it is possible for science to be fit-for-purpose retroactively. Indeed, with the evolution of the analytical methods and the permanent lowering of the laboratories' limit of detection, the re-analysis of a sample some years later under enhanced and refined science tools has permitted the establishment of anti-doping rule violations and the sanctioning of athletes years after they commit the violation. It allows science to evolve under the strict conditions it must meet and make any "cheat" obliged to wait 10 years to see whether his or her fraud is successful or not. This recognition by the law of the complexity of some science questions already has led to fruitful results.[53]

Monitoring Programme

Another support offered to science by the law is the so-called monitoring programme. As indicated previously, the responsibility of the List Expert Group to determine whether a substance or method is to be included in the Prohibited List is quite complex. Further, the Code makes it very clear that samples can be collected only and exclusively for the detection of prohibited substances or methods identified on the Prohibited List.[54] The monitoring programme makes it possible, under certain conditions, to analyse the samples to detect substances or methods absent from the List, which offers important information on trends and use, by sport disciplines or region, of some products and can lead to additional research, before making a decision whether to include a substance on the List or not. This is a very important tool for science and its required permanent adaptation.

---

[51] See article 17 of the Code

[52] See article 6.6 of the Code

[53] For example, the International Olympic Committee has a programme in place to reanalyse stored samples collected during the Olympic Games. This program is fruitful as a significant number of adverse analytical findings were reported (https://stillmed.olympic.org/media/Document%20 Library/OlympicOrg/IOC/Who-We-Are/Commissions/Disciplinary-Commission/IOC-reanalysis-programme-25-January-2017-eng.pdf)

[54] See article 6.2 of the Code. The Monitoring Program was further extended in the latest version of the Code: In addition to monitoring substances already in the monitoring program, the modification to Article 4.5 provides that WADA may monitor data pertaining to other substances in order to see if they should be included on either the monitoring program or Prohibited List

Changes to the List

Another provision provides science with some more security in its evolution. Indeed, it may well happen (and has happened[55]) that the evolution of science leads to the conclusion that the inclusion of a certain substance on the List is not justified anymore. This situation is addressed by the Code[56] to ensure that when a new List enters into force, any athlete still serving a period of ineligibility consequent to the presence or use of a substance that has been removed can be reinstated immediately.

Support to the Principle of "Related Substances"

Given the number of substances that could fall within some classes of the Prohibited List, for example, in the class of stimulants, most classes of the List deliberately remain open, which means that the list of named substances appearing in these classes is not exhaustive. The reason is simple: it would simply be impossible to list all potential substances, as new and emerging substances, legal or illegal, regularly arrive on the market. This system allows the prosecution of cases where one of the substances is not expressly included in the List, if it can be established that the substance at stake has similar chemical structure or similar biological effect(s) as the other substances included in the applicable class. The law or, more precisely, the case law has provided support to this solution, by considering that it would be totally impractical to impose that once WADA is aware of a substance that is chemically similar in structure to another prohibited substance, it must include it on the List in order for cases involving this substance to be prosecuted.[57]

Limits

The fruitful alliance of science and law has resulted many times in great advances and achievements for the anti-doping system by shaping the regulatory framework and the guiding research in their respective and parallel evolutions. Some limits do, however, appear when science is unable to provide the due explanation to meet the standard of proof required by the law. It may happen when data are still not available for the substance at stake in a case, in particular excretion studies. The principle of strict liability sets the bar quite high, as the applicable sanctions may well be career ending. The lack of data can therefore make it very challenging for the anti-doping prosecutor to verify the explanations provided by an athlete. When doubts

---

[55] With finasteride, for example, due to the evolution of analytical method, the masking effect of this substance became useless, which led to the removal of this substance from the List

[56] See article 27.6, which was an evolution proposed in the 2021 Code

[57] CAS 2018/A/5768

cannot be vacated with a quasi-certainty, hearing panels are likely to decide in a favourable way for the athlete. This issue is frequent in relation to emerging substances as these substances are generally illegal, and unlike substances put on the market by pharmaceutical companies, for which excretion studies are generally available, the lack of data is recurrent when a new substance appears. In most cases, such products have never been tested in humans before. For example, in a recent case involving ligandrol, a substance that is not yet used in any approved medication worldwide, the alleged source of the positive test was contamination through sexual intercourse with a partner using that substance. Given that the route of transmission in the conditions described by the athlete could not be excluded at the scientific level with a sufficiently high level of certainty, the panel considered that the origin was established. Further, given the lack of available data on that substance, the explanations provided by the athlete could not be verified (timing and dosage of the partner's ingestion, timing of the transmission, level detected in the athlete's sample, etc.), and no sanction was pronounced. The lack of data is also an issue in relation to substances that have already been on the Prohibited List for a long time. For example, cases involving glucocorticoids have highlighted some scientific limits over the past years. Indeed, this class of substances is only prohibited when administered via certain routes,[58] but their use by other routes was not. However, in case of a positive finding where the athlete alleges that the route of administration was not prohibited, scientific knowledge is sometimes insufficient to verify how the substance entered the athlete's body. Consequently, even if administered via a prohibited route, athletes may escape any sanction. This situation is being addressed and changes were made in the 2022 Prohibited List.[59] A third situation where the lack of available data can be detrimental to the results management of a case is when the athlete alleges that the positive finding is the consequence of the ingestion of contaminated meat. It is well known that some substances are used in some regions of the world by the cattle industry, legally or not. Data are often missing, for example, as some countries are not taking the issue seriously or simply not wanting to admit they have a public health issue. Anti-doping organizations find themselves in a complicated situation when an athlete alleges—and establishes—having eaten meat in a certain country, but where no official data are available on the use of substances in cattle in said country. Further, even if the alleged contamination relates to a country where the use of the prohibited substance by the cattle industry is officially recognized, other data may still be missing. Science is asked to determine the value for each substance above which meat contamination can be excluded as being the origin. This is possible for some of the substances used by the cattle industry, but not yet for all. However, even in a case where science is able to confirm that the level detected in the athlete's sample may be compatible with the ingestion of

---

[58] Glucocorticoids are prohibited when administered by oral, intravenous, intra-muscular, or rectal routes

[59] All systemic and injectable routes of administration are prohibited in the 2022 Prohibited List

contaminated meat, it is to date impossible to discriminate whether the low level detected is the consequence of the ingestion of contaminated meat or the lower end of the excretion following a doping practice. Both science and the law are called to evolve to address this recurrent question.[60]

Conclusion

This permanent interaction between science and law is the cornerstone of anti-doping and will continue to be as emerging substances as well as new doping techniques appear regularly. This fact will call for anti-doping science to adapt and evolve in order to maintain a fit-for-purpose Prohibited List, ensure that sufficient supporting data are available to answer the questions that may appear during any adjudication process, and also, in parallel, develop and implement the new analytical methods and techniques required, at a level sufficient to resist the numerous legal challenges that may arise. Despite significant progress, numerous complex questions remain to be addressed. Over the past years, the WADA-accredited laboratories have developed the ability to detect infinitesimal quantities of prohibited substances in athletes' samples. One may consider this improvement of the laboratories' capabilities as a great technical achievement, but the adjudication of cases involving very tiny traces of a substance is complex. At very low levels, a positive finding is possibly the consequence of the ingestion of a contaminated product or the end of the excretion period of a doping practice. Further, a very low level detected in-competition may well result from an authorized out-of-competition intake and improbably have had any in-competition effect. This distinction is key for the determination of the sanction, in particular for substances of abuse. Finally, at very low levels, it is sometimes almost impossible for the athlete, even in good faith, to provide any explanations as regards the source of the positive finding. However, the rules are clear: to get any reduction, the athlete must establish the source of the positive finding. It shall be sufficient for the prosecuting anti-doping organization to establish the presence of the substance in an athlete's sample, and if the athlete is unable to establish the origin, no reduction can be granted. Cases involving a very low amount of a prohibited substance have led hearing panels to discuss possible scenarios[61] for the positive test, and where the anti-doping organization prosecuting a case was unable to provide a likely doping scenario, hearing panels have rendered decisions in favour of the athletes, even when they could not establish the origin.[62] The discussions on possible doping scenarios take place

---

[60] A specific working group was established in 2019 by WADA to address the question of contamination. This is a complex issue as sanctioning an honest athlete whose sole fault is the ingestion of contaminated meat must be avoided, but widening the net creates a risk to let real cheats escape any sanction

[61] CAS 2011/A/2384 & CAS 2011/A/2386

[62] CAS 2017/A/5296

before hearing panels, in the form of a contradictory scientific debate. For the most part, hearing panel members are not scientists, which results in difficulties for them to determine which of the competing experts' opinions should be followed. One would normally expect that any expert brought in a case by any of the parties would provide neutral expertise and that said expertise would not be shaped with the sole interest of defending the interest of the parties which called him or her. However, the lack of procedural rules on experts and the absence of any closed list, as it exists in some public jurisdictions, has led to unnecessary confusion, groundless challenges, and some epic debates, in a world where fake news becomes a daily reality. The "forced" union of science and law is in fact a marriage of convenience, which is called to last for the good of anti-doping regulation and practice.

International Drug Control: Protecting the Health of the Athlete

Justice N. A. Tettey, Conor Crean, Asma Fakhri, and Clare Jones de Rocco

The International Drug Control System

The International Drug Control Conventions and the Welfare of Humankind

For over a century, the international community has relied on multilateral treaties to address the issue of drugs, in particular the protection of the health and welfare of people who use drugs. The first conference to discuss drugs at the international level, the Opium Commission, was held in Shanghai in 1909 to address the opium epidemic, which had led to alarming rates of addiction, particularly in China. Although the original intention was to limit the conference to the situation in Asia, it was argued that the issue could only be properly addressed through the participation of all the major producing, manufacturing and consuming nations. The Commission was eventually attended by 13 countries and represents the origin of international collaboration on drug control. In anticipation of the conference, a number of countries reported significant reforms including curbs on the trade in opium and the cultivation of opium poppies in the years prior to 1909 [1]. The Commission gave rise to the *International Opium Convention of The Hague*, signed in 1912 and effective from 1915, as the first international drug control convention, passed with the objective of stemming the shipment of drugs not intended for medical purposes. Following its establishment in 1920, the League of Nations became the custodian of the Opium Convention, and the scope of control of this treaty was expanded in 1925 to cover cannabis (The 1925 Convention). The 1931 *Convention for Limiting the Manufacture and Regulating the Distribution of Narcotic Drugs*

J. N. A. Tettey (✉) · C. Crean · A. Fakhri · C. Jones de Rocco
Laboratory and Scientific Section, Division of Policy Analysis, United Nations Office on Drugs and Crime (UNODC), Vienna, Austria
e-mail: justice.tettey@un.org

© The Author(s), under exclusive license to Springer Nature Switzerland AG 2022
O. Rabin, O. Corazza (eds.), *Emerging Drugs in Sport*,
https://doi.org/10.1007/978-3-030-79293-0_6

and the 1936 *Convention for the Suppression of the Illicit Traffic in Dangerous Drugs* were also developed under the auspices of the League of Nations. While the former focused on restricting the supply of narcotic drugs to quantities required for medical and scientific purposes, and like previous conventions regulated licit drug activities, the latter became the first international instrument to make certain drug offences international crimes. In 1946, the United Nations took over the drug control functions and responsibilities formerly carried out by the League of Nations. The Commission on Narcotic Drugs (CND) was established by the United Nations Economic and Social Council as one of its functional commissions in resolution 9(1) of February 16, 1946, to assist the Council in supervising the application of the international drug control conventions. The CND also advises the Council on all matters pertaining to the control of narcotic drugs, psychotropic substances and their precursors and is mandated to decide on the scope of control of substances under the three international drug control conventions. A number of protocols to improve the control system were signed in the post-war years, the most far-reaching of which was the 1953 *Opium Protocol* which limited opium production and trade to medical and scientific purposes. Under the auspices of the United Nations, the *Single Convention on Narcotic Drugs* of 1961, which merged all the existing conventions, was adopted. The Convention also provided for the establishment in 1968 of the International Narcotics Control Board (INCB) as the independent and quasi-judicial monitoring body for the implementation of the United Nations international drug control conventions. To underscore the need to provide adequate prevention, treatment and rehabilitation services, the Single Convention was amended by a protocol in 1972.

The *Convention on Psychotropic Substances* of 1971 was passed to address the increased abuse of psychotropic substances, such as central nervous system stimulants, sedative hypnotics and hallucinogens, which had resulted in public health and social problems in several countries. The final of the three international drug conventions which together form the cornerstones of the international drug control system, the *Convention against Illicit Traffic in Narcotic Drugs and Psychotropic Substances*, was passed in 1988. This comprehensively addresses all aspects of the illicit drug industry such as the production, manufacture, extraction, preparation, distribution, sale, importation or exportation of any narcotic drug or any psychotropic substance which, when committed intentionally, contrary to the provisions of the 1961 Convention (as amended by the 1972 Protocol), or the 1971 Convention, constitutes a criminal offence. The United Nations, recognizing that the dimensions of illicit production, abuse and trafficking of narcotic drugs and psychotropic substances in all regions of the world necessitated a more comprehensive and integrated approach to international drug control and an efficient structure to enable the organization to play a central and greatly enhanced role in this area, established the United Nations International Drug Control Programme (UNDCP) in 1991 in Vienna. The subsequent merger in 2002 of the UNDCP with the Crime Prevention and Criminal Justice Division of the United Nations Office at Vienna led to the formation of the United Nations Office on Drugs and Crime (UNODC). UNODC implements the United Nations' drug and crime programmes in an integrated manner, addressing the interrelated issues of drug control, crime prevention and international terrorism in the context of sustainable development and human security. In addition to the CND's function supervising the implementation of the drug control treaties, it continues to monitor all commitments on strengthening actions at the national, regional and international levels to address and counter the world drug problem. Notable among such commitments are the 2009 Political Declaration and Plan of Action and its 2014 review, the outcome document of the 2016 United Nations General Assembly special session on the world drug problem and the 2019 Ministerial Declaration.

The Spirit of the International Drug Conventions

The preambles of all three conventions underscore a common driving force: a concern for "the health and welfare of mankind" and the desire to make drugs ("narcotics" and "psychotropic substances" as per the Conventions) available for medical and scientific purposes, including for clinical trials, while preventing their diversion and abuse.[1] Contrary to the school of thought that they provide a basis for justifying draconian approaches to enforcement by countries, the international drug control conventions continue to provide a flexible framework for addressing the drug problem within an approach based on the principle of shared responsibility [2]. In pursuing a people-centred approach which prioritizes human health and welfare, the conventions call for the prevention of drug abuse and the treatment and rehabilitation of people with drug problems and require their signatories to "coordinate their efforts to these ends" [3]. In their efforts to protect the health and welfare of humankind, the conventions employ a scientifically guided scheduling system to define the scope of control of substances and preparations [4, 5].

Scope of Control of the Conventions

Currently, the international drug control system is based on three conventions: the *Single Convention on Narcotic Drugs* of 1961, as amended by the 1972 protocol (the 1961 Convention); the *Convention on Psychotropic Substances of 1971 (the 1971 Convention); and the United Nations Convention against Illicit Traffic in Narcotic Drugs and Psychotropic Substances of 1988 (the 1988 Convention). The 1961 Convention, as of 2020, exercises international control over 136 substances including mainly natural products such as opium and its derivatives (morphine,*

---

[1] "Drugs" are defined as any of the substances in schedules I and II of the 1961 Convention, whether natural or synthetic. For the purposes of the List of Prohibited Substances in Sports, "drugs" include narcotics (S7) and cannabis. Psychotropic substances mean any substance, whether natural or synthetic, or any natural material in schedules I–IV of the Convention

codeine and heroin), coca leaves and cocaine, cannabis and cannabis resin and also synthetic drugs such as fentanyl. The substances controlled by the convention are listed in schedules (I, II and IV)[2] based on the degree of liability to abuse and the risk to public health and welfare. Of relevance to the sports world is the overlap of substances in the 1961 Convention with the S7 narcotics (e.g., heroin, morphine and fentanyl) and S8 cannabinoids (e.g., cannabis) categories of the World Anti-Doping Code's List of Prohibited Substances and Methods (the Prohibited List) [6]. The 1971 Convention employs a sliding scale of schedules (I–IV) based on the liability to abuse (e.g., especially serious, substantial, small but still significant) and the degree of therapeutic usefulness (e.g., very limited, little to moderate and moderate to great) of each substance. Several substances prohibited in sports under the World Anti-Doping Code's Prohibited List, S6 stimulants (e.g., amphetamine, methamphetamine and cathinone) and S8 cannabinoids (e.g., delta-9-THC and other synthetic cannabimimetics) are also listed in the schedules of the 1971 Convention. The 1961 and 1971 Conventions codify internationally applicable control measures in order to ensure the availability of narcotic drugs and psychotropic substances for medical and scientific purposes and prevent their diversion to illicit channels. The 1988 Convention emphasizes the importance of precursor control at the international level and lists the substances frequently used in the illicit manufacture of narcotic drugs or psychotropic substances in the two tables of the convention. Of significance to sport is the 1988 Convention's designation of the World Anti-Doping Code's Prohibited List S6 stimulants ephedrine and pseudoephedrine as Table 1 substances in view of their use as precursors in the manufacture of methamphetamine. Since 1961, a total of 300 substances have been controlled under the 1961 and 1971 Conventions and 30 substances placed in the tables of the 1988 Convention. The substances controlled under the 1961 and 1971 Conventions include cannabimimetics, stimulants, sedative/hypnotics, classic hallucinogens and dissociatives.

The Treaty Bodies and International Scheduling

The CND, the World Health Organization (WHO) and the INCB are recognized as the "treaty bodies" under the three international conventions. The CND reviews and analyses the global drug situation, considering supply and demand reduction, and acts through resolutions and decisions. In addition, it is mandated to exercise treaty-based "scheduling" functions by considering proposals to add substances to the schedules/tables or to transfer or delete substances from the schedules/tables. The schedules/tables entail different levels of control measures. States which are party to the three drug control conventions are required to ensure that the mandatory

---

[2] Schedule III of the 1961 Convention contains exempted preparations of the drugs in Schedules I and II

control measures contained therein are applied to substances listed in the schedules/ tables which are annexed to these conventions. Under the 1961 and 1971 Conventions, a request to change the scope of control of substances can be initiated either by a state party or by the WHO. Under the 1961 and 1971 Conventions, the WHO has the role of reviewing substances for their liability to abuse, ill effects on health and usefulness in medical therapy and for making recommendations to the CND as to the scope of international control. Under the 1988 Convention, a request to change the scope of control of substances can be initiated either by a state party or by the INCB. Under the 1988 Convention, the INCB is tasked with determining whether a substance is frequently used in the illicit manufacture of a narcotic drug or psychotropic substance and whether the volume and extent of the illicit manufac- ture creates serious public or social problems, so as to warrant international action.

Role of UNODC in International Drug Control

The UNODC Mission and Mandate

UNODC serves as the United Nations central drug control entity with responsibility for leading the organization's drug control activities, providing technical expertise and advising member states on questions of international and national drug control [7]. It supports member states to implement the 17 *Sustainable Development Goals* which form the core of the UN *2030 Agenda for Sustainable Development*. The 2030 Agenda recognizes that the rule of law, in conjunction with fair, effective and humane justice systems, as well as health-oriented responses to drug use, enables sustainable development. The Agenda also recognizes the important role of sport in sustainable development, highlighting its growing contribution to achieving peace and development through its promotion of tolerance and respect. The United Nations system and its member states, international sport federations and other stakeholders are establishing frameworks for collaborative action on sport, physical activity and active play that use sport as a platform for achieving wider development outcomes rather than focusing on sport as an end in itself. These frameworks feature a wide range of goals, including personal and interpersonal social development, health pro- motion, conflict resolution, intercultural dialogue, social inclusion and economic development [8]. To further promote an integrated approach to the interrelated issues of drug control and crime prevention, UNODC is the custodian of interna- tional conventions dealing with organized crime and corruption. The *United Nations Convention against Transnational Organized Crime* is a legally binding instrument through which countries commit to taking measures against transnational organized crime including the creation of domestic offences; the adoption of new, sweeping frameworks for mutual legal assistance, extradition, law enforcement cooperation and technical assistance; and training. UNODC also oversees the *United Nations Convention against Corruption* which was adopted by the United Nations General

Assembly in 2003 and is the only universal legally binding anti-corruption instrument. Its far-reaching approach and the mandatory character of many of its provisions make it a unique tool for developing a comprehensive response to a global problem. The convention covers five main areas: preventive measures, criminalization and law enforcement, international cooperation, asset recovery and technical assistance and information exchange. In its efforts to help countries tackle the world drug problem, UNODC's work falls into three main areas, namely, normative, research and capacity building. The first relates to the implementation of the three drug control treaties whereby UNODC encourages member states to develop policies consistent with the treaties and adopt balanced, scientific and evidence-based approaches that include both supply and demand reduction. In the research domain, UNODC constitutes the global authority in the fields of drugs and crime, providing valuable knowledge and essential high-quality evidence to inform policy making in these areas. The UNODC *Thematic Programme on Research, Trend Analysis and Forensics* defines the key challenges, work priorities and quality standards, as well as the tools and services to support policy and programme development in the framework of UNODC mandates. This is done by undertaking thematic research, managing global and regional data collections, providing scientific and forensic services, defining research standards and supporting member states to strengthen their data collection, research and forensics capacities. Thirdly, working closely with governments and civil society, UNODC delivers capacity building and a wide range of tailored technical assistance through a network of over 115 field offices with a view to strengthening national responses to the world drug problem.

Addressing Emerging and Current Threats

Novel Psychoactive Substances

Over the past decade, the nature of the global drugs market has evolved rapidly and become more complex with the emergence of novel psychoactive substances (NPS). UNODC uses the term "new psychoactive substances" to refer to substances of abuse, either in a pure form or a preparation, that are not controlled by the 1961 *Single Convention on Narcotic Drugs or the 1971 Convention on Psychotropic Substances, but which may pose a public health threat. The term "new" does not necessarily refer to new inventions—several NPS were first synthesized decades ago—but to substances that have recently become available on the market. Some NPS, also known as "legal highs", "bath salts" and "research chemicals", have been associated with increased abuse, hospital emergency admissions and sometimes fatalities. A number of these substances, belonging to the classes of stimulants, hallucinogens and synthetic cannabinoids, have been encountered in sport and in food supplements. The first comprehensive UNODC report on NPS, titled "The Challenge of New Psychoactive Substances", provided the first global data in*

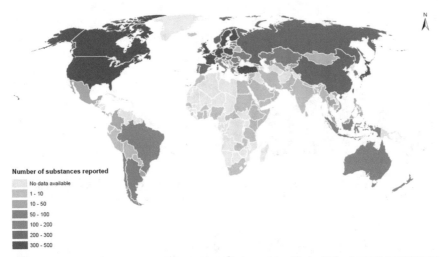

Fig. 1 UNODC Early Warning Advisory NPS Portal database. Data: Number of NPS reported by country/territory, 2020)

this area, identifying 251 individual substances in a total of 70 countries and territories (up to July 2012) [9]. Currently, UNODC is actively monitoring over 1000 different NPS that have been identified by 124 countries and territories since 2009 (Figs. 1, 2, and 3). Overall, stimulants account for the largest group of substances reported, followed by synthetic cannabinoid receptor agonists and classic hallucinogens. In recent years, reports of substances in most groups have either plateaued or even decreased following an initial rapid increase from 2012 to 2015. However, certain groups of NPS such as synthetic opioid receptor agonists continue to be on the rise with an almost fourfold increase from 2016 to mid-2020. The group of sedatives/hypnotics, including benzodiazepine-type substances, has also shown a steady increase in recent years. The effective monitoring of NPS at the global level over the past decade is a direct result of the establishment of UNODC's Early Warning Advisory on New Psychoactive Substances in 2013, further to a CND Resolution. The Early Warning Advisory allows UNODC to monitor the emergence of NPS, analyse the market trends associated with these substances, tailor support to drug analysis laboratories and support the formulation of effective measures to mitigate the problem at the international level. Early warning systems play a key role in early detection and monitoring, as well as in enabling timely responses to emerging NPS threats. Monitoring is paramount to understanding the NPS market and provides an evidence base to inform policies and responses to address the ongoing challenges posed by NPS. The UNODC Early Warning Advisory thus serves as a repository for information on NPS leading to an improved understanding of their distribution and

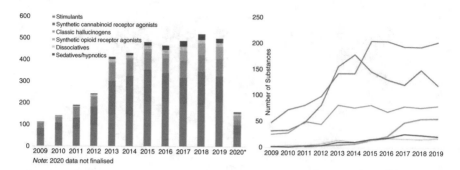

Fig. 2 Emergence of NPS by effect group reported to the UNODC Early Warning Advisory (2009–2020)

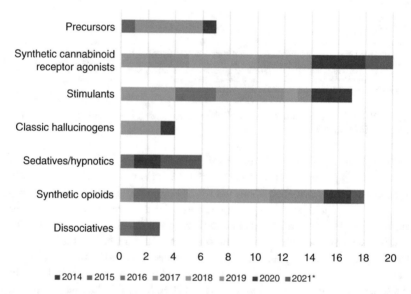

Fig. 3 Number of NPS and precursors placed under international control, 2014–2020, and considered for international scheduling in 2021

use at the global level and offering a platform for providing technical assistance to member states. NPS are characterized by geographic heterogeneity, with some being only transient in nature and others not meeting the criteria for harm which are required for international control. Consequently, in 2016 the United Nations General Assembly special session on the world drug problem adopted a pragmatic approach to prioritise the most harmful, persistent and prevalent NPS for international action. In order to collect information on the use of NPS at a global level and identify the most harmful substances, the Early Warning Advisory was expanded in 2018 to collect toxicology data in post-mortem, clinical and other casework. The information provided comes from a variety of sources, including the UNODC network of over

280 national forensic drug testing and toxicology laboratories and partnerships with international, regional and national organizations such as the International Association of Forensic Toxicologists, the European Monitoring Centre for Drugs and Drug Addiction, the US Drug Enforcement Administration and Health Canada as well as official information from member states and other sources. The information within the UNODC Early Warning Advisory is used to provide member states with the latest available global information on NPS through a variety of mechanisms and publications. These include alerts, technical reports such as the biannual "Current NPS Threats", contributions to UNODC publications such as the "World Drug Report" and "Global SMART Updates", briefings to intergovernmental bodies and the World Health Organization. The information in the Early Warning Advisory also allows UNODC's Laboratory and Scientific Service to better understand the challenges faced by forensic service providers around the world and tailor accordingly the forensic services provided. This includes a series of manuals and guidelines for forensic laboratories on recommended analysis methods as well as quality assurance support, reference materials and training. The information available in the Early Warning Advisory, in particular on the toxicology and pharmacology of NPS, has been important in providing the evidence base for prioritizing the most harmful substances for international action. Since 2015, 60 substances made up of synthetic cannabinoids (18), synthetic stimulants (17), synthetic opioids (17), classic hallucinogens (4), sedative hypnotics (3) and dissociatives (1) have been placed under international control. Most of these harmful substances are also captured under existing classes in the WADA Prohibited List such as S-6 stimulants (e.g., cathinone and its analogues such as mephedrone and MDPV, phenethylamine and its derivatives such as 25C-NBOMe), S-7 narcotics (fentanyl analogues) and S-8 cannabinoids (e.g., synthetic cannabinoids).

Addressing Emerging Challenges: From Resolutions to Results

The complexities of the implementation of the international drug control system, particularly with respect to addressing emerging challenges, are best illustrated by the response to the ongoing global opioid crisis—a far-reaching drug and public health policy issue affecting several geographical regions [10]. The opioid crisis in North America is characterized by a highly prevalent non-medical use of opioids and high rates of mortality driven by pharmaceutical opioids, heroin and synthetic opioids. In West, Central and North Africa however, the opioid crisis is characterized by a high prevalence of the non-medical use of pharmaceutical opioids, in particular tramadol. The crisis is also expanding geographically and deepening in complexity with the emergence of a new generation of NPS with opioid effects, including substances belonging to chemical structural classes which were not significantly present on illicit drug markets previously. In response to the opioid crisis,

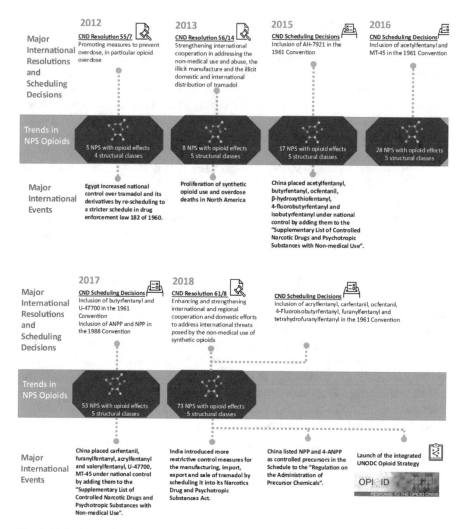

Fig. 4 Major international and national policy events in relation to the opioid crisis

the international community has taken major steps towards developing a set of balanced international and domestic responses. These efforts have aimed to balance
drug control and public health responses with adequate access to opioid analgesics
for scientific research and medical uses including pain management and palliative
care [10]. Figure 4 maps the evolution of the problem by presenting the trends in the
types and numbers of opioid-type NPS over the period 2012–2020 and outlining
various CND resolutions and decisions on the scheduling of substances which are
based on recommendations from the other treaty bodies, on narcotic and psychotropic substances from WHO and on the precursor chemicals from INCB (Fig. 4). It
also illustrates the complementary and crucial role of work at the country level, for

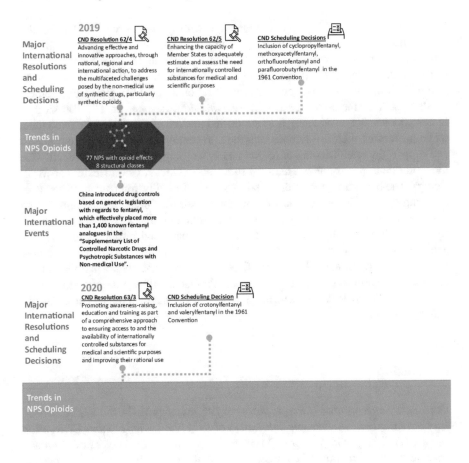

Major International Resolutions and Scheduling Decisions

2019

CND Resolution 62/4
Advancing effective and innovative approaches, through national, regional and international action, to address the multifaceted challenges posed by the non-medical use of synthetic drugs, particularly synthetic opioids

CND Resolution 62/5
Enhancing the capacity of Member States to adequately estimate and assess the need for internationally controlled substances for medical and scientific purposes

CND Scheduling Decisions
Inclusion of cyclopropylfentanyl, methoxyacetylfentanyl, orthofluorofentanyl and parafluorobutyrfentanyl in the 1961 Convention

Trends in NPS Opioids

77 NPS with opioid effects
8 structural classes

Major International Events

China introduced drug controls based on generic legislation with regards to fentanyl, which effectively placed more than 1,400 known fentanyl analogues in the "Supplementary List of Controlled Narcotic Drugs and Psychotropic Substances with Non-medical Use".

Major International Resolutions and Scheduling Decisions

2020

CND Resolution 63/3
Promoting awareness-raising, education and training as part of a comprehensive approach to ensuring access to and the availability of internationally controlled substances for medical and scientific purposes and improving their rational use

CND Scheduling Decision
Inclusion of crotonylfentanyl and valerylfentanyl in the 1961 Convention

Trends in NPS Opioids

Major International Events

Note: The "1961 Convention" refers to the Single Convention on Narcotic Drugs of 1961 as amended by the 1972 Protocol and the "1988 Convention" refers to the United Nations Convention against Illicit Traffic in Narcotic Drugs and Psychotropic Substances of 1988. "CND" refers to the The Commission on Narcotic Drugs.

Note: UNODC elaboration based on various CND resolutions and decisions, and the UNODC Early Warning Advisory on NPS. Note: The "1961 Convention" refers to the *Single Convention on Narcotic Drugs* of 1961 as amended by the 1972 Protocol and the "1988 Convention" refers to the *United Nations Convention against Illicit Traffic in Narcotic Drugs and Psychotropic Substances* of 1988. "CND" refers to The Commission on Narcotic Drugs.

Fig. 4 (continued)

example, by China and India, in achieving effective and lasting solutions on the ground. The CND continues to encourage UNODC, INCB and WHO to enhance and strengthen international and regional cooperation to address the threats posed by the non-medical use of synthetic opioids. Heeding that call, UNODC launched an integrated strategy to coordinate the global response to the opioid crisis in 2018. To equip countries with the tools needed to apply the guidance of the UNODC

Opioid Strategy and tackle problems associated with synthetic drugs, the UN Toolkit on Synthetic Drugs was developed as a one-stop shop offering multidisciplinary resources from across multiple United Nations agencies and diverse fields of expertise on a single platform (https://syntheticdrugs.unodc.org). The UN Toolkit on Synthetic Drugs also supports countries to operationalize the Strategic Development Goals to achieve the *2030 Agenda for Sustainable Development*. The Toolkit promotes policies that ensure access to controlled medicines for those who need them while preventing their diversion, strengthen prevention and treatment programmes and support the establishment of forensic early warning systems to help identify the most prevalent, persistent and harmful substances (Goal 3, Good Health and Well-Being). The Toolkit supports the establishment of quality forensic services safeguarding human rights and the rule of law (Goal 16, Peace, Justice and Strong Institutions) while promoting gender-sensitive policies (Goal 5, Gender Equality) as well as environmentally safe chemical disposal plans and resources for the safe handling of substances (Goal 6, Clean Water and Sanitation; Goal 15, Life below Water; Goal 16, Life on Land). UNODC also fosters strategic partnerships to enhance international cooperation (Goal 17, Partnerships) by promoting the use of scientific and forensic data to inform international and national policy and decision-making processes.

Conclusion

The *Single Convention on Narcotic Drugs* of 1961 as amended by the 1972 Protocol, the *Convention on Psychotropic Substances* of 1971, the *United Nations Convention against Illicit Traffic in Narcotic Drugs and Psychotropic Substances* of 1988 and other relevant international instruments constitute the cornerstones of the international drug control system. These three conventions continue to provide a flexible framework for addressing the drug problem within an approach based on the principle of shared responsibility. Their underlying principle of protecting the health and welfare of humankind; the mutually reinforcing treaty functions of the CND, WHO and INCB; and the support provided by UNODC to countries to address current and emerging threats continue to be relevant. The international response to the phenomenon of novel psychoactive substances and the related opioid crisis offers insights to the complexity of the work of the international drug control system in protecting the health and welfare of society at large, of which the sport community is an important member.

References

1. United Nations Office on Drugs and Crime (2008) World Drug Report 2008. pp 173–187. https://www.unodc.org/documents/wdr/WDR_2008/WDR_2008_eng_web.pdf. Accessed 3 Nov 2020
2. Carpentier C, Niaz K, Tettey J (2018) The international drug conventions continue to provide a flexible framework to address the drug problem. Addiction 13(7):1228–1229
3. United Nations (1977) Single convention on narcotic drugs, 1961 as amended by the 1972 Protocol. United Nations, New York, p 41 Art. 38 para. 1
4. United Nations (1977) Single convention on narcotic drugs, 1961 as amended by the 1972 Protocol. United Nations, New York, p. 17 Art. 3
5. United Nations (1977) Convention on psychotropic substances, 1971. United Nations, New York, pp 8–12 Art 2
6. World Anti-Doping Agency (2020) International Standard Prohibited List, https://www.wada-ama.org/sites/default/files/wada_2020_english_prohibited_list_0.pdf. Accessed 19 Oct 2020
7. United Nations (2004) Secretary General's bulletin, Organization of the United Nations Office on Drugs and Crime, ST/SGB/2004/6, https://undocs.org/ST/SGB/2004/6. Accessed 16 Oct 2020
8. United Nations (2018) General Assembly, Report of the Secretary-General, Strengthening the global framework for leveraging sport for development and peace, A/73/325. https://undocs.org/en/A/73/325. Accessed 16 Oct 2020
9. United Nations Office on Drugs and Crime (2013) The challenge of new psychoactive substances. https://www.unodc.org/documents/scientific/NPS_Report.pdf. Accessed 16 Oct 2020
10. United Nations Office on Drugs and Crime (2020) Global SMART Update vol. 24, The growing complexity of the opioid crisis. https://www.unodc.org/documents/scientific/Global_SMART-2020-Vol_24_web.pdf. Accessed 16 Oct 2020

Tackling New Forms of Doping: The Legal Challenges

Jean-Pierre Morand, Ross Wenzel, and Nicolas Zbinden

Introduction

When the World Anti-Doping Agency (WADA) List Committee meets on a yearly basis to determine what should or should not be prohibited, the resulting decisions are based on the knowledge of the scientific experts at that point in time. Of course, no one is able to anticipate every possible new means of artificially enhancing sports performance. It may well be that these experts are unaware of certain emerging doping practices amongst athletes. It may also be that drugs or methods start to be used only after the List of Prohibited Substances and Methods (the Prohibited List) is decided upon. This gives rise to challenges for WADA: How can one ensure that the Prohibited List is broad enough to catch as many of these new drugs as possible? What if new analytical methods, which would help detect the drugs that were undetectable at the time of the doping control, are developed later? What about the possibility of detection through markers indicating the use of a prohibited substance or method, instead of direct detection? How can investigation assist in exposing sophisticated doping cases? This chapter addresses certain tools implemented by WADA and other anti-doping organisations to tackle new forms of doping. In addition, it discusses the handling of doping violations based on novel non-listed substances in respect of sanctions.

J.-P. Morand (✉) · R. Wenzel · N. Zbinden
Kellerhals-Carrard Law Firm, Lausanne, Switzerland
e-mail: jean-pierre.morand@kellerhals-carrard.ch

© The Author(s), under exclusive license to Springer Nature Switzerland AG 2022
O. Rabin, O. Corazza (eds.), *Emerging Drugs in Sport*,
https://doi.org/10.1007/978-3-030-79293-0_7

Tools to Tackle New Forms of Doping

Prohibition by Categories

It would be not possible for the WADA List Committee to anticipate and to cover all the new doping agents in a list established at a given time. New legitimate and regulated drugs become available around the world almost every week, and this is also true for black market drugs, such as novel psychoactive substances (NPS), which remain unknown until their use is detected in an analysis or otherwise as covered in other chapters of this book. It is equally not practicable for all (known) prohibited substances to be referred to explicitly (i.e., by non-proprietary or chemical name) on the Prohibited List. This is, for example, the case for stimulants. As noted by a Court of Arbitration for Sport (CAS) Panel, "[i]t would be impractical to cite all stimulants because of the large numbers of compounds available on the market".[1] The reality is that new ones are released almost weekly and that more than 900 specific substances would have to be included for the list to be even nearly exhaustive.[2] The World Anti-Doping Code (the "Code") addresses this issue by providing that prohibited substances may be defined by categories. As per article 4.2.1 of the Code, "Prohibited Substances and Prohibited Methods may be included in the Prohibited List by general category (e.g., anabolic agents) or by specific reference to a particular Substance or Method". As a result, even if a substance is not explicitly set out on the Prohibited List, it may well fall under a relevant category in the Prohibited List and therefore still be prohibited. The Prohibited List classifies the prohibited substances or methods in different classes. There are thus nine classes of prohibited substance and three classes of prohibited methods (S1 to S9 and M1 to M3).[3] All classes of prohibited substances list specific substances. While certain classes are exhaustive (e.g., narcotics in S7), others are not. Thus, certain classes provide for a list of substances but clarify that other substances, which have a "similar chemical structure or similar biological effect(s)" as the expressly listed substances, are also prohibited (see anabolic agents (S1), peptide hormones, growth factors, related substances, and mimetics (S2), diuretics and masking agents (S5) and stimulants (S6)). In the case of stimulants, the definition is open-ended ("all stimulants [...] are prohibited" under S6).[4] The listed substances are therefore expressly provided only as examples. Although this is often not well understood, the Prohibited List is actually

---

[1] CAS 2009/A/1805 & 1847 IAAF v. RFEA & Onyia

[2] See CAS 2019/A/6574 WADA v. RANAD & Mineran, para. 62

[3] In addition, where a substance neither falls under a specific class prohibited in the Prohibited List nor has a "similar chemical structure or similar biological effect(s)" to the substances in a class, it will still be prohibited if it has "no current approval by any governmental regulatory health authority for human therapeutic use (e.g., drugs under pre-clinical or clinical development or discontinued, designer drugs, substances approved only for veterinary use)" under S0 of the Prohibited List

[4] International Standard for the List of Prohibited Substances and Methods. Available at: https://www.wada-ama.org/en/content/what-is-prohibited

in many respects an open list. However, it falls on the organisation to demonstrate that an emerging drug falls under a relevant category on the Prohibited List. This will require establishing scientifically that the drug is included in one of the prohibited classes or that it has a "similar chemical structure or similar biological effect(s)" to the substances of the classes S1, S2, S5 or S6.[5] This may not always be an easy task. In the two following examples, the CAS accepted the evidence that the non-listed substances were prohibited substance:

In CAS 2009/A/1805 & 1847 IAAF v. RFEA & Onyia (confirmed in the more recent CAS 2017/A/4984 Nesta Carter v. IOC), the question was whether methylhexaneamine,[6] which was not listed explicitly on the 2008 Prohibited List, had a "similar chemical structure or similar biological effect(s)" to tuaminoheptane, a listed stimulant. In that case, the Panel accepted that "[m]ethylhexaneamine not only has a very similar chemical structure to tuaminoheptane but it has also similar biological effects to it". This conclusion was based on WADA's evidence that "methylhexaneamine has the same molecular formula (C7H17N) as tuaminohep-tane, and the same molecular weight (115.22). It has also a very similar chemical structure". This evidence was not rebutted by the athlete. The Panel therefore confirmed that methylhexaneamine was a prohibited substance, by virtue of its similarity to tuaminoheptane.

The more recent case of CAS 2019/A/6574 WADA v. RANAD & Mineran concerned the substance higenamine. WADA submitted that this substance was to be considered as a—non-listed—beta-2 agonist, prohibited under S3 of the 2016 Prohibited List.[7] The Panel gave particular significance to a scientific report which explained that beta-2 agonists had been prohibited under the Prohibited List since 2003 (given their anabolic and stimulant properties) and concluded that there was "strong data in support of higenamine's activity through [beta2] receptors" producing similar effects.[8] The Panel concluded on this basis that higenamine, although not specifically listed (at the time of the violation), was prohibited under section S3 of the 2016 Prohibited List. The fact that substances can be prohibited by category has been challenged on multiple occasions by athletes before the CAS. Athletes typically claim that the prohibition by class breaches principles such as legal certainty, which requires prohibited conduct to be sufficiently identified in the rules in order to allow the athletes to ascertain what is prohibited or not. These arguments have been consistently rejected by the CAS.

In CAS 2009/A/1805&1847 IAAF v. RFEA & Josephine Onyia, the Panel confirmed that "[a] substance does not need to be expressly listed in the WADA Prohibited List to be considered a prohibited substance in sport".[9] "The List is an

---

[5] CAS 2009/A/1805 & 1847 IAAF v. RFEA & Onyia, para. 94

[6] Methylhexaneamine is an adrenergic drug classified as a stimulant that was used as a therapeutic nasal decongestant until discontinued in the early 1970s

[7] Whereas higenamine was added to examples of beta-2 agonists expressly set out on the Prohibited List in 2017, it did not feature on the Prohibited List up to and including 2016

[8] CAS 2019/A/6574 WADA v. RANAD & Mineran, para. 77

[9] CAS 2009/A/1805&1847 IAAF v. RFEA & Josephine Onyia, para. 90

open list. It would be impractical to cite all stimulants because of the large numbers of compounds available on the market. Further, an open list allows the inclusion of those designer drugs created only for doping purposes".[10]

In the case of CAS 2017/A/4984 Nesta Carter v. IOC, where the athlete tested positive for a stimulant that was not expressly mentioned in the 2008 Prohibited List, the Panel highlighted "that all stimulants were and are prohibited. There is a great number of stimulants, and they cannot all be listed by name. Therefore, the list of prohibited stimulants provides a list of named stimulants, which are typically the ones often detected, as well as a 'hold all basket'".[11] The Panel further explained that the athlete "was required to ensure that no stimulants were present in his bodily systems, named or unnamed. This is the legal framework which was set in order to ensure a more equal playing field to sporting competitors. It was a legal framework of which he was aware".[12]

In the more recent case of CAS 2019/A/6574 WADA v. RANAD & Mineran, the Panel referred to, and endorsed, the conclusions in the *Carter* award above and added that "the anti-doping effort would be severely obstructed if designer drugs [viz. products containing non-listed prohibited substances] were tolerated. The burden is on the athlete (which in many cases practically means team officials) to see to it, as a counterpart of the privilege of competing, that they respect the right of other athletes to a "clean" competition, i.e., a competition in which all participants manage to comply with the rules".[13] In the end, the interest of an effective fight against doping must prevail. If only specifically listed substances were prohibited and their prohibition by category was not accepted, it would be an open door to cheats, who could undermine anti-doping regulation by using substances with a slightly modified chemical structure to escape any sanction. This would render the Prohibited List almost meaningless and, consequently, an effective fight against doping practices impossible.

Prohibition of Metabolites and Markers

The prohibition of a substance does not relate only to the substance itself (i.e., the parent compound) but extends also to the metabolites or markers of the substance. Once ingested, injected or otherwise introduced into the body, a substance rarely remains intact. The parent compound is processed and—sometimes even within very short timeframes—"metabolised" and evolves into sub-substances, the so-called metabolites. Because they are *downstream* substances, metabolites may be present and detectable in the body for days or even months (in the case of certain

---

[10] CAS 2009/A/1805&1847 IAAF v. RFEA & Josephine Onyia, para. 91

[11] CAS 2017/A/4984 Nesta Carter v. IOC, para. 152

[12] CAS 2017/A/4984 Nesta Carter v. IOC, para. 153

[13] CAS 2019/A/6574 WADA v. RANAD & Mineran, para. 67

long-term or "night watch" metabolites) after the parent compound has completely disappeared. The detection through metabolites is therefore essential for the fight against doping, as it allows a longer period of detection of the prohibited substances, without which the actual detection based on punctual collection of samples would be largely ineffective. A non-listed (similar) substance may also be detected through its metabolites. If a metabolite of a non-listed substance, which has a "similar chemical structure or similar biological effect(s)" to a prohibited substance, is found in a sample, this equally constitutes a "presence" violation. While the presence of the metabolite constitutes the basis of anti-doping rule violation, this may raise a particular issue when the metabolite at stake may originate either from a prohibited substance or from a substance that is not prohibited. In this respect, according to the wording of article 2.1 of the Code, the simple presence of a metabolite of a prohibited substance constitutes an anti-doping rule violation. Based on a literal interpretation of this provision, this conclusion applies irrespective of whether the metabolite could have originated from the use of a prohibited or non-prohibited substance. In CAS 2017/O/5218 IAAF v. RUSAF and Kopeykin, the athlete sought an acquittal on the basis that the presence of trimetazidine (a metabolic modulator under S4.4 of the WADA Prohibited List) could have resulted from the use of lomerizine, a non-prohibited substance that is used for the treatment of migraines. However, WADA had issued an instruction to WADA-accredited laboratories whereby, when trimetazidine is detected, the laboratories are required to additionally test for the presence of lomerizine and its further specific metabolites. If based on this additional analysis the finding of trimetazidine could have resulted from the use of lomerizine, the WADA-accredited laboratories were instructed to report a negative finding.[14] In the *Kopeykin* case, the analytical results were not consistent with the use of lomerizine, and the athlete's claims to have used it were not accepted. In other instances of metabolites with different possible parent compounds and in the absence of additional analytical criteria allowing to objectively distinguish the source,[15] it will be up to the Panel to evaluate the analytical results in light of the respective plausibility of their sources (as well as any facts put forward and established by the parties) to determine whether it is comfortably satisfied that the metabolite originated from a prohibited substance, in which case it has to find that an anti-doping violation within the meaning of article 2.1 of the Code was committed. The problem will not arise in cases in which the alternative parent compounds of a metabolite are all prohibited substances. In this case the conclusion that a metabolite of a prohibited substance is present in the sample is in any event supported by the analytical finding.[16]

---

[14] More information is available at: https://www.wada-ama.org/sites/default/files/resources/files/tl13_trimetazidine_eng_2021_1.pdf

[15] An example is the presence of further metabolites of the prohibited substance

[16] In CAS 2016/A/4803, 4804 & CAS 2017/A/4983, when confronted with the argument that the M3 of oral Turinabol could be confused with the long-term metabolite of other prohibited substance and therefore the testing method was not valid, the Panel rejected the argument and confirmed that the detection method was a valid one "for the purpose for which it is intended, namely the detection of prohibited substances and prohibited substances only" (para. 141)

The Athlete Biological Passport

Another tool to potentially address emerging novel doping practices is the so-called Athlete Biological Passport ("ABP"). The fundamental principle of the ABP is to monitor selected variables (biomarkers of doping) over time that indirectly reveal the effect of doping, as opposed to the traditional method of direct detection. In other words, the ABP does not aim at detecting the presence of a specific substance but at indirectly detecting the effect of the administration of prohibited substances (by monitoring specific markers). The current ABP has two modules: a haematological and a steroidal one. A third module, the endocrine module, is in preparation. The haematological module, which was introduced by WADA in 2009, aims to identify blood doping, typically by use of erythropoiesis-stimulating agents (ESAs, such as erythropoietin, for instance) or blood transfusion. The steroidal module was introduced by WADA in 2014. It aims to identify the use of anabolic steroids, which may also be produced endogenously, and other anabolic agents, such as selective androgen receptor modulators (SARMS). In essence, both modules work in a similar way: samples are collected and the values of certain markers are fed into a statistical model based upon a Bayesian approach, known as the adaptive model. The adaptive model uses an algorithm that takes into account both (i) variability of such values within the population generally and (ii) factors affecting the variability of the athlete's individual values (including gender, ethnic origin, age, type of sport, and instrument-related technology). The selected biological markers are monitored over time. On this basis, a longitudinal profile is created that establishes an athlete's upper and lower limits within which the athlete's values would be expected to remain, assuming normal physiological conditions (i.e., the athlete is healthy and has not been doping). Where a value is not within the expected range, it is considered as an outlier. In case of outliers (or even in the absence of an outlier where the variations remain within the parameters but appear suspicious for other reasons), the passport is submitted to a panel of experts. Based firstly on the sole review of the profile, the experts have to determine on an anonymous basis whether the profile is likely to have resulted from doping in the absence of any (medical or other) explanation for the abnormalities. If this is the case, the athlete is given an opportunity to provide explanations for the abnormalities. If the experts consider, even in light of the athlete's explanations, that doping remains the likely cause of the results observed in the profile, the experts will issue a final conclusion of "likely doping". The matter will then normally proceed for decision before a hearing panel, which will have to decide whether an anti-doping rule violation is established.[17] When the

---

[17] This is normally happening in results obtained with respect to the haematological module. So far the steroid module has mainly served to target potential analytical cases. Before a case is referred to a panel of experts, the data obtained serves to identify suspicious samples. The results are subject to an Atypical Passport Finding Confirmation Procedure Request (ATPF-CPR). In other words, the suspicious sample will undergo an analytical procedure (in particular IRMS). If such additional analysis identifies the presence of a prohibited substance, the case then proceeds as a usual case based on the presence of a prohibited substance. In this context, the ABP actually serves

ABP is involved, the relevant anti-doping rule violation is qualified as "use" of a prohibited substance or method under article 2 of the Code, which can be established by any reliable means (including conclusions drawn from longitudinal profiling).[18] The CAS has confirmed on multiple occasions that the ABP is a reliable means to establish "use" violations.[19] Therefore, the ABP is a further tool at the disposal of anti-doping organisations to indicate the use of novel substances which may be missed in an analysis, for example, because a reference substance is not available yet.

Re-analysis

Effective detection of prohibited substances is a difficult and arduous task. While anti-doping authorities and laboratories are unlikely to be able to fully understand what the sophisticated doping cheats are up to, those same cheats may well have an insight into the detection capabilities. They can therefore manage their doping practices in terms of content and timing to minimise the risk of detection. However, anti-doping science evolves, and the detection capabilities improve over time, sometimes drastically. Enabling the long-term storage of samples creates an opportunity to subject them to new and improved analysis and thus to catch dopers who initially escaped prosecution. Improvement in detection is sometimes achieved through wholly new detection methods. The validation of the IRMS analysis in 1998 which allowed laboratories to distinguish exogenously applied from endogenously produced testosterone (which replaced or rather completed the crude method based on T/E ratio) and the direct detection of the erythropoietin in the urine in 1999 were amongst the most important examples thereof.[20] More often than not, significant improvements occur in the detection of substances which were already detectable but not necessarily in an efficient manner. Since metabolites often remain in the body long after the parent compound has disappeared, it should not come as a surprise that advances in detection were often linked to the identification of new

---

as a targeting tool and brings supporting evidence. Although the possibility exists, no case has so far proceeded solely on the basis of an abnormal steroidal profile in the absence of confirmed analytical results

[18] See Comment to article 2.2 of the Code, which specifically refers to the ABP

[19] See, for instance, CAS 2012/A/2773 IAAF v. SEGAS & Kokkinariou (para. 13): "Systems which make use of these longitudinal profiles have evolved to become widespread and highly effective means of detecting EPO doping"; CAS 2014/A/3614 & 3561 IAAF & WADA v. RFEA & Ms. Marta Dominguez (para. 278) – "the ABP Model is a reliable and a valid mean of establishing an ADRV"

[20] For another example of new methods amongst others: CAS 2018/A/5654 & 5655 Zemliak & Povh v. UAF & WADA. Of note, the analytical method had not been approved by WADA yet. The CAS found that it could be relied upon to establish an anti-doping rule violation. The fact that a method is not validated only means that it does not benefit from a presumption of validity under article 3.2.1 of the Code, which did not exclude it being used as reliable evidence

long-term metabolites, which thus considerably lengthened the potential window of detection after use of the substance. This was particularly important in relation to steroids. Steroids are typically used in advance of, and in preparation for, important competitions. Sophisticated dopers will cease using them sufficiently in advance of competition so that they cannot be detected in in-competition doping controls. For a long time, the window of detection for the concerned products went from a few hours to a few days. Consequently, it was relatively easy for doping cheats to take this into account in their doping strategy and optimise the effects of the doping substance up to the time of the competitions. When, however, long-term metabolites extended this window of detection to weeks or even months, this was a real game changer. As cautious as doping cheats might be, they could not anticipate the radical change in the detection window, which the new long-term metabolites brought with them. Typical examples in this respect are the progress made through newly identified metabolites for the detection of widely used steroids like stanozolol or dehydrochlormethyltestosterone (oral Turinabol). Since the so-called long-term metabolites are often found at very low levels, advances in this respect were linked to another very relevant factor in the improvement of detection in anti-doping, namely, the considerably improved sensitivity of the equipment. In this respect, a significant progress was notably achieved around 2010, when a new generation of mass spectrometers brought the capability for laboratories to detect at much lower levels, the limit of detection being brought down from the ng/ml range to a low pg/ml range. Technological progress of that magnitude is in itself a game changer. Re-analysis assumes that samples remain available for re-analysis. According to the Code, samples which returned initially negative analytical results may be destroyed after 6 months. This has a valid and sound practical and logistical reason. The storage in preserved conditions of all the samples collected worldwide over the years would represent disproportionately high costs. However, the possibility to dispose the samples shortly after the first analysis does not exclude the alternative of keeping them for potential re-analysis. The Code thus provides for the possibility of long-term storing samples for the purposes of re-analysing them at a later stage.[21] The only limitation to the re-analysis is the statute of limitation. Indeed, as per article 17 of the Code, "[n]o anti-doping rule violation proceeding may be commenced against an Athlete or other Person unless he or she has been notified of the anti-doping rule violation [...] within ten (10) years from the date the violation is asserted to have occurred". An anti-doping organisation can therefore store samples for as long as they may be used for anti-doping purposes. The International Olympic Committee was the first organisation which stored samples long term. It did so already back in 2004 with the samples collected on the occasion of the 2004 Athens Olympic Games. Thereafter, the samples collected at all subsequent Olympic Games were systematically preserved and stored. They were eventually subjected to re-analysis,

---

[21] See article 6.6 of the Code: "After a laboratory has reported a Sample as negative, or the Sample has not otherwise resulted in an anti-doping rule violation charge, it may be stored and subjected to further analyses for the purpose of Article 6.2 at any time exclusively at the direction of either the Anti-Doping Organization that initiated and directed Sample collection or WADA"

at first in a targeted sampling approach (Athens 2004/Torino 2006) and then massively (Beijing 2008/London 2012). Major International Federations followed, notably but not only in respect samples collected at major events such as World Championships. Presently, a long-term storage and re-analysis strategy is part of the anti-doping strategic planning of all major anti-doping organisations. The importance of re-analysis has been notably demonstrated in the re-analysis of the samples collected on the occasion of the Beijing and London Olympic Games. From 2016 to 2020, thousands of samples were re-analysed. This led to a spectacularly high number of positive cases, well over a hundred. The main reason for this flood of positive cases was that significant advances had been made since 2008 and even 2012 in the detection of substances, including ones which were widely used at the time, in particular dehydrochlormethyltestosterone and stanozolol. These two substances were found, in isolation or even in combination, in the vast majority of the positive re-analysis cases of Beijing and London. They were, at the time, substances of choice amongst dopers because they are both effective and were thought to be low risk in view of their relatively short windows of detection. Initially, this doping strategy succeeded. These athletes went undetected through the initial analysis performed on the occasion of the Olympic Games. Eventually, however, this feeling of "safety" proved ill-conceived. Through a combination of the identification of new long-term metabolites and a decisive improvement of the sensitivity of the equipment, the detection window of these two substances increased massively. This caught the dopers off-guard and led to well over a hundred positive cases, an unprecedented result in anti-doping. Without the long-term storage of the concerned samples and their re-analysis, none of these anti-doping rule violations would have been established, and all the dopers that were ultimately caught would still enjoy the Olympic results they took away from their competitors. It is unlikely that the results of re-analysis of samples collected at the Olympic Games will ever be as spectacular. These results were also linked to particular circumstances with regard to both the doping practices and the evolution of the detection capabilities. These exceptional results sent, however, a resounding message to athletes who might be tempted by doping: "You will never be safe". It is to be hoped that this message will be heard. In this perspective, re-analysis, even if it will probably return more modest results in the future (and hopefully so), will then fulfil another useful purpose: the verification a posteriori that sport is evolving in a sounder direction with regard to doping.

Other Evidence

The "use" of a prohibited substance or method can be established by any reliable means. This does not only include analytical evidence (such as analytical data or the conclusions drawn from the ABP) but also any other evidence, such as admissions or witness testimony. Conscious of the decisive importance of these other evidentiary elements, WADA has developed tools to promote them. In terms of admissions, athletes who come forward can thus benefit from a reduction in their sanction.[22] A reduction can also be obtained by athletes who provide substantial assistance to the anti-doping organisation. The assistance must result in inter alia the anti-doping organisation being provided with elements allowing it to bring forward an anti-doping rule violation against another person.[23] Where a person, who has not committed any anti-doping rule violation, brings relevant information, this person can benefit from the whistle-blower programme, which WADA put in place to protect the integrity of the whistle-blower, who may be at risk of retaliation. In the 2021 Code, it is now a specific anti-doping rule violation to engage in such acts of retaliation (article 2.11). Where the use of an emerging drug is involved and this use is not established analytically, an anti-doping rule violation can therefore also be established through the admission of the athlete, or the testimony of another athlete (or other person) providing substantial assistance or acting as a whistle-blower. For example, in CAS 2004/O/645 USADA v. Montgomery & IAAF, the "use" of tetrahydrogestrinone (THG) by the athlete was established by the (uncontroverted) testimony of a fellow athlete (Kelly White), who confirmed that the athlete had admitted the use of the substance to her. Even in cases where testimony alone might not always be sufficient to establish a "use" to the required standard of "comfortable satisfaction", it is at the very least a crucial element of intelligence on the basis of which a case can be investigated and built by an anti-doping organisation, which might have otherwise gone undetected. Lance Armstrong is maybe the most spectacular illustration of the crucial importance of other evidence, including testimonies. Despite being tested throughout all his career, Lance Armstrong never officially returned a positive control. Based initially on the revelations of Floyd Landis, a former teammate of Armstrong's, the US Anti-Doping Agency conducted an extremely thorough investigation into Armstrong's case. This investigation which included interviews of a number of other former teammates ultimately resulted in a lifetime ban being imposed on Armstrong, as well as disqualification of results since 1998 (which included his seven victories in the *Tour de France*). Another example of a whistle-blower leading to the conviction of athletes (and other support personnel) is the case of Yuliya Stepanova. Yuliya Stepanova recorded and filmed conversations that she had with other athletes and her entourage, during which she discussed in detail the use of prohibited substances. Based principally on this evidence, charges were brought against a number of Russian athletes and support personnel, and all were sanctioned for doping (or administration of prohibited substances).[24] More recently, the revelations of the former director of the Moscow Laboratory, supported by documentary evidence, led to the discovery of a centrally administered doping and anti-detection scheme that was in operation over the course of years in Russia.

---

[22] See in particular article 10.7 and 10.8 of the Code

[23] See article 10.7.1 of the Code

[24] See, for instance, CAS 2016/A/4486 IAAF v. Poistogova, CAS 2016/O/4488 IAAF v. ARAF & Bazdyreva, CAS 2016/O/4481 IAAF v. ARAF & Savinova-Farnasova (as well as on appeal: CAS 2017/A/5045), CAS 2016/O/4504 IAAF v. ARAF & Mokhnev, CAS 2016/A/4480 IAAF v. ARAF & Kazarin, CAS 2018/A/4487 IAAF v. Melnikov, CAS 2016/O/4575 IAAF v. ARAF & Portugalov

The Impact on the Sanctioning Regime

General Framework

The ordinary regime applies with respect to sanctions irrespective of whether the substance is novel and/or expressly listed or not. In principle, an anti-doping rule violation of "use" or "presence" is subject to a 2- or 4-year period of ineligibility. The Code distinguishes between specified and non-specified substances or methods[25] and provides for a system of inverted burden in respect of the determination of the length of the applicable sanction. If the substance or method at stake is non-specified, the athlete will be subject to a 4-year period of ineligibility, unless he/she can demonstrate that the violation was not intentional.[26] If the substance or method is specified, then the basic sanction will be 2 years of ineligibility. In this case, the burden is on the anti-doping organisation to establish that the violation was intentional if it wants to seek a higher sanction.[27] In principle, the distinction between non-specified and specified substances and methods in the Prohibited List is made by class. For example, anabolic agents (class S1) are all non-specified. The same applies to peptide hormones, growth factors, related substances and mimetics (class S2). On the contrary, beta-2 agonists (class S3), diuretics (class S5), narcotics (class S7), cannabinoids (class S8) and glucocorticoids (class S9) are all characterised as specified substances.[28] With respect to hormones and metabolic modulators (class S4), the determination is made by sub-classes. More specifically, the substances in S4.1 (aromatase inhibitors) and S4.2 (anti-estrogenic substances) are specified, and those in S4.3 (agents preventing activin receptor IIB activation) and S4.4 (metabolic modulators) are non-specified. For non-listed substances the same logic applies. These substances are deemed to be specified or non-specified depending on their classification into a class (or sub-class with respect to S4). There exists a specific classification rule for class S6 (stimulants). In this case, there are two distinct lists, one for specified and one for non-specified stimulants. The Prohibited List provides explicitly that "[a] stimulant not expressly listed in [the list of non-specified stimulants] is a Specified Substance". In other words, non-specified stimulants are exhaustively listed in the Prohibited List with the consequence that non-listed stimulants will always be categorised as specified. Another issue of interest in respect of sanctions applicable to anti-doping violations based on non-listed substances is the

---

[25] Comment to article 4.2.2 of the Code clarifies that Specified prohibited substances or methods are "simply Substances and Methods which are more likely to have been consumed or used by an Athlete for a purpose other than the enhancement of sport performance"

[26] Article 10.2.1.1 of the Code

[27] Article 10.2.1.2 of the Code

[28] In addition, the Code provides for another category of substances, i.e. the Substances of Abuse (article 4.2.3 of the Code), which are subject to a more lenient regime of sanctions (article 10.2.4 of the Code). The Substances of Abuse are those "frequently abused in society outside of the context of sport" and include, for instance, cocaine or THC

question of aggravating circumstances. As per article 10.4 of the Code, if the anti-doping organisation can establish that the violation was committed with aggravating circumstances, the period of ineligibility otherwise applicable will be increased by an additional period of up to 2 years depending on the seriousness of the violation and the nature of the aggravating circumstances. The Code gives a definition of aggravating circumstances, which may include the fact that the athlete used multiple prohibited substances, or used prohibited substances on multiple occasions, or the fact that the performance-enhancing effects of the use would likely extend beyond the end of the otherwise applicable period of ineligibility. The potentially relevant element in respect of non-listed substances specifically is the aggravating circumstance that the athlete "engaged in deceptive or obstructive conduct to avoid the detection or adjudication of an anti-doping rule violation". The deliberate use of a non-listed sophisticated prohibited substance, which could not be detected through the analytical methods in use, could conceivably constitute an aggravating circumstance.[29]

Potential Reductions

On the other hand, the use of non-listed prohibited substances might also be the result of an inadvertence. Indeed, it might be that an athlete did some diligence and cross-checked all the ingredients of a product that he/she was using against the Prohibited List and—since the substance was not indicated—assumed that the use of the product was safe. Should this be taken into consideration when a sanction is imposed? Articles 10.5 and 10.6 of the Code provide for reductions where the athlete can show that he committed the anti-doping rule violation with "No Fault or Negligence" or "No Significant Fault or Negligence", respectively. In the case of No Fault or Negligence, no period of ineligibility is imposed. In the case of No Significant Fault or Negligence, the sanction can be reduced down to 1 year of ineligibility (if the violation involved a non-specified substance), or a reprimand and no period of ineligibility (if the violation involved a specified substance or a contaminated product[30]). Before any reduction in the period of ineligibility can be awarded to the athlete, a prerequisite is that the athlete will have to establish how the prohibited substance entered his/her body. In other words, the athlete will be required to establish the source of the positive finding. As per the CAS case law, this requires the athlete to provide "actual evidence" rather than mere speculation or protestations of innocence.[31] In addition, the athlete will be required to demonstrate, on a balance of probabilities, that he/she used the product in question but also that it

---

[29] See article 10.4 of the Code

[30] A contaminated product is defined in the Code as a product "that contains a Prohibited Substance that is not disclosed on the product label or in information available in a reasonable Internet search"

[31] CAS 2014/A/3820 WADA v. Damar Robinson & JADCO, para. 80

could have caused the specifics of the analytical result, in particular in terms of pharmacokinetics.[32] Having established the source of the positive finding, the second step for the athlete will be to demonstrate that he committed the violation with No (Significant) Fault or Negligence. In other words, the athlete will have to show all the verifications that he/she conducted in order to avoid the anti-doping rule violation. These verifications may include checking the ingredients on the Prohibited List, through Internet searches, consulting a doctor, having the product analysed for prohibited substances, etc. As the CAS case law shows, whether the substance is listed on the Prohibited List is ultimately only one of the parameters, which may be taken into account when assessing the athlete's overall level of fault. For example, in CAS OG 12/007 ICF v. Sterba, as stated earlier, the violation involved methylhexanamine, which is a stimulant (at the time) not listed on the Prohibited List. In that case, it was unchallenged that the athlete did not intend to cheat by using a supplement containing this substance. To determine the level of reduction to be awarded to the athlete, the Panel carefully assessed the diligence conducted by the athlete. In this case, it was accepted that (1) he had cross-checked the ingredients in the product against the Prohibited List, (2) he sought specific advice from a qualified practitioner (who confirmed that the product was safe), and (3) he disclosed his use of the product on the doping control form. The Panel, therefore, found his level of fault to "be so small that it justifies the full reduction of the period of ineligibility to no period, and the sanction of a reprimand".[33] In reaching this conclusion, the Panel did also take into account the fact that methylhexanamine was not expressly listed on the Prohibited List: "the use of the substance by the Respondent, in light of the steps that he took in order to check whether it was safe for him to use, could have been avoided if indeed the substance had been expressly included on the Prohibited List or in any other data base that can be easily accessed with modern technology and the internet".[34] The Panel ultimately found that "[t]his, of course, does not change the fact that the Anti-Doping violation occurred, but the Panel considers this fact to be important and relevant in respect of assessing and examining the level of the fault of the Respondent and the consequential sanction".[35] On the other hand, if the diligence conducted by the athlete is inexistent or not appropriate, the fact that the substance was not listed should not have any impact on the sanction at all especially when, by exercising a minimum of diligence, the athlete could have found out that the substances at stake were prohibited (even if not listed). In CAS 2019/A/6574 WADA v. RANAD & Mineran, the Panel thus observed that "by a basic Internet search" the athlete could have found out that the substance was prohibited. In addition, the Global DRO database, which "provides athletes and support personnel with information about the status of particular substances", already

---

[32] See CAS 2010/A/2277 La Barbera v. IWAS, para. 31; see also CAS 2017/A/5369 WADA v. SAIDS and Gordon Gilbert

[33] CAS OG 12/007 ICF v. Sterba, para. 40

[34] CAS OG 12/007 ICF v. Sterba, para. 37

[35] CAS OG 12/007 ICF v. Sterba, para. 37

explicitly set out that higenamine was a prohibited beta-2 agonist. The Panel excluded any reduction of the sanction. In line with this precedent, the conclusion must be the following: if an athlete does not exercise diligence in checking the ingredients of products that he/she takes, the fact that the prohibited substance at stake is listed or not will have little or no impact on the applicable sanction.

Conclusion

As we have seen, the issues raised by novel and/or non-listed substances and methods are quite complex. They constitute an opportunity for novel doping practices, and it is in the nature of things that the cheats may often try to be one step ahead. The challenge for anti-doping organisations, in particular WADA, is to ensure that an adequate countermeasure can be organised if not immediately at least a posteriori. This has required WADA and other anti-doping organisations to constantly seek to establish and adapt the rules and the means used to fight against doping. The use of a regularly adapted and "open" list of prohibited substances or methods, the use of the ABP to detect indirect markers of doping, the re-analysis of samples, non-analytical investigations and the promotion of (self)denunciation are all amongst the instruments that the Code includes to that end. If the anti-doping fight is to continue and to be efficient, these and other instruments must continue to be developed to address the further developments of doping practices, including emerging drugs, which the future will bring.

Part III
Towards a Doping Society?

Olympism and the Idea of Anti-doping: Between the Thick and Thin Interpretations of Sporting Progress

Sigmund Loland and Mike McNamee

Introduction

Olympism is a term of art. It is used widely. Yet its meaning is often opaque to the very people who use it. Some refer to it in exulted terms, as a "philosophy"—specifically the philosophy of the Olympic Movement in its totality. Others, Olympic critics, typically from the human sciences (taken to include some—but not all—historians, sociologists, philosophers, political scientists) have usually referred to Olympism as a form of "ideology" in the sense of a set of beliefs and values used to legitimize the Olympic Movement and justify its actions and policies. In this essay we critically review the conceptual landscape of Olympism and identify the relations it has with the anti-doping world, in relation to the World Anti-Doping Code (WADC) and, more specifically, the rationale for global anti-doping efforts under the umbrella of the World Anti-doping Agency (WADA).

S. Loland (✉)
Institute for Sport and Social Sciences, Norwegian School of Sport Sciences, Oslo, Norway

Swedish School of Sport and Health Sciences, Stockholm, Sweden
e-mail: sigmundl@nih.no

M. McNamee
Faculty of Movement and Rehabilitation Sciences, KU Leuven, Leuven, Belgium

School of Sport and Exercise Sciences, Swansea University, Swansea, Wales, UK
e-mail: mike.mcnamee@kuleuven.be

© The Author(s), under exclusive license to Springer Nature Switzerland AG 2022
O. Rabin, O. Corazza (eds.), *Emerging Drugs in Sport*,
https://doi.org/10.1007/978-3-030-79293-0_8

Olympism

Olympism, like all complex ideas, has a history [1, 2]. That history is not quite as archaic as one might think, and it certainly cannot be attributed to ethos of the ancient games whose value system reflected the "warrior-politician" ethic of the time. Conceived in the late nineteenth-century Europe and influenced by increased international communication, technological and scientific innovation, a growing peace movement and "vitalistic" visions of human potential, the French Baron Pierre de Coubertin developed the ideas of Olympism as philosophy of moral progress [3, 4]. Of course, the word "philosophy" here is intended in an older sense of that word, a way of conceiving something or some activity behind which lies some reasoned basis. Moreover, Olympism is typically referred to as the philosophy of the Olympic movement, that is to say all the official entities and actions carried out by the International Olympic Committee (IOC) [5]. It is often also alluded to by National Olympic Committees in the same vein. It was clear that Coubertin's conception—though it boasted continuity with an ideologically pure ancient Olympic legacy—was a highly moralized conception. For him sport was intrinsically ethical in nature. Of course, a legion of critical commentators has challenged the moral superiority entailed in his claim that Olympic sport was a religious enterprise [6]. Nevertheless, it is true that there is continuity between the first explicit espousal of Olympism and the various revisions that have taken place.

Fundamental Principles of Olympism

In contemporary times, we find the following explicit articulation of Olympism, espoused by the IOC [7]. The first four so-called fundamental principles and the sixth (from a list of seven) are particularly illuminating in this respect:

1. Olympism is a philosophy of life, exalting and combining in a balanced whole the qualities of body, will and mind. Blending sport with culture and education, Olympism seeks to create a way of life based on the joy of effort, the educational value of good example, social responsibility and respect for universal fundamental ethical principles.
2. The goal of Olympism is to place sport at the service of the harmonious development of humankind, with a view to promoting a peaceful society concerned with the preservation of human dignity.
3. The Olympic Movement is the concerted, organized, universal and permanent action, carried out under the supreme authority of the IOC, of all individuals and entities who are inspired by the values of Olympism. It covers the five continents. It reaches its peak with the bringing together of the world's athletes at the great sports festival, the Olympic Games. Its symbol is five interlaced rings.

4. The practice of sport is a human right. Every individual must have the possibility of practising sport, without discrimination of any kind and in the Olympic spirit, which requires mutual understanding with a spirit of friendship, solidarity and fair play.
5. The enjoyment of the rights and freedoms set forth in this Olympic Charter shall be secured without discrimination of any kind, such as race, colour, sex, sexual orientation, language, religion, political or other opinion, national or social origin, property, birth or other status.

In recognition of their heterogeneity and purpose [8], one thing we can surely say is that the principles of Olympism are not exclusively ethical in character [9]. Considerable moral and political content is enshrined therein. Principle 1 espouses a balanced conception of the human person within a balanced way of life. It recognizes that Olympism is an educational conception of sport (a point de Coubertin stressed since the beginning) that promotes role modelling of athletes. It claims to espouse a conception of sport based on universal moral principles—an idea that has been under threat from philosophers and sociologists in late modernity. Finally, it espouses the idea that there is joy to be found in the kinds of efforts athletes make, a point rarely commented upon by critics and acolytes alike [10, 11]. Other specific and substantial ethical content is listed in Principle 2 where Olympic sport is said to have the goal of contributing to a peaceful society. Importantly too, Olympism is specifically associated with the right to human dignity. This can be linked directly to Principles 4 and 5, which embody a rights-based rejection of all forms of discrimination.

Summing up, there is in Olympism, as a philosophy or an idealized conception of sport, a strong and explicit commitment in an ethical conception of athletic endeavour and sport administration and officiating where, if practiced according to the ideals of fair play and just meritocracy, sport serves noble goals beyond itself: it is believed to relieve social tensions and solve conflicts between individuals, groups and even between nation states peacefully and based on mutual respect. Throughout his many writings [12], Coubertin emphasized the value of sport in the promotion of what he referred to as "enlightened patriotism" as opposed to "aggressive nationalism" [13]. The Olympic rings, designed by Coubertin himself, symbolize the five continents interconnected in a harmonious form.

Olympism is not a strict and consistent philosophical system, however, as it includes, too, clear views on the significance of dynamic and never-ending development and transcendence. The official Olympic motto is *Citius, Altius, Fortius:* faster, higher, stronger! As Kreft [14] observes, this better coheres with Roman bread and circus excesses than the Greek ideal of balance and harmony captured in the concept of *Kalokagathia* [15]. Coubertin's vision of the Olympic athlete was not *mens sana in corpore sano* primarily: a healthy mind in a healthy body, but the vitalistic *mens fervida in corpore lacertoso*—a burning soul in a well-trained body [16]. In one speech, Coubertin compared the function in Olympism of the sport record with the force of gravity in Newtonian mechanics: it was the eternal axiom. One may summarize this point by observing that Coubertin may have been no scholastic philosopher, that there are tensions and contradictions in his oeuvre, but one cannot fail to be impressed by his zealous promotion of an explicitly ethical conception of sport.

In the institutions of the Olympic Movement itself, similar tensions are found in many ways and at many levels between ideals of harmony and peace and beliefs in competitiveness and infinite progress and transcendence. On the one hand, the Olympic Movement promotes a vision of ethically sound development, exemplified with its humanitarian efforts, its solidarity funds and its recent emphasis on a sustainable development and, in symbolic and ritual expressions, as with the Olympic rings and as in the ritual in the Olympic Games closing ceremonies where athletes march into the stadium without any distinction by group or nationality. On the other hand, Olympic competition cultivates extreme perfectionism expressed in spectacular performances in an elite system in a constant pursuit of even more efficient means and methods in the quest for success and victory. These tensions can be found, too, in the views in elite sporting systems on sporting progress with implications for the use of performance-enhancing drugs (PED). We turn now to discuss two positions in this respect: what we will refer to as the thin and the thick interpretation of the Olympic vision of sporting progress.

Views on Sporting Progress and the Use of PED

The development of the WADC has legitimated—both with the world of sports and also with national governments in nearly every country of the world—the vision of doping-free sport. One may wonder why it is necessary to further discuss its justification. As is evident from recent anti-doping violations, among them extensive and systemic violations as in the case of Russia, public acknowledgement does not necessarily reflect true agreement and action. Moreover, the scholarly community has not taken the vision and policy of anti-doping for granted. Indeed, this is still a deeply contested affair. Before diving into the contested terrain, there is need for preliminary contextualization.

Most anti-doping rule violations, that is, cases involving the use of banned PEDs or their presence in athlete samples, involve the intentional violation of rules to get an exclusive advantage. Although psychological, sociological, cultural and also political explanations of these violations require complex analyses, ethically speaking, intentional rule violations are relatively straightforward. Cheating is wrong by definition [17]. Cheaters depend upon others' rule adherence to reach exclusive advantages, and they are the free riders of the sporting system and enjoy the benefits of others´ cooperation without doing their fair share. The challenging ethical discourse relates to whether the anti-doping regime and its regulations are justified at all or whether a situation of no regulation is preferable compared to the current situation of a PED ban.

This is where what Loland calls the "thin" and the "thick" interpretations of sporting progress follow different paths [18]. The thin interpretation has a brute expression in so-called doping doctors such as the notoriously famous Michele Ferrari allegedly claiming that "if it doesn't show up in the doping control, then it's not doping" [19]. Ideas of the inadequacy of the PED bans are given more complex and philosophical justification in various ways by authors such as Savulescu, Miah and others [20, 21]. The argument is that the doping ban is an expression of more or less arbitrary and anachronistic fears about the medically assisted pursuit of non-medical or health-related goals. There is a shared interpretation here of elite sport as a sphere of human transcendence. Interpreting the Olympic motto *Citius, Altius, Fortius* in direct ways and "thin" in the sense of downscaling its larger historical, social and cultural context, the nature of Olympic sport is considered a quest for constantly challenging existing human performance limits. Sporting progress is seen as it's most clear in typical record sports in which performances are measured in exact mathematical-physical entities: track and field, swimming and weightlifting. Sporting games such as soccer and basketball measuring team success in goals and points respectively, and in wins and losses, bear witness of progress, too, but in less accurate ways.

Thin interpretations are often combined with the position of technological optimism. The idea is that humanity has entered a new stage of development in which we, to a larger extent than before and with the help of biomedical technology, can control our biological destiny [22]. We can modify and enhance ourselves to be able to live longer, more productive, more harmonious and happier lives. Just as the Formula 1 class in car racing is a test zone for new automotive technologies, elite sport becomes a front zone for developing the new and bio-technologically enhanced human being; and, just as the amateur rules in Olympic sport that prevented participation by professional athletes have become an anachronistic reminder of elitist discriminatory norms and values of the past, the anti-doping rules will fade and eventually disappear as unnecessary restrictions. In fact, anti-doping is not just unnecessary but can be counter-productive in the pursuit of a healthier, more honest and more impressive elite sport.

The implication of the thin view of sporting progress is straightforward. Competitions are designed to measure, compare and rank competitors according to relevant performance [23]. Reliable and valid evaluations depend upon rule adherence and fair play. Outside of competition, however, there should be no regulation on performance-enhancing means and methods. If based on informed consent, athletes should be able to choose whatever performance-enhancing strategy they find appropriate. Thus, anti-doping in its current form should be abandoned.

Thin interpretations have merits. They challenge traditional understandings of sport adopted more or less uncritically by sporting institutions and society, they articulate in systematic ways views and opinions held in some sporting countries and communities, and they relate sport to actual and possible enhancement technologies that might have beneficial consequences in the future. However, thin positions are also exposed to criticism from alternative viewpoints, both pragmatic and more principled in kind. Pragmatically speaking, critics point out that elite sport is an immensely contested field of human endeavour and involves tough struggles over prestige and profit between extensive sporting systems through individual and team glory. If PED regulations are lifted, athletes and teams end up in vulnerable positions to be exploited and exposed to harm. History, for instance, of the systematic use of PED in former German Democratic Republic, or of the creative use of designer PED in North American sport such as in the so-called BALCO scandal, teaches relevant lessons in this respect. To critics, the anti-doping slogan of "protecting the athlete" makes sense indeed. From a principled point of view, proponents of what we refer to as the thick interpretation follow a markedly different line of reasoning.

Naturally, as with the thin interpretation, fairness and rule adherence in competition are also considered a necessity. Rule violators and cheaters corrupt performance evaluations and rankings by their actions and thus detract meaning and value of sport. Contrasted with the thin interpretation, however, thick interpretation proponents reject a medicalized vision of sport. One might imagine, as representatives of the thin position sometimes do, an ideal position in which athletes and teams engage in biomedical enhancement practices under fully informed consent and within systems of responsible risk management. The reason is that in thick interpretations sport is interweaved to a larger extent in the historical, social and cultural traditions in which it has found its form and accept therefore further regulations and restrictions outside of competition.

The departure point of this principled criticism is the internal logic of sport itself. In a thick interpretation, the emphasis is not simply on faster times, higher jumps or stronger lifts. Rather, as the philosopher Bernard Suits [24] has argued, there is a logic of inefficiency at play, a gratuitous logic [25, 26]. The argument belongs to the sport philosophical theory of formalism [27]. The constitutive rules of a sport do not only define the nature of the activity but make the securing of goal(s) of the sport challenging; they rule out the most inefficient ways of achieving the end by prohibiting the most efficient means. Thus, the quickest way to cover 100 m in a sprint, or to jump over 2.5 m bar or lift 500 kg in a squat is to use some form of mechanical assistance. Of course, this is ludicrous. Equally, an alternative and highly efficient way to secure victory on the field of play is to bribe an official or one's opponents. Yet these are not the kind of test and contest we seek for athletic endeavours. So too, it could be argued, the paradigmatic forms of anti-doping rule violations (such as ingestion of prohibited substances, or the masking of them) pursue a form of efficiency that challenges the gratuitous logic of sporting competition.

The thick view of sporting progress rests its argument on further consideration about how ethical norms are woven into this logic. A closer look at sporting rules systems demonstrates several operationalizations of fairness. All sports have rules to enable as equal external conditions as possible. Soccer teams switch pitch halves at half time, tennis players switch court halves after every second game, and skiers who perform individually and one by one get their starting number, at least in part and within their performance group, in a lottery. For similar reasons, there are rules on athlete and team classification. Men and women compete in separate classes in sports in which men, statistically speaking, have stronger predisposition for performance and heavy boxers do not meet lightweight boxers as boxing fights are not to be determined by body size but by performance in "the noble art of self-defence".

More generally, then, the common logic in all sports is guided by the ideal of fair equality of opportunity: to eliminate or compensate for inequalities upon which competitors cannot exert control or impact in any reasonable way [28]. What is to be achieved by this common, structural characteristic of sporting rules? The reason seems to be that the relevant inequality that must be evaluated, i.e., inequality in *sport* performance, is one within the sphere of control and impact of the individual athlete and team. Sporting rule systems, it is argued, are set up to cultivate performance as the outcome of athlete and team talent developed with athletes' and team's effort and hard training. Along these lines, we may talk of sport performances as genuine and authentic expressions of individual athletes, of their history and of their efforts and struggles in developing and expressing their own unique potential and talent.

Murray [29] summarizes the main idea:

> The meaning and value we find in sport comes from our sense of wonder at the natural talents displayed, and our admiration for the dedication required to bring those talents to their highest expression.

At its best, sport can cultivate more general moral virtues such as resilience, courage and also a sense of fairness and mutual respect. In this way, an athletic performance can be admirable, not just as a narrow expression of physical or psychological excellence but, at its best, of human excellence per se; and this is where the issue of PED cuts deepest. Most PED use involves the aspiration to maximum efficiency where significant risk of harm is seriously invited. Even if PED can be used in medically responsible ways, efficient performance-enhancing use overruns the adaptive capacities of the human body (talent) and requires and relies upon medical competence and expertise [30]. Compared to training and own effort, PED-enhanced performance is less the outcome of efforts on the athlete's side and to a larger extent the responsibility of a supporting system. In that sense, it is less authentic, less admirable and of lesser moral relevance.

From the thick interpretation perspective, this is the core of the PED problem: extensive PED use drains sport of cultural and moral value. Thus, a thick interpretation of sporting progress supports the vision of a doping-free sport and hence a ban on PED.

WADA, Olympism and the Spirit of Sport

A full consideration of the ethical rationale is beyond the scope of this article [31]. Nevertheless, we sketch the ethically relevant contours of the WADC and establish its link with Olympism and the thick interpretation of sporting progress outlined above.

Since its first publication in 2003, the WADC has been the principled anti-doping policy document in the world of sport. It is one among several policies including international standards for the globalization of anti-doping and the harmonization (perhaps better: interoperability) of anti-doping organizations that range from national organizations, event organizers (e.g., Olympic Games, FIFA World Cup, Grand Slam Tennis tournaments) and even to states that have criminalized doping actions. The Code sets out 11 Anti-doping Rule Violations (ADRVs) of which, in the mind of the general public and perhaps most sportspersons, and although there is no hierarchy among the ADRVs [32], Article 2.1 is probably the paradigmatic understanding of doping: "Presence of a Prohibited Substance or its Metabolites or Markers in an Athlete's Sample". The determination of candidates for the list of prohibited substances and methods (in short the Prohibited List, PL hereafter) is a critical rampart of anti-doping policy and is intimately related to the justificatory arguments above.

Criteria for Including Substances and Methods on the Prohibited List

WADA shall consider the following criteria in deciding whether to include a substance or method on the Prohibited List:

- 4.3.1 A substance or method shall be considered for inclusion on the Prohibited List if WADA, in its sole discretion, determines that the substance or method meets any two of the following three criteria: World Anti-Doping Code 2021 PART 1 Doping Control;
- 4.3.1.1 Medical or other scientific evidence, pharmacological effect or experience that the substance or method, alone or in combination with other substances or methods, has the potential to enhance or enhances sport performance;
- 4.3.1.2 Medical or other scientific evidence, pharmacological effect or experience that the Use of the substance or method represents an actual or potential health risk to the Athlete;
- 4.3.1.3 WADA's determination that the Use of the substance or method violates the spirit of sport described in the introduction to the Code [33].

The criteria, two of which at least need to be satisfied to consider a substance or a method as a candidate for the PL, have been the subject of extensive scholarship and criticism. Scholars and scientists have not always acknowledged the kinds and degrees of performance enhancement and the normativity of the concept of health (criteria 4.3.1.1 and 4.3.1.2 are also open to serious contest). Most contested however has been the presence of the explicitly normative criterion concerning the spirit of sport [34]. Broadly the views divide into two camps that we have characterized above as the thin and the thick interpretations of sporting progress.

The spirit of sport criterion (4.3.1.3) links directly to the WADA's own rationale for anti-doping. Indeed, it is tied specifically to it by that clause, in which it is necessary to quote in full:

The spirit of sport is the celebration of the human spirit, body and mind. It is the essence of Olympism and is reflected in the values we find in and through sport, including:

- Health
- Ethics, fair play and honesty
- Athletes' rights as set forth in the Code
- Excellence in performance
- Character and education
- Fun and joy
- Teamwork
- Dedication and commitment
- Respect for rules and laws
- Respect for self and other participants
- Courage
- Community and solidarity

The spirit of sport is expressed in how we play true. Doping is fundamentally contrary to the spirit of sport [35].

The opening clause is undeniably vague and prescriptive. Whether it is excessively vague is a point that scholars dispute [36–40]. That is to say, it is not especially precise but harks back to the idea of *Kalokagathia* as a harmonious human ideal and links it to the concept of Olympism. It makes a further move in highlighting a list of values that has also been the object of critical scrutiny. Whether it is problematically prescriptive is a different question. Clearly, policy documents do not always lay out their justificatory position in detail. Rather, they prescribe them. Few would deny that the list of values prescribed have a role to play in identifying and maintaining the ethical status of sports.

Critics complain about their operationalization. But our concern here is their relation to Olympism. In short, it asserts (i.e., prescribes) that the spirit of sport is the essence of Olympism. What kind of claim is this? One might argue that this is a kind of historical claim. Perhaps it is even an extension of a historical claim. Just as Coubertin, dubiously, asserted, continuity between the ancient games and their modern revival, so too WADA's anti-doping armoury of policy tools, seeks valorization by alignment with that heritage.

This is not a strong foundation. As Ritchie observes: "Coubertin sought to establish a 'mythology of continuity' between the ancient Games and his proposed modern ones in his attempt to make his version appear to stand above the crass materialism of industrial capitalism" [41]. Ample historical evidence refutes this naïve or politically motivated claim [42]. There are other possibilities, however. Thick interpretations of sporting progress are dynamic and sensitive both to historical traditions and current challenges. McNamee [43] has argued for an ethical equilibrium between the internal goods (i.e., those elements of intrinsic value) in sports and the external goods (i.e., the extrinsically valuable things that elite sports secure) that have always been associated with it. These points, however, do not wholly detract from the moral aspiration of Coubertin: as custodians of sport's best traditions, resistance to the ravages of commercialization—and the commodification of sport via media that promotes the myth of never-ending progress in terms of doping-fuelled world records or transcendent performances—these are proper ethical concerns.

Ritchie fails to acknowledge this when he asserts:

> ...WADA's Code reflects Coubertin's legacy perfectly, defending anti-drug rules based on the 'intrinsic value [of] 'the spirit of sport.'... But such notions, it should be realized, are as sociologically and historically vacuous as we now know Coubertin's to have been a century ago... The competitive events themselves are social practices embedded in a broad and complex network of activities and ideas that constitute and reconstitute a highly competitive, increasingly commercialized and professionalized, and often exploitative international system. *The use of banned substances and performance-enhancing practices in high-performance sport is an integral component of the human activities that currently constitute the entire international, high-performance sport system* [44]. (emphasis added)

We do not challenge Richie's descriptive points. Socially and politically structured institutions have always and simultaneously structured and exploited social practices like sports. And there is undeniably a strong relationship between the *Citius, Altius, Fortius* mentality and the commercialized and commodified forms of elite sport that have driven athletes to dope.

What is not valid, however, is Ritchie's conclusion that this is somehow an integral part of the "entire international, high-performance sport system". The point to be made in part defence of Coubertin and the proponents of thick interpretations of sporting progress is this: anti-doping is representative of ideals of sport structured in line with the fair equality of opportunity principle and conceived of as an ethical enterprise. Athletes, conforming to limitations on the means of their preparation, performance and recovery, struggle against these challenges to perform to their optimal capacities. We admire the struggles—in part at least—precisely because of those limitations. That is not to say that some limitations are arbitrary. Why sprint 100m not 125? Why play soccer for 90 minutes not 95? Why throw the baseball towards the strike zone that does not include the batter's physical and spatial location? We could overthrow or revise any and all constitutive rules. But we have to do so within a human framework that celebrates the authenticity of the athlete and the team and not to the same extent their biomedical and technological support systems. Providing Murray's [45] vision of sport at its best with an Olympic anchoring, Nussbaum puts the point particularly well:

> ... the Greeks ... praise outstanding athletic performance as a wonderful instance of human excellence. ... But clearly, such activity has point and value only relatively to the context of the human body, which imposes certain species-specific limits and creates certain possibilities of movements rather than others. To excel is to use those abilities especially fully, to struggle against those limits especially successfully. [46]

The human body is an important starting point for ethical reflection regarding sport's value and the normative shape of sporting progress that we defend. Anti-doping efforts seek to retain the humanity of athletic performance and progress even in extremis as we witness marathon runners and triathletes collapse over the finish line or boxers embrace each other after periods of mutually reciprocated battery.

And the complex of this ethical admiration is protected by normative strictures relating to excessive or unnecessary harms, courage under fire, solidarity and sacrifice. But not any means adopted to achieve victory commands admiration. To the extent that modern Olympism and WADA's "spirit of sport" criterion hark back to a conception of balance, it is a normative one. Its historical authenticity is one thing, and its normative value is another.

There is a sense in which these general normative arguments do not attract a new bioethics of sports. This is sometimes a claim made by libertarian scholars of human enhancement who adhere to what we have called the thin theory of sporting progress. The posture is superficially appealing. Do not new biotechnologies offer new means of human enhancement that may transform identity? At the radical end of that posture, the cyborg athlete, it is quite possible that new ethical norms must be advanced, and argued over, to account for radical shifts in human ontology.

These are not the kinds of enhancements that the authors of this book advance. Rather, they discuss modifications on a well-trodden theme of human longing: the transcendence of known human limits. Technology is ambiguous per definition. Its application requires careful consideration and adjustment in order to realize human values and goals. To this extent, a dynamic interchange between general bioethics and sport ethics is needed in the patient consideration of normative aspects of biotechnological innovations. And that is a narrative consistent with the questions asked by Plato in the education of the would-be gardens of his utopian city state. As McKenny observes: "...his underlying question is how the pursuit of health can be so managed that medicine service rather than hinders or dominates our moral projects." [47].

Conclusion

Anti-doping is a ubiquitous feature of elite sport in practice and in policy. It is also a burgeoning field of scientific research and scholarship. It is remarkably multidisciplinary. Nevertheless, all arguments and experiments concerning the prohibited substances and methods of doping rest upon or presuppose a clarification of the normative justification of the field itself. We have attempted to clarify part of that conceptual geography and to link it specifically to the idea of Olympism.

Two points serve as a summary for this account. First, the thick interpretation of sporting progress that we support does not naïvely idealize sport as a moral ideal. Ritchie's descriptive account of a harsh and to a certain extent immoral reality of Olympic sport has to be taken seriously. On the other hand, sport, too, has the potential of realizing values at the other and admirable end of the moral scale. Good competition requires mutual respect between participants in a setting of fair and equal opportunity and can, as Olympism claims, be an embodied expression of human virtue and excellence. To recall an Olympic slogan in which sport participation is considered a significant means: "Be the best that you can be!" This, then, is the main rationale of sport ethics: elite sport is morally ambiguous, and we need critical and systematic analyses on its potential values underpinning the organization and policies of sport, among them WADA's anti-doping regime.

A second comment relates to future challenges related to Olympic values and anti-doping. In the quest for performance enhancement and record-breaking, innovative and powerful biomedical technologies offer means that can change the very nature of sport. With the help of genetic technologies (among them gene-editing techniques with the potential of germline design of an individual with particularly favourable predispositions for a sport (to the extent that such genetic profiles can be identified), we may imagine future elite athletes who adapt easily to training, are less injured, experience mastery and joy in their sports and perform fairly. We extend here the sphere of specific sport ethics and move into the broader and increasingly important bio-ethical field of human enhancement. This fusion of sport and bioethics must be conducted, as it always has been, in reference to a humane conception of the inviolable moral status of all committed athletes, Olympian or otherwise.

References

1. Chatziefstathiou D (2011) Paradoxes and contestations of Olympism in the history of the modern Olympic Movement. Sport Soc 14(3):332–344
2. Chatziefstathiou D, Henry I (2012) Discourses of Olympism. From the Sorbonne 1894 to London 2012. Palgrave Macmillan, New York
3. MacAloon J (1984) This great symbol. Pierre de Coubertin and the Origins of the Modern Olympic Games. University of Chicago Press, Chicago
4. Loland S (1995) Coubertin's ideology of Olympism from the perspective of the history of Ideas. Olympika 4:49–78
5. Reid H, Austin MW, Torres CR (2012) The Olympics and philosophy. University Press of Kentucky, Lexington
6. DaCosta L (2006) A never-ending story: the philosophical controversy over Olympism. J Philos Sport 33(2):157–173
7. https://stillmedab.olympic.org/media/Document%20Library/OlympicOrg/General/EN-Olympic-Charter.pdf#_ga=2.135429681.1631003973.1610646112-1014900725.1610646112. Accessed 14 Jan 2021
8. DaCosta L (2006) A never-ending story: the philosophical controversy over Olympism. J Philos Sport 33(2):157–173
9. McNamee M (2006) Olympism, Eurocentricity, and transcultural virtues. J Philos Sport 33(2):174–187
10. Cléret L, McNamee M (2012) Olympism, the values of sport, and the will to power: De Coubertin and Nietzsche meet Eugenio Monti. Sport Ethics Philos 6(2):183–194
11. Loland S (2012) A well-balanced life based on 'The Joy of Effort': Olympic hype or a meaningful ideal? Sport Ethics Philos 6(2):155–165
12. Coubertin P de (2000) Olympism. Comité International Olympique. Lausanne, IOC (Editor: N. Muller)
13. Loland S (1995) Coubertin's Ideology of Olympism from the Perspective of the History of Ideas. Olympika 4:49–78

14. Kreft L (2012) Sport as a drama. J Philos Sport 39(2):219–234
15. Martinkova I (2001) Kalokagathia: how to understand harmony of a human being. Nikephoros 14:21–28
16. Loland S (1995) Coubertin's Ideology of Olympism from the Perspective of the History of Ideas. Olympika 4:49–78
17. Russell JS (2014) Is there a normatively distinctive conception of cheating in sport (or anywhere else)? J Philos Sport 41(3):303–323
18. Loland S (2002) Technology in sport: three ideal-typical views and their implications. Eur J Sport Sci 2(1):1–11
19. Fouché R (2018) Game changer. The techno-scientific revolution in sports. Johns Hopkins University Press, Baltimore
20. Savulescu J, Foddy B, Clayton M (2004) Why we should allow performance enhancing drugs in sport. Br J Sports Med 38(6):666–670
21. Miah A (2010) Towards the transhuman athlete: therapy, non-therapy and enhancement. Sport in Soc 13(2):221–233
22. Savulescu J, Bostrom N (eds) (2009) Human Enhancement. Oxford University Press, Oxford
23. Loland S (2002) Fair Play: A Moral Norm System. Routledge, London
24. Suits B (2014) The grasshopper: games, life and Utopia, 3rd edn. Broadview Press, Peterborough, CA
25. Loland S (2018) Morgan, the 'gratuitous' logic of sport, and the art of self-imposed constraints. Sport Ethics Philos 12(4):348–360
26. Morgan WJ (1994) Leftist theories of sport: a critique and reconstruction. University of Illinois Press, Chicago
27. Kretchmar RS, McNamee M, Morgan WJ (eds) (2015) Routledge Handbook of the Philosophy of Sport. Routledge, London, pp 11–22
28. Loland S (2002) Fair play: a moral norm system. Routledge, London
29. Murray TH (2018) Good sport: why our games matter—and how doping undermines them. Oxford University Press, New York, p 15
30. Loland S, Hoppeler H (2012) Justifying anti-doping: the fair opportunity principle and the biology of performance-enhancement. Eur J Sport Sci 12(4):347–353
31. Loland S, McNamee MJ (2019) The 'spirit of sport', WADAs code review, and the search for an overlapping consensus. Int J Sport Policy Politics 11(2):325–339
32. McNamee M (2015) The spirit of sport and the World Anti-Doping Code. In: Møller V, Waddington I, Hoberman J (eds) Routledge Handbook of Drugs in Sport. Routledge, London, pp 41–53
33. https://www.wada-ama.org/sites/default/files/resources/files/2021_wada_code.pdf. Accessed January 21, 2020 pp 33-34
34. Obasa M, Borry P (2019) The landscape of the "Spirit of Sport". Journal of Bioethical Inquiry 16(3):443–453
35. https://www.wada-ama.org/sites/default/files/resources/files/2021_wada_code.pdf. Accessed January 21, 2020 p 13
36. de Hon O (2017) The redundancy of the concept of "spirit of sport" in discussions on the prohibited list of doping substances. Int J Sport Policy Politics 9(4):667–676
37. Gleaves J, Llewellyn ML, Lehrbach T (2014) Before the rules are written: navigating moral ambiguity in performance enhancement. Sport Ethics Philos 8(1):85–99
38. Kayser B, Mauron A, Miah A (2007) Current anti-doping policy: a critical appraisal. BMC Med Ethics 8(1):1–10
39. Kornbeck J (2013) The naked spirit of sport: a framework for revisiting the system of bans and justifications in the world anti-doping code. Sport Ethics Philos 7(3):313–330
40. McNamee MJ (2012) The spirit of sport and the medicalisation of anti-doping: empirical and normative ethics. Asian Bioethics Rev 4(4):374–392
41. Ritchie I (2012) The 'Spirit of Sport'. Understanding the cultural foundations of Olympism through anti-doping policies. In: Problems, Possibilities, Promising Practices: Critical

Dialogues on the Olympic and Paralympic Games. London, Ontario, International Centre for Olympic Studies, pp 78–82

42. Young DC (2008) A brief history of the Olympic games. Blackwell, Malden, MA
43. McNamee M (1995) Sporting practices, institutions, and virtues: a critique and a restatement. J Philos Sport 22(1):61–82
44. Ritchie I (2012) The 'Spirit of Sport'. Understanding the cultural foundations of Olympism through anti-doping policies. In: Problems, Possibilities, Promising Practices: Critical Dialogues on the Olympic and Paralympic Games. London, Ontario, International Centre for Olympic Studies, pp 78–82
45. Murray TH (2018) Good Sport: Why Our Games Matter—and How Doping Undermines Them. Oxford University Press, New York
46. Nussbaum MC (1992) Love's knowledge: essays on philosophy and literature. Oxford University Press, New York p 372
47. McKenny GP (1997) To relieve the human condition: bioethics, technology, and the body. SUNY Press, Brockport, NY p 1

Emerging Trends in Doping: Investigations and Field Operations

Gunter Younger, Meike Younger, and Sebastien Gaillard

Introduction

As a member of the Independent Commission we had contact with high-profile sports officials who were alleged to have protected doped athletes. One interview took less than 5 minutes, as the interviewee stated: "Who are you? Who do you think you are that you can summon me to this interview? What do you think will happen after your report gets out? There will be a media outcry for a couple of days and then we will continue as usual as there will be no consequences". This arrogance was shocking for me, the confidence that nothing can happen and that there will be no consequences for wrongdoings. I wanted to change that! We teach our children to be fair and honest in all their doings and try to raise them with a correctly calibrated moral compass. If their sporting heroes are only achieving greatness through dishonest means, then they are only role models for corruption and duplicity. I wanted to do my part to level the playing field.

– Gunter Younger, October 2016

One of the greatest emerging trends to arise in the fight against doping in sport in recent years is the recognition of the value of the information brought forward by "whistleblowers" and the resultant investigations thereafter. Until January 2015, the World Anti-Doping Agency (WADA) had no powers of investigation. This changed with the 2015 World Anti-Doping Code that granted authority to WADA to proactively pursue investigations into allegations of doping practices. The first case was already waiting. In December 2014, the German broadcaster ARD aired a

G. Younger (✉)
Intelligence and Investigations Department, World Anti-Doping Agency (WADA), Montreal, QC, Canada
e-mail: Gunter.Younger@wada-ama.org

M. Younger
International Investigations Expert, Auckland, New Zealand

S. Gaillard
Interpol, Lyon, France

© The Author(s), under exclusive license to Springer Nature Switzerland AG 2022
O. Rabin, O. Corazza (eds.), *Emerging Drugs in Sport*,
https://doi.org/10.1007/978-3-030-79293-0_9

documentary "Geheimsache Doping: Wie Russland seine Sieger macht" that used whistleblower evidence to expose government-sanctioned, systematic doping and corrupt practices in Russia and at the International Association of Athletics Federations (IAAF). Two independent investigations[1] were launched as a direct response to the ability to investigate. The outcome of both commissions shocked the sport world, but also demonstrated the value of investigations in sport. The sport community further realized that testing alone is not enough. If you consider that less than 2%[2] of all tested samples produce an adverse analytical finding (AAF), and add to that the fact that detection methods used at WADA-accredited laboratories are by nature predictable, it became clear that new tools needed to be implemented to complement traditional detection methods. Many doping substances are perceptible for only a short period of time or "micro-dosed" to avoid detection, enabling cheaters to stay ahead of the curve. New and analog substances, novel ways of using and the level of certainty that is expected in order to proceed with an AAF mean that intelligence gathering and investigations provide not only a big advantage in the toolbox for fighting for clean sport, but also a retrospectivity that only human intelligence can provide. Whether doping is considered as a crime varies greatly from country to country. In those jurisdictions where it is a crime, competing for resources against departments dealing with, for example, organized crime, terrorism, cybercrime and drugs, usually means that doping is not considered as a priority, and consequently local authorities are not sufficiently resourced to proactively follow up cases. Additionally, as most sport investigations have an international aspect, and are usually complex and time-consuming, this further reduces the ability of law enforcement agencies to allocate resources to investigate. Add to this the relatively mild sanctions applied to such offences, and it is easy to understand why criminals are drawn to this lucrative niche market and the legal vacuum that has developed. After the Pound and McLaren Investigations and the significant costs they incurred (almost $4 million USD combined), it became apparent that WADA needed to reduce costly third-party commissions and enhance its in-house investigative capabilities. Therefore, in 2016, WADA created its Intelligence and Investigations Department (I&I), an entity that, although an integral part of WADA, is at the same time independent. This independence ensures that the matters handled by I&I are concluded without outside influence or interference. Moreover, an independent supervisor has been appointed to audit the department's work on an annual basis, providing an assurance that the work performed by I&I is conducted in accordance with its investigation policy.[3] WADA then proceeded to hire skilled professionals with either law enforcement background or profound analytical skills to develop

---

[1] Independent Commission (Pound Commission) was created in January 2015 to investigate the allegations raised by the ARD documentary. In May 2016, following allegations by Dr. Rodchenkov, the former Director of the Moscow Laboratory, WADA appointed Prof. Richard McLaren to investigate further

[2] According to the 2018 Testing Figures Report, only 1.42% of tested samples worldwide (344,177) produced adverse analytical findings (4,896)

[3] WADA Investigation Policy (https://www.wada-ama.org/en/what-we-do/investigation-trafficking/investigative-process)

analytical, investigative and source handling capabilities. A further key aspect of the establishment of the I&I Department is in its name: "Intelligence and Investigations". An often-overlooked aspect of the investigative field is the role played by Intelligence. The gathering, quantifying and cogent application of information into a comprehensive intelligence cycle prior to its application in an investigative context is invaluable. We will also highlight the essential role held by whistleblowers and informants because of the limited powers of non-law enforcement investigations. Since 2016, none of the investigations conducted by the I&I Department would have been possible without whistleblowers. Unfortunately, these brave people must share this arena with malicious whistleblowers whose intent is to defame, distract or confuse. To distinguish the two is not always easy and thus due diligence when assessing information and its source is an important step in every investigation. The bravery of these genuine people in coming forward and the psychological and material impact upon them cannot be underestimated and therefore requires professional source handlers to give them the utmost possible care.

Investigation Process

Most anti-doping organizations have no enforceable law enforcement powers (e.g., the power of search and seizure), so interactions with the respondent largely happen on a voluntary basis. Thus, investigators can only apply methods and techniques that do not intrude on an individual's rights. The main techniques employed are therefore whistleblower information, open source research and interviews. This proves challenging as hard evidence is rarely exposed on the Internet, and respondents are reluctant to voluntarily disclose evidence in interviews. Recruitment of whistleblowers and informants, therefore, greatly increases the success rate of cases. Take note, this chapter is not a "how-to" guide for performing anti-doping investigations. Excellent information, resources and courses are readily available that can effectively communicate that. What this chapter will attempt to do is to serve as an aide-memoire and point out common pitfalls and traps as well as to highlight emerging trends with case examples.

Organization

WADA has purposefully created a distinct separation between its whistleblower management and investigation functions for the twofold purpose of ensuring that the whistleblower and informant confidentiality and/or anonymity is protected and for preserving the integrity of ensuing investigations and the judicial processes that may follow. By removing the direct contact with the information source from the investigation function, an information barrier is built that also brings an element of impartiality to an investigation that may be lost when an investigator is also managing the source. Furthermore, this both safeguards the anonymity of the source and protects

Case Decision Matrix for the INTELLIGENCE & INVESTIGATIONS DEPARTMENT of WADA

EVIDENCE

	Sports entourage (except Doctors, Coaches)	Athlete	Group of Athletes/Team	Coaches, Doctors	Reported by Media	Organization (ADO, IF)	Crime (Bribery, corruption)
Irrefutable evidence (video, audio, computer)							
Evidence (documents, statements) from multiple sources							
Evidence (documents, statements)							
Multiple similar detailed allegations from known sources							
Detailed allegation from known source							
Multiple similar allegations from known sources							
Allegation from known source							
Anonymous allegation							
Hearsay from known source							
Anonymous hearsay							
Assumption							

RED: WADA I&I Department investigates
Orange: WADA I&I Department considers to investigate
Green: Case to be forwarded to respective ADO / IF

SOURCE

Source Evaluation	Information Evaluation	Handling Code
A=always reliable D=Unreliable	1=Known to be true without reservation 4=Cannot be judged	WA=WADA LA=Law enforcement
B=mostly reliable X=Untested Source	2=Known personally to source 5=Suspected to be false/malicious	NA=NADO OT=Others
C=sometimes reliable	3=Not personally known to source but corroborated	IF=International Federations

Fig. 1 Case decision matrix for the Intelligence and Investigations Department of WADA (WADA Investigation Policy (https://www.wada-ama.org/en/what-we-do/investigation-trafficking/investigative-process)) (used with permission from WADA)

the investigator from perjury in the event that they may be required to give evidence and therefore be compelled to disclose their source during a judicial process. A "case decision matrix" is helpful to ensure that an objective view of the information and source is taken, as well as to help establish priorities and allocate resources (Fig. 1). Resource limitations often mean that not every case is able to be followed up immediately, and a case decision matrix provides a reasonably objective justification for your decision that may be referred to in the future. For matters that are reported but not taken further, an often-overlooked aspect is the documentation of this and the reasoning for not proceeding to investigation. You never know when further allegations of the same or a similar nature may come to light or further corresponding information may be received that can change a case's priority assessment. Consider how information that has been received and your responses to it are stored. Is it searchable and retrievable, and is there a secure solution in which to store information that oftentimes contains personal data? Who else has (or may obtain) access to this information? Can IT access it? Is regular penetration testing performed to ensure the data remain safe from hacking? Best practice scenario is for all information pertaining to whistleblowing and investigations to be stored in a secure, encrypted environment to which access is strictly limited to those that need to know.

Consider implementing a whistleblowing platform or hotline such as WADA's *Speak up!*. Established in March 2017, the following 3 years gave rise to more than

900 reports. If such a communication platform is established, then it is imperative to have experts in place who can follow up on the received messages in a timely manner. WADA I&I has created its own unit (Confidential Information Unit) for the sole purpose of managing, guiding and representing whistleblowers throughout an investigation.

Collecting Information

Collecting information is the first step and quite possibly the most crucial one in any investigation. The decision to pass on information is not one that is made lightly, for that reason, we need to make it as simple and straightforward as possible for that person to find where and how they can confidently give information. Reliability, confidentiality and trust are key elements to receiving relevant information. We must be committed (and able) to provide all three throughout all stages of the process of managing whistleblowers and informants. Following receipt of information, the first stage must be to qualify and quantify the information provided and (where possible) the source. Consider the plausibility of the information provided; and ask yourself: Is it a reasonable allegation provided by a credible source? What is the motivation of the source? How did the source gain access to this information? Is it first-hand information or did they get it from somebody else (hearsay)?

Speak up! and the Role of Whistleblowers and Informants

WADA has provided an online solution called *Speak Up!* for those looking to pass on information in a secure, confidential and anonymous way. *Speak Up!* is an easily accessible platform that functions like an email exchange in that a person may (if they choose) remain anonymous but continue a dialog with WADA about the information provided. This has proven extremely helpful as the whistleblower (or informant) may have overlooked pertinent details when giving their original statement. Furthermore, these people are often still active in the environment for which they are providing information and may be able to continue to elaborate upon details as situations evolve. Providing a whistleblowing solution is, in itself, a redundant exercise if the organization does not then equip itself to be able to competently follow up and follow through with the information provided. It is a very courageous step for a whistleblower to come forward, and thus it is important that during the first contact they know that they still control their information until they feel confident enough to share. Even if a source ultimately decides not to disclose, respect their decision. There are many reasons why a source may change their mind. It is not up to us to pass judgement on them or their situation. If they trust you and they themselves feel trusted and respected, they may return later. To this end, in the first contact explain the reasons why the whistleblower can trust you. Describe the measures you have in place to keep their identity and information confidential. Be transparent with them about what they can expect throughout the process; they should be provided with enough information to make an informed decision about their role. This brings us to another important aspect. What would you do if the whistleblower or informant has provided you with compelling primary evidence but using this evidence would disclose the identity of the source? Where possible, use the evidence as guidance for the investigation.

Case Example:
In one case example, we were provided with direct evidence that would have endangered the confidentiality of the whistleblower if we had used it. We showed the evidence to the investigators and asked them to source this information during their investigation. They did so, and the allegations were verified. Evidence can be like the proverbial needle in a haystack; if somebody tells you in which corner to look, then it is much easier to find it.

Finally, it is worthwhile here to touch upon source credibility and motivation. The provision of a service such as *Speak Up!* may empower persons with malicious intent to provide erroneous or untrue information with the distinct purpose of defaming or discrediting an individual or organization (mala fide allegations). In order to identify and carve out malicious assertions, it is important to also enquire into the motivation and credibility of your source. Keep in mind, however, that detailed and direct questions may irritate forthcoming whistleblowers as they may feel they are not taken seriously or trusted. Be honest with your source and explain that cooperation is built on mutual trust. One of the main objectives of a source handler is to support, protect and guide a whistleblower throughout the investigation process. Explaining that this is standard procedure and clarifying why these questions are important, in most cases, will allow a genuine whistleblower to understand.

Case Example
A senior sport official was alleged of involvement in the sourcing and trafficking of prohibited substances. The information was originally sent to WADA's I&I Department via its Anti-Doping hotline, "Speak up!". The Source then agreed to speak directly to a member of the department and proceeded to share screenshots of chat conversations that they were in possession of. The messages were assessed, and an investigation ensued. During the investigation, additional information was obtained that brought the original messages into question. The veracity of this "evidence" was reassessed, and, in collaboration with another anti-doping organisation, I&I was able to determine that the messages had been fabricated. This example serves to highlight that we should continue to reassess not only the information provided by a source but also the source themselves, as motivations may change throughout the lifetime of an investigation.

Intelligence Process

The Intelligence process describes the management of information from collection to interpretation and then development of a hypothesis. Throughout this process, information is subject to a perpetual cycle of reexamination until there is no doubt about its veracity. Hypotheses help investigators to develop investigative strategies for the overt phase. There are two approaches towards the intelligence process. The first one is the inductive approach. In this approach, a whistleblower reports about misconduct perpetrated by a singular person or organization. The epicentre of the intelligence process is therefore a singular entity. The analyst will then collect information from multiple sources that either corroborates or contradicts the hypothesis. This process continues until there is no doubt about the accuracy of the information. The "enquiring mind" so often referred to as essential for any good investigator is equally important in a skilled analyst. An analyst must continue to question provided information and enquire into what may contradict it. Only once doubt has been removed can the information be considered reliable intelligence. The deductive approach is the second method and one where you start with a hypothesis and then collect and analyse information to support or refute the hypothesis. An abundance of information that can be whittled down to singular entities is preferred, as this further confirms the hypothesis (if proven) due to the probability of having a greater number of instances that support it. As an example of this approach, see the following case study.

Case Study: Operation Arrow

In 2018, the WADA I&I Department received allegations that doped athletes in a specific sport were using "doppelgänger" or look-alikes during out-of-competition sample collection. Later in the year, a former Olympic medallist was caught using their sibling as a doppelgänger during a test. The case inspired the I&I Department to have a closer look at the methodology and whether this was an extraordinary case or whether it was a prevalent evasion method. Further information collected throughout 2019 strengthened the hypothesis that doped athletes might be using a "doppelgänger" to provide samples to Doping Control Officers. Based on this hypothesis, a comprehensive data collection plan that included all athletes of a specific sport for a defined time period was concluded. By using scientific techniques and consulting with experts in this field, data from around 60,000 samples were reduced to 35 samples of interest. DNA examination was conducted on all available samples, and from there 26 samples, representing 18 athletes, were identified as being highly likely to have been substituted. These individual cases were then followed up by investigators. The intelligence that was gathered formed the hypothesis, that led to the investigative strategy, that finally identified 18 cheaters.

Collate, Integrate and Interpret Information

Collation is the process whereby information is stored and cross-referenced so it can be retrieved easily. It may also be referred to as knowledge management. All information gathered must be stored and secured in a database as the efficiency and value of the analysis can be seriously affected if the collation process is poor. Relevant information should be easily cross-checked and retrievable from internal databases, external partners or open sources. These days, as almost everybody is connected to at least one social network, open source information is of great value to investigations; however, it may not remain readily retrievable in its original (online) format. Consideration should therefore be given to how to collect and store this information (e.g., screenshot the information as well as copying the URL). The *integration* part is an exciting part when an array of information coalesces and suddenly takes on a meaning. It can be compared to a puzzle; a singular piece doesn't mean anything, but once you put multiple pieces together in the right order you can see the bigger picture. Visualization tools for complex networks or relationships also help us to understand and communicate the big picture. Once the picture is revealed, the *interpretation* of it is crucial for the overall process and for the development of the investigation strategy. Of special consideration here is if three people look at the same picture, they all may return different opinions about the content. Embrace this, as it helps to prepare for every eventuality. Only an investigation that has considered all possibilities and probabilities and from that point confirms or disregards them, can be considered a complete investigation.

Investigation

Often seen as the most exciting part of a case, the success (or otherwise) of this phase of the process is largely determined by the investment in the prior stages. What has likely up until now been covert activity, generally changes to overt as during this phase the investigator will need to make contact with persons who can provide information relevant to the matter. This includes witnesses as well as the person(s) alleged of the misconduct. When putting together a team for this phase, consider strengths. Not everybody is a good interviewer or analyst. Investigations are complex. Some are good interviewers, some good in developing strategies. Take ownership out of the equation and compose the best team for the challenge.

Interviews

An integral part of any case, an interview—whether it be of a witness or an alleged person—can be a pivotal point. Interaction with the concerned subject is crucial, but careful consideration should be given to the timing of this contact. Here two methods can be considered, "inside out" or "outside in". The traditional course of action is "outside in", that is, to speak with all other sources of information prior to interviewing the alleged. However, the "inside out" technique should not be overlooked. By interviewing the alleged person first, it may set off other events and interactions relevant to the case, or others may feel more inclined or empowered to speak up. Whichever method is chosen, remember to learn as much as you can about the interviewee, their motivation and accessibility to information and evidence, and consider your ability to cross-check or corroborate facts presented by them. Be prepared (the previous phase will have readied you for this) and keep an open mind—but at the same time do not believe everything you are told! Remember, the final report on the matter will be based on facts and corroborations; anything that cannot be proven or disproven should not be included (but may be taken into the intelligence cycle). Of particular note here are the challenges presented by our ever-changing world. The COVID-19 global pandemic brought the challenges associated with interviewing subjects and witnesses in-person into sharp focus. As the world sat in lockdown, international travel was reduced to near-extinction, and face-to-face contact became an alien experience, we were forced to reevaluate our previous expectations on how to conduct interviews. This was a new environment to work in, but one that is not unique to a pandemic. Geographical distance, civil unrest or simple things such as budget restrictions can all affect our ability to be physically present at all stages of an investigation. As much as the benefits of in-person interviews should not be dismissed, when the option is to do a video interview or none at all, then video must be explored.

Collaboration with Law Enforcement

At any stage of the investigation process, there may come a point where suspicion arises that a criminal act has been committed. At this point it is recommended to reach out to either a local law enforcement agency or an international police organization, such as Interpol or Europol, for support. Law enforcement agencies have far more powerful tools to obtain evidence and therefore the facts. This approach has been very successful for WADA's I&I Department. Since its inauguration in 2016, more than 10 law enforcement agencies have been contacted and important information shared. Although WADA holds no law enforcement powers, the knowledge and expertise they bring to the fight against doping have proven to be very advantageous for law enforcement agencies. To use these synergies while remaining respectful of each other's boundaries has been a game changer for sport investigations and supports the common objective of both organizations: to catch cheaters. With the establishment of international anti-doping conventions (Council of Europe-1989/UNESCO-2007), many countries decided to bring doping and doping-related crime into the scope of law enforcement for the protection of public health. In this context, and given that the crime world rarely confines itself to within a single nation's borders, Interpol worked to develop important links with major anti-doping actors, culminating in the 2009 signing of a Memorandum of Understanding (MoU) with WADA. Interpol's primary mandate is to facilitate and coordinate the work of police investigations involving the 194 member countries of its organization and to connect them in the fight against transnational criminal issues. In order to support its member countries in international investigations, Interpol's anti-doping team continues to develop an expert network with high-level partnerships and innovative projects. One such example is project Energia in which Interpol, the University of Lausanne and WADA worked hand-in-hand. Created in 2015, the project aims to tackle international performance-enhancing drug (PED) trafficking by analysing PED seizures carried out by Interpol's member countries and undertake profiling of the physical (e.g., packages and labels), chemical (e.g. liquid chromatography) and context of the seizures (e.g., circumstances of seizure, modus operandi) in order to identify patterns of criminal activities. In addition, identification and monitoring of websites selling PEDs was conducted to learn more about their accessibility. In today's online world, the Dark Web is believed to play an increasing role in PED manufacturing, trafficking and purchasing on account of its anonymity. Moreover, the different online markets attract criminals from all over the world due to the volume of potential customers and manufacturers. Law enforcement investigations in this field are complex, and consequently few criminals are caught. Cooperation between law enforcement agencies and sport organizations is necessary to achieve greater impact on these PED networks. In this respect, WADA discovered new avenues of cooperation together with universities and law enforcement agencies. Such joint projects enable us to gain further insight into not only anti-doping but also criminal networks or new substances that we would not normally have access to.

Project Energia
This multifaceted proactive approach to tackle international PED trafficking was proposed in partnership with the School of Criminal Science of the University of Lausanne (UNIL) and has allowed Interpol to identify 271 cases (3,575,348 seized products) with more than 200 producing PEDs. Additionally, more than 14 million URLs were gathered during the monitoring process from 2016 to 2019. This has led to the detection of 4,170 distinct hostnames categorized by the types of products sold: 3170 websites were classified as doping websites.

In addition to the research facet, Interpol has also provided key support to operational activities such as Operations Augeas[4] and Barium.[5] The international expertise and network that Interpol brings to the table as the only global law enforcement player are invaluable.

Case Studies

Operation Augeas

Interpol facilitated a meeting between WADA's Independent Commission and the French authorities where the Commission's findings related to alleged doping, corruption and extortion involving the former president of the IAAF were shared. This is considered one of the biggest corruption cases discovered by WADA. The French authority brought charges against the main actors.[6]

Operation Barium

Interpol's anti-doping team worked with the US Federal Drug Control Service to stop the illicit production and distribution of doping products in more than 80 countries. Intelligence on raw material purchasers from the US clandestine market were collected and led to a significant disruption of illicit production and distribution of PEDs. The operation—supported by WADA's I&I Department—resulted in the seizure of millions of bottles and tablets, led to the arrest of more than 30 individuals and dismantled four state-of-the-art clandestine laboratories.

Another important international law enforcement partner is Europol. It supports 27 EU member countries in their fight against serious and organized crime. In its latest situation report about the involvement of organized crime groups in sports corruption,[7] Europol highlighted the importance of tackling this crime on an international level, including doping as a very common method to influence the result of sport competitions. Operation Viribus,[8] coordinated by Europol, clearly demonstrated the involvement of organized crime groups in doping practices. The excellent cooperation between the two organizations, coupled with the success of the

---

[4] https://www.cbc.ca/sports/olympics/summer/trackandfield/doping-trial-corruption-diack-iaaf-world-athletics-1.5617092

[5] https://www.Interpol.int/en/Crimes/Corruption/Anti-doping

[6] Six people, including the former President of the International Association of Athletics Federations (IAAF, today World Athletics), Lamine Diack, were sentenced on 16 September 2020 for corruption linked to the Russian doping scandal. (https://www.wada-ama.org/en/media/news/2020-09/wada-welcomes-decision-of-french-court-in-diack-case)

[7] For more information: https://www.Europol.europa.eu/publications-documents/involvement-of-organised-crime-groups-in-sports-corruption

[8] https://www.Europol.europa.eu/newsroom/news/keeping-sport-safe-and-fair-38-million-doping-substances-and-fake-medicines-seized-worldwide

operation, has led to WADA and Europol agreeing to sign a Memorandum of Understanding underscoring their combined commitment to clean sport.

> **Case Study: Operation Viribus**
> *In July 2019, led by Europol through IPC3 (Intellectual Property Crime Coordinated Coalition), this operation was aimed at countering the smuggling of counterfeit sports food supplements, the illegal trade of doping substances and, in general, the commerce of a large variety of illegal and dangerous substances. It concerned 33 European countries with the involvement of a number of private entities, including WADA I&I. Described as the biggest crackdown against PED manufacturing and trafficking, around 3.8 million illicit doping substances and counterfeit medicines were seized, 17 organised crime groups dismantled, 9 underground laboratories disrupted, 234 suspects arrested, 839 judicial cases opened and almost 1000 individuals reported for the production, commerce or use of doping substances.*

Reporting

All cases—including those that are not taken up, or not taken further—should be concluded with a comprehensive report that details all steps taken, draws conclusions on the alleged misconduct and proposes recommendations (or reasons why a case was not taken further, e.g. insufficient evidence). All conclusions should be based on facts, and careful consideration should be given to whom the report is shared. The privacy of persons alleged of misconduct always remains a priority, and in most jurisdictions, laws are in place to protect individual's right to retain their privacy. For this reason, it is prudent to redact or anonymize reports. It is important to review the report through the eyes of your whistleblower. Is there anything in the report that might endanger or disclose their identity or role? If so, make sure that it is amended or removed. Once the report is published, there is no way back. For this reason, WADA's I&I Department has put procedures in place where the responsible whistleblower manager reviews the final report and intervenes if they identify anything that would disclose the identity of their source. An often-overlooked point at the conclusion of an investigation is the follow-up of recommended actions to ensure remediation is implemented. This follow-up may not lie with one department, person or organization, and for that reason a follow-up evaluation plan that brings all involved parties to one table is strongly recommended (e.g. by a working group).

Conclusion

The emergence of new drugs and usage methods in sport is a continually changing landscape, and, if we do not endeavour to try to stay ahead of the curve by embracing new methods and technologies, we will be doing a great disservice to the true and clean athletes. It is our strong belief that strategic alliances with like-minded partners animated by similar global objectives are essential tools to combat those who seek to gain dishonest advantages. These partnerships may in some ways be considered unconventional (whistleblowers) while others are often overlooked (law enforcement and international organizations), but each brings a different element to the table, and together they have a greater capacity to truly make an impact in the field. Invest in creating a strong and effective Intelligence and Investigations capacity; where this is limited, look to form alliances and partnerships, share knowledge and efforts, reach out to other organizations and form networks. Anti-doping agencies do not have to work in a vacuum; law enforcement agencies, national and international organizations, and international federations all have equally committed to contribute to this battle. Finally, the biggest asset in all investigations are the whistleblowers. It is a courageous step to come forward and not an easy decision to make. Unfortunately, many brave whistleblowers are still treated as traitors and do not get the credit that they deserve. It is our responsibility to listen to and protect them. There are many out there who want to speak up; the best example is the Stepanovs,[9] who gave up everything they loved, family and friends, left their country and even gave up their sport and jobs because they believed that a change in Russia's sport was necessary. Collectively, we need to be serious in our efforts. Only by committing sufficient resources and experts can we guarantee the confidentiality, trust and reliability we need to make progress in this field. In this respect we need to continue to strengthen Intelligence and Investigation capabilities at all relevant sport organizations. It is our responsibility to support and encourage whistleblowers to come forward by demonstrating our professionalism and passion to create a level playing field for all clean athletes. At WADA I&I, we are striving to understand and then dismantle the bigger picture. It is not enough anymore to simply catch cheating athletes during competition with doping controls. We are looking for the facilitators, the organizers, the suppliers and the organized criminal networks that have been going unpunished for years, as athletes are found and then sanctioned, while their conspirators then move on to the next athlete. It's time to shift our focus and look beyond the short-term "success" of catching one doped athlete. At the end, the fight can only be won together, and even with a small investigation team, you can achieve big results for clean sport. Every small victory for us is a big victory for the clean athlete.

---

[9] In the ARD Documentary "How Russia makes its winners" aired in Germany on 4 December 2014, Yuliya and Vitaly Stepanov were instrumental in revealing an institutionalized doping scheme in Russia. Their statements triggered the Independent Commission investigation set up by WADA

Anti-doping Stories Narrated by a Law Enforcement Investigator: Mind the "Good Guys"!

Renzo Ferrante

Introduction

I have been working the frontline in the fight against doping-related crime for the last 25 years of my life. I believe doping is a "monster" that devours professional sportsmen and amateurs' health and ethics and endangers the lives of ordinary people. I have witnessed before my eyes many stories of elite athletes falling from the podium straight into hell, because of unscrupulous individuals manipulating science for their own interests. I see the struggle of the "good guys", such as scientists, investigators, anti-doping organizations and educators to be always a step ahead of the "bad guys". Human beings are always looking for new substances to boost their performance regardless of their dangers. Such an ever-increasing demand fuels a huge criminal business. In this chapter, I will share some stories of this endless challenge through some real cases that I had to face in my busy working life.

Sugaring the Pill

Spain, International airport, Summer of 2005: the sliding doors of the Arrivals are opening. Among the just-landed passengers, there is a young athlete, who just stepped off the plane and drags his luggage full of clothes and hopes of success. His new personal "wizard" chosen by his team is waiting for him in a beautiful convertible car: that's not the first doping wizard he meets but will be the last one, because

R. Ferrante (✉)
Carabinieri, Comando Carabinieri Tutela Salute, Nucleo Antisofisticazioni (NAS), Florence, Italy
e-mail: renzo.ferrante@gmail.com

the storm is going to hit on all of them ending their careers ingloriously. However, in this very moment, none of them knows about it or can imagine how their lives are going to change in a matter of minutes.

Due to a medical check, "the doctor" reassures his new follower—"You're in the right place, we have everything you need to fly, you cannot fail!". He recommends a long list of banned substances and makes them available to him. Then totally unexpectedly, he pulls a blister of tablets from the pocket of his shirt and offers them to the "boy" as if it was a pack of candies. He explains that it is something brand new, a powerful anabolic steroid that comes from the East and that, above all, is invisible to doping controls. The young man is now frightened and decides that this is too much, even for him who relied upon chemical help since the beginning of his competitive career. He refuses.

It might sound like a movie scene, but unfortunately it isn't. And it is not even the weirdest deposition I have heard from an athlete. During my career I have met hundreds of them, practicing all sport disciplines at every level, each one ready to tell his story full of half-truths, or sensational lies, to defend a respect that is now lost. Many of them were famous athletes, who were more used to signing autographs than police interview reports!

The Spanish anecdote had particularly impressed me as it brought to my mind a detail of my childhood. When I was a child, once I was ill and my father took me to the doctor; then, we went to the pharmacy to take the medicines that the doctor prescribed for me. These were available in the form of pills, syrups (with a horrible taste!) or injections. My father consoled me by taking from the counter display a pack of fruit candies that would have "sweetened" the taste of medicines. Fifty years have passed, but those sweet candies still exist, in their attractive colourful boxes and with their fruit flavours; they still serve to make the taste of pills less bitter. It's a perfect metaphor for me to describe the psychological link between substance and consumption, in sport or in everyday life: there's always something bitter to swallow; there's always a way to make it less bitter! If the bugaboo is fatigue, or defeat, there is doping; if the everyday life is too unbearable, or even just boring, deprived of stimuli and unsuccessful, there are recreational drugs. These are two sides of the same coin.

Such a craving for drugs generates a multibillion business and continuously feeds the search for new substances. While I am writing this chapter, the last international operation against pharmaceutical crime has just been completed. It's known as the Operation SHIELD, coordinated by Europol in cooperation with Carabinieri as a partner, which also involved the trafficking of performance-enhancing drugs (PEDs).[1] Among the new trends identified by Operation SHIELD, there are the increased trafficking of anticonvulsants or antiepileptics (e.g., clonazepam) and synthetic opioids (e.g., tramadol and fentanyl) and underground laboratories producing medicines, anabolic steroids and narcotics. The number of seizures, arrests

---

[1] https://www.europol.europa.eu/newsroom/news/medicines-and-doping-substances-worth-%E2%82%AC73-million-seized-in-europe-wide-operation

and judicial proceedings triggered by Operation SHIELD really shows the great joint effort to put a barrier against this cancer that undermines modern society. However, this is not enough. Investigations on underground laboratories show that the primary objective of the "criminal science" is to jeopardize the action of international bodies, governments and law enforcement agencies by modifying the chemical composition of known substances or creating new ones every day. As far as I see it, the aim is threefold: to create increasingly powerful and effective substances; to bypass the lists of controlled substances making the existing laws and regulations unenforceable; and to cheat analytical monitoring systems, especially anti-doping testing. The health and safety of those taking these substances are of no concern to these unscrupulous manufacturers. For them, it is important to create a product that can feed physical and psychological addiction. Sometimes, as I will show you in this chapter, only the psychological aspect is satisfied. I will share cases of fake products capable of causing only one effect, the placebo effect.

The search for the latest product is, therefore, one of the leitmotivs in the business of substances. In the sport environment, the latest trends are peptides, "designer steroids" and the selective androgen receptor modulators (SARMs), the latter being linked to the industry of food supplements; in the recreational environment, the latest trend are the novel psychoactive substances (NPS). But it's not a new trend. I had the opportunity to observe its development throughout my career, especially with regard to PEDs. I can state that each season had its own totem, be it a specific substance or a category of substances.

When I dig into my memories, what comes to mind is an unbelievable case that turned out to be an absolute fraud instead of an attack on public health. The case dates back to 2001, at the time of an investigation called "Quadrifoglio"[2] against the use of doping substances in professional cycling. As a result of an intelligence operation, my office was monitoring the behaviour of some people suspected of supplying drugs to several professional cycling teams. In May, we had the *Giro d'Italia*, one of the main road cycling events included in the Union Cycliste Internationale world calendar: on May 27, we performed a covert inspection in the hotel rooms just after the teams departed to ride from Montecatini Terme to Reggio Emilia. Among the waste left in the rooms, or in the waste bags abandoned by the athletes' support personnel, we found hundreds of medical devices (syringes and phlebotomy equipment) used for injections and intravenous infusions, but not even a single vial or package of medicine. It was clear that someone took them away because it was not appropriate to leave them behind and risk to reveal the type of drugs taken by the cyclists.

The prosecutors at the Public Prosecutor's Office in Florence, who led the investigation, considered this selective removal the final evidence of the massive use of doping substances among cyclists. In December 2000, the Italian Parliament had just enacted a new anti-doping law, Act number 376, which classified the use of doping by athletes as a criminal offence. It was no longer considered an

---

[2] "Four-leaf clover" in English

administrative offence simply sanctioned at disciplinary level but a real crime against the health and the fairness of sports competitions. Magistrates in charge of the case decided to issue a search warrant for all the teams involved in the Giro d'Italia during the night from 6 to 7 June in San Remo, near the French border.[3] On June 6, at around 9:00 p.m., more than 160 NAS investigators raided the hotels hosting the cycling teams. The scale of this police action makes it hard to forget. Inside an athlete's room, investigators seized some vials filled with a transparent liquid substance, labelled as a drug based on synthetic haemoglobin still in clinical trial; we learned later that the trial had been stopped in phase three, during the testing of the drug on participants to assess its efficacy and safety. Later, the rider confessed he had paid the price of 800,000 liras per vial (approx. 400 €). The same year those vials began to appear in several places during several police raids; we also seized some of them at the Women's *Giro d'Italia*. Experts appointed by the prosecutor's office immediately expressed their doubts about the composition of the liquid contained in the vials as the synthetic haemoglobin was notoriously red in colour and this liquid was not. Such doubts were later confirmed by analytical testing which proved that athletes were self-injecting just a very expensive physiological saline solution with no substance. At least they didn't risk their health, but they remained victim of a fraud and allegations for attempted use of doping.

Years later in April 2010, we found a mysterious and dangerous red substance. The scene took place again at an airport, during another doping investigation involving professional cycling. Some athletes had been under surveillance for months because they were suspected of using prohibited substances. We discovered that a network of people was operating on their behalf, hiding PEDs and helping them to avoid the risk of being caught in possession of such illicit substances.

These accomplices followed them during races and cycling training camps, staying in the same hotels. In April, two athletes reached Belgium to compete in the Spring Classics; this time their wives were in charge of smuggling the PEDs and for delivering them to the accomplices once they arrived in Belgium. We decided to stop and search them at the airport while they were leaving Italy to fly to Brussels Charleroi. Inside their luggage we found some albumin, used as physiological plasma expander to mask blood doping when tested and a large unlabelled glass vial with an intense red-coloured liquid inside, different from anything we had seen before. Unfortunately, the magical device able to identify any kind of substance exists only in cartoons; we had the task (a very difficult one!) to give experts some hints on a possible range of substances to look for, but it was so new to us that we had no clue. Luckily, we obtained some hints from one of our most reliable informers who directed the analysis for liquid PFC. The acronym PFC stands for perfluorocarbon, a class of fluorine and carbon-based chemical compounds. We heard about it in the 1990s as a "synthetic blood" with boosting effect to carry oxygen to the muscles. It was massively used during the Wars in Chechnya to front

---

[3] For more information on the blitz, view https://www.repubblica.it/online/giroditalia/albergo/albergo/albergo.html (in Italian)

haemorrhagic shocks in severely wounded soldiers. The use of PFC was considered a very dangerous practice. In May 1998, it was implicated in a serious disease of a Swiss cyclist, who probably used it during the *Tour de Romandie*, and was hospitalized for 10 days in intensive care. The athlete had suffered respiratory failure, severe pain, gastroenteritis and disseminated intravascular coagulation.[4] I remember that the forensic expert who analysed the content of the vial and identified the substance was shocked by the red colorant added to the substance as so dangerous that only a fool could inject it! I always thought that by seizing it, we might have saved lives!

A year later, a new case emerged; this time it was the seizure of a dietary supplement for athletes, which was made from bovine colostrum and produced in the United Kingdom. Colostrum, also called "first milk", is a yellow serous liquid, very rich in class A immunoglobulin, secreted by the mammary glands during pregnancy and the first days after birth. Its constituents are mainly water, proteins (especially immunoglobulins), fats, minerals and carbohydrates. This substance is known in nature for its nutritional value and sought after by athletes to boost their performances.

The seizure confirmed the existence of new trend, which was already known to us as our intelligence constantly monitors the commerce of supplements. In this case, the supplement in question was legally advertised and sold on the manufacturer's website as a restorative for damaged muscle and immune system stimulator.

However, thanks to some documents in our possession, we were aware of the potential adulteration of the supplement with anabolic steroids (DHEA and androstenediol). This was later confirmed by laboratory analysis.

The possible links between the use of colostrum and the gain in sports performance had been for a long time subject of scientific debate; there were various studies in the literature, carried out in particular on cyclists undergoing intensive training after colostrum administration, which had produced contradictory results.

During the investigation we found no evidence that athletes who bought the supplement were aware of anabolic steroid adulteration. Alternately, they were not informed about the risks associated with their intake, including that of testing positive for IGF-1. Colostrum became popular among athletes despite WADA discouraging its ingestion back in 2008, as potentially related the presence of IGF-1 and other prohibited growth factors that may influence the anti-doping testing results. However, such WADA recommendation, instead of dissuading athletes from using it, seemed to have produced the opposite effect, as a sort of reverse advertising. The seized product was then analysed by an expert appointed by the prosecutor who found traces of IGF-1, expressing at the same time a highly doubtful opinion about the effectiveness on the performance considered the oral intake. The expert in charge explained that the preferred route for the administration of active substances of peptide or protein origin was undoubtedly the systemic administration; ingesting them generally tends to degrade the proteins due to the destructive action of the protease enzymes activated during digestion inside the gastrointestinal tract,

---

[4] https://www.nytimes.com/1998/10/18/sports/a-new-threat-in-blood-doping.html

hindering or increasing the absorption and the passage in the blood circulation. Therefore, athletes accepted the risk for a very doubtful ergogenic help: the placebo effect was guaranteed.

The following case also regards sports dietary supplements as well and goes back several years: an Italian athlete, a member of a national team participating in the Winter Olympic Games in Sochi, Russia, from 7 to 23 February 2014, had been found positive for an anti-doping test for the stimulant dimethylamylamine (DMAA). He was immediately banned from the Olympic Games and subjected to disciplinary procedures.

DMAA is an aliphatic amine with stimulating properties. In the past, it was used as a supplement in diets (for its thermogenic and appetite-reducing effect), also combined with caffeine, as well as in nasal decongestant drugs for hypertrophic or hyperplastic oral tissues. Due to its pronounced adverse effects, it is now banned worldwide.

In Italy the DMAA molecule, despite its similarities to amphetamines, is not included in the list of narcotic substances. In 2009, WADA included it by name in the list of prohibited substances (class S6—stimulants); the substance ban was later adopted by Italian legislation by the inclusion among the biologically or pharmacologically active substances considered as doping according to the Anti-Doping Law, nr. 376 of 2000. In the United States, the substance was banned by the Food and Drug Administration (FDA) in 2012 due to its dangerous effects.

At the Winter Olympics in Sochi in 2014, an Italian athlete, a Lithuanian hockey player and a German cross-country skier and biathlete were found positive for DMAA.

After returning to his home country, the Italian athlete filed a complaint declaring that the hypothesis that he voluntarily used a stimulant substance such as DMAA during the Olympic Games was an illogical and insane gamble, leading to an unwanted and hard-to-accept "professional suicide". He carried out his own investigations, delivering samples of the food supplements he used to take at the time of the Games to the University of Turin in Italy. Results from the chemical tests confirmed the undisclosed presence of DMAA in supplement products containing a *Tribulus terrestris* extract that he bought in the United States; consequently, the use was to be considered unintentional. The athlete also provided evidence of purchase from a specialized US website along with other food supplement samples shipped from the same source.

He claimed he had bought the supplement under investigation other times before, facing no problem with anti-doping testing. A few months after his first complaint, he presented to us an addendum, enclosing additional documents related to a new online purchase of the same supplement from an Italian website. This new sample had been analysed by the WADA-accredited Anti-doping Laboratory in Rome, Italy, on behalf of NADO ITALIA; the laboratory attested in its report the presence in the sample of 4-methyl-2-hexaneamine (analog name of DMAA), with concentrations of hundreds of micrograms per tablet, such that it could potentially cause adverse analytical findings for 4-methyl-2-hexaneamine in urine.

The intelligence we gathered about the Italian importer allowed us to uncover that it was the case of a company managed by some individuals with criminal records for doping-related crimes. This led to a major operation during which 420 packages of the supplement from the same batch as the one analysed by the laboratory in Rome were seized. As per procedure, a technical expert was appointed by the public prosecutor, who extracted a total amount of 128 tablets from the 420 packages according to the statistical criterion of hypergeometric distribution and the indications outlined in the "Guidelines on representative drug sampling United Nations Office on Drugs and Crime, 2009". The analyses confirmed that DMAA analyte was present in all seized tablets, and its concentration was randomly distributed—with a variability ranging from a minimum of 5.00 µg/g up to a maximum of 36.71 µg/g.

We thus had positive analytical evidence emerging from different sources and operations:

- The first, on April 2014, resulting from the tests carried out on behalf of the athlete by the University of Turin on an open pack of the supplement, with DMAA present in relatively high quantities
- The second, at the end of May 2014, resulting from the tests carried out by the WADA-accredited laboratory in Rome on behalf of NADO ITALIA Anti-doping Prosecutor's Office on a package of the same supplement—DMAA was detected in concentrations of hundreds of micrograms per tablet, such that they can potentially cause adverse analytical results in urine
- The third, assessed by the technical adviser appointed by the public prosecutor, carried out on packages from the same batch of those analysed by the Anti-doping Laboratory in Rome, with the aforementioned result.

The undisclosed presence of DMAA was therefore confirmed in different batches, always in variable quantity, even between tablets, with potentially dangerous effects on the health of users. The lack of a systematic and standardized criterion for the illicit production of these products was evident. The risks were further enhanced by the fact that the supplements were available not only for the athletes but also for the general sporting population, thus leading to a major public health issue. Therefore, we had enough material to conclude that the case was not an isolated accident but a major fraud in the manufacturing and packaging activities in the United States. Carabinieri worked in close cooperation with the Rapid Alert System for Food and Feed[5] (RASFF) and used the EU Food and Feed Safety Alert System, a key tool to enable a rapid reaction when public health risks in the food chain are detected. Created in 1979, the RASFF enables information to be efficiently shared among its members (national food safety authorities of EU member states, European Commission, EFSA, ESA, Norway, Liechtenstein, Iceland and Switzerland) and provides a 24-hour service to ensure that notifications are sent, received and answered collectively and efficiently. As a result of a query we made in the public

---

[5] https://ec.europa.eu/food/safety/rasff_en

register of reports (reachable through this link[6]), we were able to find 47 reports alerting the presence of DMAA mainly in US-produced food supplements during the previous 2 years. This could have occurred as a result of a cross-contamination during the production/processing phase of one of the active ingredients contained in the supplement or, on the other hand, as an intentional adulteration act by the American manufacturer. It is undeniable that the presence of a stimulant increases the energizing effect of the supplement and can therefore increase its popularity among consumers, particularly those who practice strenuous sports activities. Anyone who is familiar with online fora and social networks for athletes or fitness enthusiasts knows that the best advertising for these products are consumer reviews, especially if they are specialists in the field such as personal trainers or famous athletes/body builders. It was not surprising to find out that the US manufacturer under our investigation had already been reported on the RASFF in 2012 by the Spanish authorities as a result of an official test over another food supplement sampled in commerce, which received a warning for "unauthorised substance 1,3 dimethyl-amylamine (DMAA) in food supplement from the United States, via the Netherlands". Also similar to our case, the content of DMAA was not declared among the ingredients. Therefore, if it could not be established beyond reasonable doubt that the manufacturer consciously added DMAA, somehow the substance continued to enter into the production process (illegally because it is also banned in the United States and was not declared on the label). To solve the case, Carabinieri had to work in partnership with the Office of Criminal Investigation of the US FDA of the District of Los Angeles (US FDA—OCI) with jurisdiction over Southern California. While carrying out a joint investigation, we found out that the FDA, in the framework of its regulatory function, had also identified DMAA as an ingredient illegally contained in some food supplements often advertised as a "natural" stimulant. DMAA, especially in combination with other ingredients such as caffeine, was considered a risk to the health of consumers because it could raise blood pressure and cause cardiovascular problems like shortness of breath and sense of tightness in the chest as well as heart attacks. Food supplements containing DMAA were considered illegal, and the FDA was doing its best to take these products away from the market. In 2012, the FDA sent warning letters to the companies notifying them that the products with DMAA had to be withdrawn from the market or reformulated to eliminate this substance. Most of the notified companies had complied but obviously not all of them did.[7] The US website where the Italian athlete had purchased the supplement for the first time had been previously sentenced to pay a fine of seven million US dollars by an American state court for selling supplements containing anabolic steroids undeclared on the label.

Over the years, Carabinieri for Health Protection HQ and Nucleo Antisofisticazioni (NAS) faced many other cases like the ones described in this chapter, just as the

---

[6] https://webgate.ec.europa.eu/rasff-window/portal/?event=searchForm&cleanSearch=1

[7] See also: https://www.fda.gov/food/dietary-supplement-products-ingredients/dmaa-products-marketed-dietary-supplements

volume of illicit products circulating in the world every day continues to increase. We were particularly challenged by the proliferation of NPS, an emerging market linked predominantly to drug consumption in a recreational rather than a sport-related context. However, both respond to the same logic that I mentioned at the beginning of this chapter. In the case of NPS, the creativity of the "drug designers" is far more enhanced as, in most of the cases, there are no barriers imposed by the anti-doping test to pass.

Operations against such an illicit commerce helped to raise the level of social alarm. During a 3-year-long and astonishing investigation called "Flying Dutchman",[8] carried out by the Operations Department of Carabinieri for Health Protection HQ in Rome and concerning an illicit trafficking of "NPS" (mainly synthetic cathinones) from the Netherlands, 22 people were arrested, and 200 shipments with a total of 3.2 kg of NPS were seized, with a market value of about €700,000, as well as some "classic" narcotics (cocaine, marijuana and hashish). This demonstrates the proximity of distribution channels and networks between these substances. Raw materials used for production of NPS, which since 2010 caused dozens of deaths and severe intoxications in consumers throughout Europe (50 cases were identified in Italy alone), were mainly imported from China and packaged in the Netherlands. Final products were advertised online via fora and dedicated websites and sold as "pure", "uncut" powders. They reached Italy by express courier or postal service from the Netherlands, Spain, England, Germany and the Philippines. Among the seized substances, some of which have not yet been included in the forbidden narcotics list, the very dangerous 6-APB—chemical name 6-(2-aminopropyl) benzofuran—also known as "Benzofury", which had caused many deaths in Sweden, was identified.

In conclusion, it is clear that the phenomenon described in this chapter cannot be solved by the action of law enforcement alone. In my opinion, it is necessary to create a strong common alliance among science, education and law enforcement authorities; otherwise, the "good guys" could easily lose the game. Not only do police forces need new laws and investigative instruments to eradicate the related illicit business controlled by Organized Transnational Crime, but their action also must be supported by more effective and harmonized legal frameworks at the international level. PED-related illicit businesses operate across countries, and it's very difficult—and sometimes impossible—to contrast them effectively, if what is illegal in one state is lawful in many others or if there is no common and shared awareness of the seriousness of the issue. We all together have to persuade people, and especially young people, to say "no!" to those who profit from pushing them into the abyss of addiction and turning them into slaves of the "fake chemical paradise".

---

[8] See also: http://www.salute.gov.it/portale/news/p3_2_1_2_1.jsp?lingua=italiano&menu=notizie&p=nas&id=593

The Performance Enhanced: Clinical Relationships Between Performance- and Image-Enhancing Drugs, Physical Exercise and Mental Disorders

Pierluigi Simonato, Angela Scoppettone, Francesco Saverio Bersani, and Silvia Rossato

Introduction

The use of performance- and/or image-enhancing drugs (PIEDs) has grown exponentially over the last decades [1, 2]. The concept of PIEDs includes a variety of substances used with the aim of enhancing human skills, such as muscles' structure and function, body image, cognitive functioning and sexual and social behaviours [1, 3, 4]. Prescription medicines, certain nutraceutical supplements and illicit substances may be considered as PIEDs to the extent that they are used without medical indications, can lead to addiction and/or to adverse health effects and are taken by users in order to increase their own skills and abilities [5, 6]. Several factors play a role in the increased use of PIEDs, including (i) a social drive towards achieving unrealistic models of bodily perfection, (ii) inappropriate legislative and regulatory systems, which may not adequately address the rapid spread of novel forms of psychoactive substances, (iii) the emergence of low-cost pharmaceutical manufacturing capacity in certain countries, which can provide chemicals at affordable prices, and (iv) globalisation and the Internet, which facilitate the international trade of substances [1]. At the psychiatric level, attention is usually paid to the use of "traditional" substances (e.g. heroin, cocaine, cannabis, alcohol), while the use of novel

P. Simonato (✉)
Department of Clinical, Pharmaceutical and Biological Sciences, School of Life and Medical Science, University of Hertfordshire, Hatfield, Hertfordshire, UK

Dual Diagnosis Unit, Clinica Parco dei Tigli, Padua, Italy
e-mail: pierluigi.simonato@gmail.com

A. Scoppettone · S. Rossato
Dual Diagnosis Unit, Clinica Parco dei Tigli, Padua, Italy

F. S. Bersani
Department of Human Neurosciences, Sapienza University of Rome, Rome, Italy

© The Author(s), under exclusive license to Springer Nature Switzerland AG 2022
O. Rabin, O. Corazza (eds.), *Emerging Drugs in Sport*,
https://doi.org/10.1007/978-3-030-79293-0_11

psychoactive substances (NPSs) and PIEDs is often underestimated [7]. However, data suggest that NPSs and PIEDs may lead to psychopathological symptoms and may play a role in the etiopathophysiology of certain mental illnesses [3, 6, 8, 9]. Furthermore, different psychopathological constructs such as eating disorders, intended as "disturbed attitudes towards weight, body shape and eating" [10]), exercise addiction (i.e., attitudes towards exercise characterised by tolerance, withdrawal, lack of control, intention effect, reduction in other activities, continuance [11]), body dysmorphic disorder (BDD), a mental disorder characterised by a "distressing or impairing preoccupation with imagined or slight defects in appearance" [12], body dissatisfaction (i.e., "negative thoughts and feelings about one's body" [13]) and muscle dysmorphia (MD, a "pathologic preoccupation with muscularity and leanness" [14]) may have a link with the use of PIEDs and with physical exercise. In this chapter we present case reports showing connections between mental disorders, certain sport-related habits, substance addictions, behavioural addictions and use of PIEDs.

Case Reports

The patients described here were recently admitted to the Dual Diagnosis Unit of the "Casa di Cura Parco dei Tigli" (www.parcotigli.it). The Parco dei Tigli Clinic is located in Padua, Italy, and offers a unit specialised in the assessment and treatment of patients with comorbid psychiatric disorders and substance use, with special attention to NPSs and PIEDs. The clinical team includes medical doctors (with specialisations in psychiatry, toxicology and internal medicine), psychologists and nurses, providing a high specialised integrated multidisciplinary care. Hospitalisation usually lasts 30 days, during which all patients (i) follow a detoxification programme and undergo specific pharmacological treatments, (ii) receive comprehensive psychiatric and psychological evaluations, (iii) participate in rehabilitation programmes with individual and group cognitive-behavioural psychotherapy focused on addiction, and (iv) are involved in psychomotricity and art therapy programmes. The clinical team works in collaboration with addiction and mental health services located in all Italian regions.

Case 1

Arrival at Our Unit

The patient arrived at our unit at the age of 33 years, with a stimulant use disorder (cocaine) in the absence of a history of previous psychiatric disorders. He was clinically followed by the local addiction service; before admission he privately consulted a psychiatrist who prescribed him valproic acid (300 mg/day) and alprazolam.

Anamnestic Information

There were no major medical conditions. The patient referred that recreational use of substances (cannabis, alcohol, MDMA [3,4-methylenedioxyamphetamine], LSD [lysergic acid diethylamide] and ketamine) began at age of 15; the use of substances gradually increased until he was 20 years old, and at this age he started using cocaine (insufflated and smoked).

Assessment, Intervention and Treatment

During hospitalisation he underwent various assessment tests (Addiction Severity Index [ASI], Symptom Checklist-90-R [SCL-90], Beck Depression Inventory [BDI-II], Alcohol Use Disorders Identification Test [AUDIT], Structured Clinical Interview for DSM-5 [SCID-5-PD] and MMPI-2 [Minnesota Multiphasic Personality Inventory]), and he followed the aforementioned pharmacological and rehabilitation programmes. At the end of hospitalisation, his treatment was with vortioxetine (20 mg/day) and trazodone (150 mg/day). During this hospitalisation certain features were identified, including (i) an important role of physical training in the patient's daily life, which made him at risk of exercise addiction, (ii) the presence of BDD, diagnosed according to the criteria of *Diagnostic and Statistical Manual of Mental Disorders, 5th Edition* (DSM-5) [15] and (iii) the use of PIEDs, mainly supplements and steroids, without any kind of medical supervision.

About Physical Exercise, BDD and Use of PIEDs

BDD is a mental disorder characterised by a "distressing or impairing preoccupation with imagined or slight defects in appearance" [12]. This disorder causes severe emotional distress and difficulties in daily functioning; intrusive thoughts about the perfect body may occur for several hours a day and may be followed by repetitive behaviours; the DSM-5 mentions this condition in the section of obsessive-compulsive and related disorders [15]. In this case report, the patient had serious concerns regarding the appearance of his body: the first concern was to not be tall enough (he was 160 cm), and the second was to not be sufficiently muscular (this idea first emerged in response to bullying problems during the adolescence that persisted into adulthood). The concern of not being sufficiently muscular is identified by DSM-5 as MD, a specification of BDD [15]. Evidence from studies on the topic raises the possibility that BDD and/or MD is common among body-building athletes [16–19]. In the present case, the patient began increasing exercise and the use of PIEDs in order to pursuit muscle-related body image ideals: at the age of 15, he began practicing high-intensity sports (including boxing, mixed martial arts and lastly body-building), although he never reached professional levels. At the time of hospitalisation, he trained four to five times a week for 1–2 h. On the one hand, the family members of the patient considered his sport activity a "safe" phenomenon as it kept the patient away from cocaine-related environments, but on the other hand, they identified it as a core problem (patient's father once said: "I will know that my son will be healed when he removes the mirror from his wardrobe"). At the time of hospitalisation, the patient took several PIED products, including:

- Supplements (e.g., proteins, amino acids and creatine), a product containing niacin, citrulline, red pepper extract, hawthorn extract, pterostilbene, pomegranate fruit, grape seed extract, trans-resveratrol, black pepper extract and creatine. He used this product very often, three tablets a day for 2 months; he described it as an effective pre-workout product.
- Anabolic androgenic steroids (AAS): after a period of intense use of cocaine, he perceived himself "skinny" and started using steroids in order to increase his muscle mass. He started using testosterone propionate, stanozolol and nandrolone with so-called "cycling", "stacking" and "pyramiding" methods [20]. The patient specified that he felt adequately informed about the use of such substances (he mentioned that he had not received medical supervision but rather that he had received information from his personal trainer), that he underwent blood tests every 3 months to check his liver functioning and that he never experienced any side effects.

Overall, cases like this, in which intense physical exercise and the use of PIEDs are at least partially a consequence of mental disturbances related to body image, contribute to raise awareness of the potential reciprocal connections between apparently distant phenomena such as BDD, MD, use of stimulants, use of PIEDs without medical supervision and certain forms of physical exercise.

Case 2

Arrival at Our Unit

The patient was a 32-year-old man who was admitted to our dual diagnosis unit (30-day programme). He complained of stimulants and alcohol use disorders associated with mood disturbances.

Anamnestic Information

The patient was described by his family as a hyperactive child but without any specific psychological or psychiatric diagnosis and without clinical follow-ups during childhood. At the age of 12, he started consuming alcohol, and then, at the age of 15, he started using cannabis recreationally. At the age of 18, he increased his consumption of alcohol and cannabis, and he also occasionally took MDMA and ketamine. He stopped using cannabis at the age of 19 years, and, at the same age, he started using cocaine (insufflated). At the age of 29, he started to be clinically followed at the local addiction service. The patient worked as a financial broker as well as a manager in a fitness-related business and as a personal trainer at a gym.

Assessment, Intervention and Treatment

During the hospitalisation the patient underwent several assessment tests (ASI, SCL-90, BDI-II, SCID-5-PD, AUDIT) and followed the aforementioned pharmacological and rehabilitation programmes. He was diagnosed as follows: narcissistic personality disorder, stimulant and alcohol use disorders and unspecified bipolar disorder. The presence of training habits was observed in the patient's routine (four to five times a week, for 1–2 h). At the end of the hospitalisation, his treatment was with aripiprazole 15 mg/day.

Physical Exercise and Use of PIEDs

The patient has been involved in intense sports activity since childhood: at the age of 3, he started playing soccer, basketball, karate and skiing. At the age of 5, he already practiced skiing and karate at competitive levels. Until the age of 15, he kept practicing karate and skiing as well as other sports (basketball, tennis and soccer); during the summer he used to spend 3 months performing intensive workouts. When he was 15, he stopped playing sports at competitive levels, but he continued to train and to practice various activities (including mixed martial arts). At the age of 29, he started to practice at the gym at increasing levels (three to four workouts per week, 1–2 h/day). During hospitalisation, the patient described his daily use of various supplements, and he insisted on taking them. He claimed that a proper supplementation and a balanced diet were important to him and that he used to recommend specific products to other gym customers. He reportedly used to select the products in absence of medical supervision choosing the brand according with the "chemical purity". These are some of the products he mentioned:

- Proteins in powder form, 30 g at a time. He considered them useful for post-workout and for sleep.
- Glutamine in powder form: he mixed 5 g with 200 mL of water and took it once a day, during the day or after physical activity.
- Conjugated linoleic acid, three capsules/day: he used it to burn fat.
- Branched-chain amino acids in powder: he mixed 5.5 g with 150 mL of water that he consumed once a day before or right after training or competition; he said

that such products can be taken five times a day with an action on muscle regeneration and mental performances.

- Capsule products containing l-tyrosine, green tea, cocoa seeds, theobromine, bitter orange fruit, synephrine, caffeine; he took two capsules/day, preferably before meals, and he reportedly experienced strong effects on mood along with some physical side effects (mainly gastrointestinal).
- Acetyl l-carnitine: he suggested to use one tablet in the morning, two tablets pre-workout and one tablet in the evening; he said that such substance can provide a "sprint" effect on physical activity.
- Phosphatidylserine one capsule/day; he used such substance in order to achieve improved neuronal transmission level.
- Creatine monohydrate in powder form, 3.5 g before workout; he reported a good effect on repetitive, high-intensity and short-duration activities.

Overall, cases like this, among other things, raise awareness of individuals who use several PIED products and act as information and tip providers on their use to other people in the absence of appropriate education in the field. Furthermore, the described patient had disorders related to personality, mood and addiction (i.e., he had the DSM-defined diagnoses of narcissistic personality disorder, stimulant and alcohol use disorders, unspecified bipolar disorder) associated with extensive use of PIEDs which, therefore, (i) can be at least partially considered as a consequence of his psychopathological disturbances and (ii) may have played a role in the clinical worsening of such psychopathological disturbances. It is known, in fact, that individuals with bipolar disorder can experience increased energy, increased activity, increased impulsivity and increased involvement in potentially harmful circumstances [15], with such symptoms potentially being causally related to increased misuse of substances; furthermore, studies have observed that several exogenous substances can worsen or exacerbate severe psychopathological episodes related to bipolar disorder, as well as complicate the overall course of the disease [3–8–21].

Case 3

Arrival at Our Unit

The patient arrived at our unit at the age of 25 with a previous diagnosis of bipolar disorder and cocaine use disorder; he was undergoing psychiatric pharmacotherapy based on valproic acid, duloxetine and olanzapine.

Anamnestic Information

He reported having experienced psychological disturbances since the age of 13. Around that time, he developed a form of body dissatisfaction, and he began stealing and using various products (including supplements, AAS, sexual enhancers and antidepressants). All compounds were stolen from a pharmacy where he occasionally worked as warehouseman and were used with the aim of improving his own appearance and performance. The patient also used to undergo intense physical activity at the gym (three to four workouts per week). At the age of 19, he started using cocaine, and, later, he occasionally used cannabis, LSD and ketamine. When his thefts were discovered, he got banned from the pharmacy, which lead him to develop severe episodes of mood disturbances. In the months preceding the arrival at our unit, he began experiencing persistent auditory hallucinations.

Assessment, Intervention and Treatment

During hospitalisation the patient underwent several assessment tests (ASI, SCL-90, BDI-II, SCID-5-PD, AUDIT) and followed the aforementioned pharmacological and rehabilitation programmes. He was diagnosed as follows: BDD, narcissistic and antisocial personality disorders, cocaine use disorder, unspecified bipolar disorder and unspecified psychotic disorder. At the end of hospitalisation, his treatment was with aripiprazole 15 mg/day, valproic acid 800 mg/day and asenapine 15 mg/day.

Use of PIEDs

The following products have reportedly been used by the patient without medical supervision:

- Arginine, cysteine and glutathione (the first products he took).
- Vitamins (including vitamins C, E, B6, B1, folate).
- Carnitine powders.
- T4 thyroid hormone: he used this compound with a maximum dosage of 150 mcg in order to lose weight.
- Tyrosine: he used this compound to "increase the blood levels of T4".
- AAS: he started using AAS (including testosterone) as the amino acids he previously consumed did not build his body enough; he searched online the way to use AAS and applied "cycling" and "pyramiding" methods [20]. The substances reportedly had both physical and psychological effects (they induced good mood in the short term and dysphoria in the long term).
- Human growth hormone (hGH).
- Ornithine was used in order to increase the levels of GH.

- Sexual enhancers (tadalafil, sildenafil, vardenafil) were used from the age of 16.
- Antidepressants (fluoxetine, clomipramine, paroxetine) were used to obtain delayed ejaculation.
- Barbiturates.

Overall, cases like this raise awareness on, among other things, subjects who undergo intense physical activity and use PIEDs in the context of multiple psychiatric diagnoses. The described case highlights how the unidentified condition of bodily dissatisfaction at a young age can contribute to lead to the uncontrolled use of PIEDs as well as to the emergence of full mental disorders. Furthermore, it is relevant to observe that certain environmental circumstances, in addition to individual features, may increase the risk of substance misuse: the described patient worked in a pharmacy, which made it easy for him to use PIEDs and difficult to control such use. This is consistent with evidence suggesting that certain professionals (e.g., health professionals working in the field of anaesthesiology) are at increased risk of drug misuse due to easy access to psychoactive agents [6–22].

Conclusion

The described cases suggest that special attention should be paid to the complex reciprocal relationships linking mental disorders, certain sport-related habits, substance addictions, behavioural addictions and use of PIEDs. From a clinical point of view, mental health professionals nowadays often face multifaceted circumstances in which novel compounds (e.g., PIEDs) and novel forms of behavioural addictions interact with pre-existing biological, psychological and social vulnerability factors leading to psychopathological manifestations. Dysfunctional forms of physical activity may play a role in this complex phenomenon, which deserves specific consideration. We believe that future studies aimed at developing a more substantial set of empirical and epidemiological data on the topic should be strongly encouraged and that protocols aimed at increasing knowledge on the field among athletes, professionals working with athletes and healthcare providers should be implemented in order to develop more targeted interventions for at-risk individuals.

References

1. McVeigh J, Evans-Brown M, Bellis MA (2012) Human enhancement drugs and the pursuit of perfection. Adicciones 24:185–190
2. Rowe R, Berger I, Copeland J (2016) No pain, no gainz? Performance and image enhancing drugs, health effects and information seeking. Drugs: Education, Prevention and Policy, pp 1-9
3. Bersani FS et al (2015) Adverse Psychiatric Effects Associated with Herbal Weight-Loss Products. Biomed Res Int 2015:120679
4. Napoletano F et al (2020) The Psychonauts' World of Cognitive Enhancers. Front Psychiatry 11:546796
5. Corazza O et al (2014) "Spice," "kryptonite," "black mamba": an overview of brand names and marketing strategies of novel psychoactive substances on the web. J Psychoactive Drugs 46:287–294
6. Bersani FS, Imperatori C (2018) Misuse, recreational use, and addiction in relation to prescription medicines. In: Corazza O, Roman-Urrestarazu A (eds) Handbook of Novel Psychoactive Substances. Routledge, New York
7. Simonato P et al (2018) Novel psychoactive substances as a novel challenge for health professionals: results from an Italian survey. Hum Psychopharmacol 28:324–331
8. Schifano F, et al (2019) New emerging psychoactive substances and associated psychopathological consequences. Psychol Med 2019:1–13
9. Schifano F et al (2015) Novel psychoactive substances of interest for psychiatry. World Psychiatry 14:15–26
10. Treasure J, Duarte TA, Schmidt U (2020) Eating disorders. Lancet 395:14–20
11. Freimuth M, Moniz S, Kim SR (2011) Clarifying exercise addiction: differential diagnosis, co-occurring disorders, and phases of addiction. Int J Environ Res Public Health 8:4069–4081
12. Bjornsson AS, Didie ER, Phillips KA (2010) Body dysmorphic disorder. Dialogues Clin Neurosci 12:221–232
13. Quittkat HL et al (2019) Body dissatisfaction, importance of appearance, and body appreciation in men and women over the lifespan. Front Psychiatry 10:864
14. Leone JE, Sedory EJ, Gray KA (2005) Recognition and treatment of muscle dysmorphia and related body image disorders. J Athl Train 40:352
15. American Psychiatric Association (2013) Diagnostic and statistical manual of mental disorders, 5th edn. American Psychiatric Publishing
16. Mosley PE (2009) Bigorexia: bodybuilding and muscle dysmorphia. Eur Eat Disord Rev 17:191–198
17. Longobardi C et al (2017) Muscle dysmorphia and psychopathology: Findings from an Italian sample of male bodybuilders. Psychiatry Res 256:231–236
18. Cerea S et al (2018) Muscle dysmorphia and its associated psychological features in three groups of recreational athletes. Sci Rep 8:8877
19. Corazza O et al (2019) The emergence of Exercise Addiction, Body Dysmorphic Disorder, and other image-related psychopathological correlates in fitness settings: A cross sectional study. PLoS One 14:e0213060
20. NHS Website (2020) Anabolic steroid misuse. Available from: https://www.nhs.uk/conditions/anabolic-steroid-misuse/#:~:text=Do%20a%20combination%20of%20both,before%20starting%20the%20cycle%20again
21. Strakowski SM et al (2000) The impact of substance abuse on the course of bipolar disorder. Biol Psychiatry 48:477–485
22. Bryson EO, Silverstein JH (2008) Addiction and substance abuse in anesthesiology. Anesthesiology 109:905–917

Part IV
Winning at Any Cost: Doping Experiences of World-Class Athletes

Faster and Dirtier for Russia: The Story of Yuliya Stepanova

Yuliya Stepanova (née Rusanova)

Introduction

Yuliya Stepanova (née Rusanova) is a former world-class 800 m track runner for Russia, who competed in multiple world-level competitions. During her peak competitive years (2010–2014), she was part of an institutionalized doping programme established by officials for Russian athletes. In this chapter, she shares her insights on the doping programme she was exposed to while competing for Russia. It is a rare testimony providing the unique view of an athlete's approach to her love for running and her personal performance with the perspective on how this is integrated into a global doping system.

My Fight Against Doping in Russian Sports

"I love running, I love competing and I hope that my admittance of doping can somehow help the fight against doping and make athletics a better sport".

– Yuliya Stepanova (née Rusanova)

These are the words that I shared in my statement to the World Anti-Doping Agency (WADA) in 2013, when I decided to collaborate in the fight against doping and joined my husband, Vitaly Stepanov, in the fight against doping in Russian sports.

I would like to begin this chapter by apologizing about my doping past. Unfortunately, I cannot change it. As an athlete, an 800 m runner, I cheated. I now changed and want to help make sports cleaner.

Y. Stepanova (née Rusanova) (✉)
World Anti-Doping Agency (WADA), Montreal, QC, Canada
e-mail: Olivier.Rabin@wada-ama.org

© The Author(s), under exclusive license to Springer Nature Switzerland AG 2022
O. Rabin, O. Corazza (eds.), *Emerging Drugs in Sport*,
https://doi.org/10.1007/978-3-030-79293-0_12

When I was 14 years old, I watched the 2000 Olympics in Sydney, Australia. Like many people in the world, I watched it on TV. Seeing the Russian athletes in the competition made me feel very emotional. I looked at them as superior human beings, almost as gods. I was crying when they were losing and felt happiness when they were winning. I felt a lot of respect for our country and the people who compete in the Olympic Games. Back then, I could not imagine that one day I would also represent Russia in international competitions. I was convinced that to be a professional athlete, you would need to train since your childhood. I was already 14 and I felt I could only watch and admire these "athletic heroes".

At the age of 17, I went to a college in my hometown Kursk in Russia, and like many teenagers in my physical education class, I had to pass a standard running test. I always did better than most of my classmates. I was faster. During a running competition between colleges, a couple of students and I were chosen to compete for our college. Although I came in third, I did not receive a medal. Only the winner received the medal. This pushed me to find a coach, to train, with the aim to win the same competition the following year. It was when my sports career started.

I was sure that after a year of supervised and intensive training, I could get a medal and then quit. But it did not turn out to be like that. I started to like training. I was getting faster and faster. Despite the college competition that I was training for was cancelled that year, I still was able to become one of the top 3 runners in my city and region. I started going to national competitions, but I was always far away from medalling. The girls from my age group were running a lot faster than me. I knew I could not compete with them because I had not trained enough yet. About the same time, my running friends started telling me that they heard those girls were running so fast not because they were more talented, or because they trained more, but apparently because they were taking some prohibited pills that they got from their coaches.

After training for another 3 years and continuing to lose at national competitions, I decided to ask my coach for those pills. He thought it was too early for me as my level of competition did not require the use of pills. I followed his advice, and for the first 2 years I did not take any medicine or dietary supplement at all. At my third year, I started taking multivitamins, extra iron, vitamin B12, inosine, ascorbic acid, carnitine, actovegin, mildronate, potassium orotate and glucose. Some of those medications were injected by my coach.

In March 2006, I got very sick and was diagnosed with tuberculosis. Even though many people around me were telling me that I will not be able to run again, I kept dreaming that I will get healthy and be able to run again. I just loved running so much that I could not imagine my life without it. I felt lucky. My doctor turned out to be a very good man and supported and promised me that I would have been able to run again.

When I came out from hospital, I slowly started running again and, during the first 6 months or so, I was only taking the pills that were prescribed to recover from tuberculosis. The following Winter I was offered to take testosterone propionate to boost my performance. I was told to take a 2 mL ampoule divided in seven equal parts and to inject subcutaneously every third day. I was also informed that the substance was detectable by anti-doping tests for 5 days after the last administration. However, I only became aware in 2011 that testosterone injections are good only when the ampoule was freshly opened, and there was no point in dividing the ampoule in seven parts as only the first fraction was actually efficacious, and also that testosterone is used for intramuscular injection only, among other things that turned out to be incorrect and put my health at risk. It also became harder to tell at that point of my career whether my result was getting better because I trained more or because I used some medicine or if it was a placebo effect, as I knew I was taking some medicine and therefore I was running much faster. Before doing testosterone injections wrongly, my personal record in 800m was 2:13; after injections it lowered to 2:08.47.

In Summer 2007, I was given for the first time dehydrochloromethyltestosterone pills (oral Turinabol) and erythropoietin (EPO) injections. My personal record lowered to 2:03.47 in 800 m. I was seventh in the Nationals for my age group. Dehydrochloromethyltestosterone was taken daily for 15 days in May 2007. I did EPO injections (1000 IU) subcutaneously every other day in early June. As I was concerned with doping controls, the whole preparation (training and intake of prohibited substances) was carefully calculated in such a way that I was clean while competing in the National Championships. In Winter 2008, I took dehydrochloromethyltestosterone pills every day in two cycles between mid-October and end of December. My EPO injections started in January. I did testosterone injections the same way as during the previous Winter. I also took non-prohibited substances. My personal record lowered to 2.01.96. I won the National Championships in the 20- to 23-year-old age group and became a member of the Russian National Team.

The following few seasons, my preparation did not change much. I took new anabolic steroids such as oxandrolone and trenbolone. The more I trained, the more pharmacological help my body needed to boost my performance. Because of the drugs, my muscles were sometimes very stiff and I just could not run. Sometimes, also, my blood was getting very thick. Despite this, I had to carry on training as I thought that all athletes were going through the same side effects. Finally, by the time I was competing at the National Championships without taking anything prohibited, my body and my muscles were beginning to act normally, and I was able to compete well. I discovered later that most athletes did not go through the same problems as I did, but my coach was not knowledgeable enough about the best ways to avoid such problems. I continued my training while taking prohibited substances, but by the time I was competing again at the National Championships I was clean and I never failed an anti-doping test during a competition. Being from the Kursk region, I could only dream about winning and qualifying for European or World Championships. I was taking the prohibited substances just as others were doing, but I still could not win.

Everything became clearer when national head coaches and managers finally noticed my results and decided to take me under their wing. During the 2010 Summer National Championships, athletes were competing to qualify for the European Championships. Since Mariya Savinova already qualified, only two other 800m runners could qualify. I was running in the final and finished third, losing by just 0.01 second to Svetlana Klyuka. It was only then that I finally started to be taken seriously. About a month before the National Championships, I was asked to compete at European Athletics Outdoor Classic Meeting "Znamensky Memorial" near Moscow, and some cash was paid in order to avoid my doping test. I was also given the opportunity to be trained for the 2011 Winter season, while the doping experimentation continued with other pharmacological preparations designed to boost athletic and sport performances that I was asked to take. These included a combination of dehydrochloromethyltestosterone and oxandrolone, which was detectable for about 35 days. I was advised to start with a pill per day and eventually increase to 1.5 pills. I took oxandrolone for several days in December 2010 before deciding to go for a lower dosage. My past doping at high dosages already had an impact on my tense muscles, and my body could not take it any longer. I also knew I had to stay clean when competing at the European Indoor Championships.

When I came back from Portugal training camp in December, I was asked to do three injections (1/2 ampoule each) of testosterone. I thought that this was just way too much for me, but since I always listened to my coach, I did as he said. I was also given oxandrolone for 3 weeks. It was from mid-January that I was given low doses of EPO each day. I was informed to take iron sucrose with EPO. My blood results on 19.01.2011 were Hb, 156; Ht, 47%; Ret, 0,25; Fe, 11,2. Later my values were even higher. On February 6 while running 600m at IAAF Permit Meeting "Russian Winter" in Moscow, I was very close to breaking a world record—1:24.04. Later that evening, I was asked to do an ampoule of testosterone and not to do any hard workouts for 3 days as I could tear my muscles. I also did more EPO injections early in February. My blood results on 11.02.2011 were Hb, 165; Ht, 50%.

On February 16 and 17, I competed at the Russian National Indoor Championships. I won my heat with the time 1:59.98 and won the final with the time 1:58.14. After the final, I was tested by the Russian Anti-Doping Agency (RUSADA). Once I exited the doping control station, I sent an SMS with the code number of my sample to my coaches. I still have today all the pink duplicates of my doping control forms. Like many others that were preparing directly for the European Indoor Championships, my sample was clean. One week before the European Championships, RUSADA tested us again. This is called "away" doping control. On February 25, 2011, my blood results were Hb, 164; Ht, 50%. As I realize now, those advising me on doping did not understand the whole concept of blood passport and kept preparing people the old way as their main goal was to make sure that the sample was clean by certain dates.

In France on March 3, 2011, I gave blood for my blood passport for the first time. My results were Hb, 161; Ht, 48.5%, Re, 0.31; Off-score, 127.6. Those were abnormal results, and I probably could have been or should have been sanctioned then. But I continued competing. Preparing for the Summer 2011 was similar to the Winter 2011. I was doing everything that I was told to do: oxandrolone, EPO, competing dirty at the Russian National Championships. I ended up finishing third at the European Championships, and this generated a lot of disappointment. So, in the Summer of 2011, I was competing "dirty" again at the Nationals, and I arrived second in the final—1:56.99—losing by a few hundredths of a second to Savinova.

During the Summer training, I realized fewer people were willing to train me. I suspected this was because of my husband Vitaly. He used to work at the Russian Anti-Doping Agency (RUSADA) from 2008 to 2011 and really tried fighting doping and many people including those working with me. Vitaly did not want to be a part of the corrupt doping system.

When I first started training, athletes used much stronger steroids, sometimes without even knowing it. In general, Russian coaches are preparing athletes the same way as they did back in the 1980s and the 1990s as they do not know any other way! The faster they run, the more they are getting paid. I was lucky that my coach did not hide from me what I was taking and did not really push me with running faster when I just started training. In the Spring of 2012, I was injured at a training camp in Portugal and was not able to compete during the whole summer season. As I continued training, the injury got worse during the next training camp in Kyrgyzstan. I was hoping that the pain would disappear and I would be able to compete in the Russian National Athletics Championships in order to qualify for the 2012 Summer Olympic Games in London.

When I came back home to Russia, I understood that I could not continue to run. I felt pain even when walking. My coach kept pushing for a faster recovery, and I was advised to do infusions with creatinolfosfate sodium and tolperisone. I knew some cases in Russia where athletes became very sick because of those infusions, and hospital care was required to save them. I did not have any allergies, and I thought that there was no reason for me to be concerned. First, I infused creatinolfosfate sodium and then tolperisone. Shortly after, my heart rate started to increase rapidly. My heart was beating stronger and stronger with every second. I was scared that my heart would simply stop beating in the end. I asked Vitaly to call an ambulance and my coach. I thought that I would die. The ambulance came quickly, and they injected something to get my heart rate down. My heart had withstood the effects of these drugs and I stayed alive.

After this incident I started being afraid of injections and infusions on my own. Is the Olympic medal worth taking all these risks? Right before the 2012 Olympic Games, I decided to change my coach but faced some opposition as I was considered to be a very problematic person, with a husband who "did not fit in the system".

Right after the Olympic Games, I started training with a new coach. We started having discussions about pharmacological preparation. He did not change much of what I was advised to use but was very surprised that I did not use any human growth hormone. He considered that it could be a big plus in the future as I still had room for improvement. In November 2012, when I was supposed to start taking oxandrolone and methenolone tablets, it turned out that my blood passport results were not considered normal and that I could be sanctioned sooner or later.

I was advised that the best way for female athletes to avoid this was disqualification for being pregnant. Under the Russian law, in fact, a pregnant woman or a mother with a small child cannot be fired. So, it means that if I was able to become pregnant fast enough, then I could probably still receive salaries even if I was sanctioned and be able to come back in 2 years, just in time for the main international events, including the 2016 Summer Olympic Games in Rio de Janeiro, Brazil.

However, when I found out about my sanction, the world that I imagined for myself collapsed in front of my eyes. It was hard for me to realize that I was the only one paying for this, while those behind such a corrupted system continued to prepare athletes the same way. Why should I be punished, when they are not? I thought that my sports career was over and people will be angry at me. However, people around me were not angry, and at the end they supported me.

I understand that by telling my story I might not be able to change anything in a better direction. Probably for a good change, many, many years must go by, and my confession will not change a well-organized doping system of preparing athletes.

In 2013, I wrote to WADA that my husband Vitaly and I would love to make athletes cleaner and we were willing to do anything to try to make a change in a better direction. I felt that maybe the most that I could do was to share my story with others. Vitaly and I married in October 2009. Our marriage was terrible until February 2013. I have no explanation how we managed to stay together through that difficult time. Since February 2013, Vitaly and I have a goal that unites us. We hope to make sports cleaner. This goal made our marriage stronger and our relationship better.

I would like to end this chapter by apologizing again about my doping past. I am sorry. Unfortunately, I cannot change my past. I was in the Russian doping system, I used doping and now I am writing about it. I still bear the physiological and physical scars of doping. My health could be at risk. It has been almost 8 years since I started whistleblowing about the doping problems in Russia. I regret not speaking up sooner, but I am thankful to the WADA Code for giving athletes a second chance. Vitaly and I could never imagine that we would get this far in raising our concerns about the doping situation in Russia. We were not able to find much support inside of Russia, but we were happy to see that most Russian sports officials were not right. Not every country's goal is to cover up doping use by athletes of their own country. In fact, rules do matter, and ethics matters in sports.

Conclusion

It was the encounter with her now husband, Vitaly, that encouraged Yuliya to find the courage and the forces to go against the Russian doping system and ultimately decide to share information with WADA. The information and testimonies they jointly provided were not only essential in bringing first-line information to anti-doping authorities but also pivotal in the decision by such authorities to significantly modify world anti-doping rules, in particular giving WADA and other anti-doping organizations the legitimacy and capabilities to investigate doping cases and participate in field operations. As a result, two independent commissions were established by WADA to investigate doping in Russia. All conclusions led to expose the institutionalized doping programme in Russia and triggered major sanctions on several Russian athletes and officials, including the inability for the country to host international sport events or banning the presence of Russian officials at some major events, including Olympic Games or World championships. Yuliya's testimonies contributed to expose what is considered to be the biggest doping scandal in the history of sport. Today, Yuliya lives far from her motherland, had to give up on her Olympic dreams, is perceived as a traitor by some people she helped expose, but in the end followed her true love for sport, continues running and contributing to the protection of clean sport like few people did in the history of sport and as such should be seen as a true hero for the cause of clean sport. She may have never won an Olympic medal, but her contribution to sport goes far beyond and undoubtedly holds a place for her on the podium in the hall of fame for true sports fans.

Is It Worth Winning a Race If You Lose Yourself in the Process? An Interview with Olympic Champion Tyler Hamilton

Honor D. Townshend

Introduction

Tyler Hamilton is a former US pro-cyclist. His career spanned over a decade which saw him master some of the most notoriously difficult races in the sporting world. He won a Tour de France stage despite riding with a broken collarbone, he travelled the world competing, and he was lieutenant in what came to be cycling's most notorious team. Having won an Olympic gold medal, Tyler returned it after having tested positive for performance-enhancing drugs. He went on to release a book, *The Secret Race*, which won the William Hill Sports Book of the Year title in 2012. The book was a no-holds-barred exposé into the world of performance enhancement in cycling, and the fallout began. Now a financial advisor, sport coach and bike packer, who works keenly with multiple sclerosis (MS) charities in his spare time, Tyler has long left the drop-bar bikes of his cycling past behind him. Nearly a decade on from the release of his life-changing book, Honor Townshend talked with Tyler to discuss everything from his entry into the world of professional sport, his introductions to doping, reflections on this period of his life and what he has learned since.

Where Did Your Desire to Become an Athlete Come From?

I was a bit of an introvert and a bit quiet when I was young, so I would always say that I let my legs do the talking. Ever since I was a kid, I was really good at sports. I did fine to pretty well in school, but in sports, I was always at the top of my class.

H. D. Townshend (✉)
Department of Criminology, School of Law, University of Hertfordshire,
Hatfield, Hertfordshire, UK
e-mail: h.townshend@herts.ac.uk

Growing up, I played a lot of soccer and baseball. And I was fortunate to have gone to a school with a great ski programme, which led me to become a downhill ski racer. Ski racing gave me some good building blocks for the sport of cycling later, because ski racing required a lot of dedication. It also keeps your body and your legs in shape. My family was also extremely supportive. For them, it wasn't about results. For them, it was about doing your best and then congratulating your competitors afterwards. Hard work and dedication to your passions was the mantra I grew up with. Becoming a professional athlete happened kind of by accident. I was a downhill ski racer at the University of Colorado, and during my sophomore year, I broke my back while training with the Ski Team. When I got out of bed, they said I could ride a road bike to aid recovery. Being there in Boulder, Colorado, a huge cycling town, I was soon riding with some of the best riders in the world. So, lucky for me, and I got to learn from some of the best. But even though that kind of fell into my lap, I worked really hard at my ability. Cycling is a lot about suffering, and for whatever reason I had the ability to dig really deep for that, and so that was a huge asset. I became the collegiate National Champion in 1993, and eventually I left university to take the opportunity to ride with the United States National Team and travel all over the world. It was a steep learning curve, but I excelled at it pretty quickly. I was on the US National Team for 1 year and then went professional in 1995. Two years later, I was on the start line of the prestigious Tour de France. The transition to cycling professionally was exciting. My life changed really fast, and each year, it felt like I was taking big steps. Looking back, those were the most exciting years – being the underdog, proving people wrong and surprising people, including yourself. You don't really know enough to even worry about the future, so you just go out there and do your best. Because of the speed of it all, I didn't even set any specific achievement goals. It was only when I got up to the Tour de France level that I started to see where my talent was compared to the best cyclists in the world. That's when I started setting goals, or maybe other people started setting them for me. At that point, with coaches and managers around, I started to set the bar a little higher and putting pressure on myself.

When Did You First Become Aware of Doping Occurring in Your Sport?

In 1997, it was my third year of professional cycling. Up to that point, I had heard rumours about doping occurring in European teams at the highest levels, but it wasn't really spoken about. There were small signs though, like certain riders being handed white lunch bags after a race to take home with them. Later I learned that these bags were full of vitamins, injectable vitamins and some performance-enhancing drugs. I remember not getting one. Next, I started hearing people speaking about me, referring to me as "Pan Y Agua", a Spanish term meaning "bread and water". I figured out eventually that it was a comment that I wasn't using any PEDs – though eventually I got invited into that fraternity, so to speak.

Can You Explain the Events that Led Up to You Beginning to Dope Yourself?

Introduction to Doping

During the 1997 season, I had just finished a really hard week-long stage race in Spain. One of the team doctors came into my room, and we had what was my first open conversation about PEDs. I was told it was time to start taking better care of my body, to "start acting professionally", and I was handed like a little red testosterone pill. He was a well-respected doctor who had worked with big champions for years, and I was told it was for my health. For me, it was an honour just having him in my hotel room and talking to me, and so when I was told to "take this", I really didn't think about it. I just swallowed it. Instead, I thought about it later. That was just the start of my introduction into doping, and my crossover to the dark side. The doctor's presence as a medical professional, especially one so well-respected within the cycling community, had a big impact on my willingness to trust him. And there was also a feeling of not wanting to rock the boat and along with the fear of exclusion from opportunities due to not going with the flow. It was only after that moment when I thought about the potential consequences, both of the use itself, but just generally of not telling the truth, too. I was brought up to know the difference between right and wrong, and I knew what I was doing was wrong, which brought up a lot of internal conflict. But from that point on, there was a progression into other forms of doping. The next step was when they administered an injection of EPO [erythropoietin] during a night off mid-way through a race in order to increase my red blood cell count. In any kind of endurance sport, EPO is a real game changer with regard to performance and recovery, which is why it has been such a highly abused performance-enhancing drug, particularly in the sport of cycling. At the time, the presence of a needle made this feel like a very sinister step into my own involvement of doping. But over the years of cycling, this became somewhat normalized, and I accepted it as just a part of the life of a professional cyclist at the highest elite level. It was only a number of years later that I took an even further step into doping, which was through blood doping methods. This came up due to changes in testing for EPO by sport and anti-doping authorities, which led cycling teams to "re-evaluate" methods for the upcoming Tour de France. Methods like autologous blood doping, which involves the removal of some of your own blood, for it to then be re-injected into your body a few weeks later. It has a huge impact on your hematocrit levels almost immediately after transfusion, which dramatically increases your capacity to transport oxygen to your muscles and ultimately gives you a huge advantage in endurance sports.

Pressures to Engage in Doping

My introduction to doping was not something that I readily discussed with people outside of the cycling community and rarely within it too. Within the community, it was only upon my own involvement that I became privy to a lot of conversations about it. At that point though, I felt pressure from those already engaging in doping to continue doing so. I noticed an attitude that this was just the way things were done, so I should just get used to it and not complain. Although there was the presence of a few individuals on my team that I knew to not be doping, it was presumed that this was only because they were towards the end of their professional career at that level. I felt a certain amount of disappointment from them, but due to it not being an openly discussed activity, it was only in more recent years that I have spoken with and apologized to them for my part in it. When you're young, and unsure what the next step in life is going to be, that's sometimes when we make poor choices, and doping was mine.

Risks and Concerns

Although I naturally had concerns about the potential impacts of doping on my health, I was consistently reassured by team doctors that all the substances I was using were not going to impact on my health. The advice of older veteran teammates and team directors also added to a feeling of minimal risk regarding health and doping in general. The doctors justified the use of testosterone in particular to us, by saying that the levels of exertion we were doing meant that our natural testosterone levels were depleted. So, any use of testosterone was just to get us back to normal, "natural" levels and would actually help to avoid injuries and any other health risks caused by depleted natural hormone levels. If you hear this enough from team doctors, directors and teammates, you start to believe it. Because of that reassurance, my biggest concern about doping was getting caught, and the truth coming out. This became a pretty consistent worry throughout my career, as it felt like too big of a secret for it to not come out, which obviously it eventually did. Because I thought that everyone at the top level of the sport seemed to be doping, ethical considerations were less concerning. Right and wrong paled out of context when confronted with what seemed like an inevitable reality.

> "For a long time, keeping this secret made it feel as though I was living a double life and waiting to go back to my true self".

In 2004, When You Originally Tested Positive for Doping Supplements, You Denied that You Had Intentionally Used Any Substances. Why Did You Do This?

I was simply not ready to tell the truth. By that point in time, I had been doping for a long time, and I had no intention to stop. I did not see an end in sight to doping in cycling, and so I had resigned to the fact that this would be the process of my life until retirement. It was also a lot to deal with all at once. From being an Olympic champion to my cycling career being over in a matter of months, it is a lot to process and does not allow a lot of time for real reflection and thought. There were a lot of people I wanted to protect from the truth, too. Not only myself but a lot of ex-teammates, too. Despite no longer being on the US Postal Team, I knew that had I come out with the truth that eventually questions were going to be asked of me that would implicate dozens of others, and I was not ready to take that responsibility for others. There was a code of silence around doping within the sport, and I felt the external pressure from the community, as well as internally to "take one for the team". And for myself, I did not want to let down the support networks around me. My family, friends, even sponsors. So, I decided to fight it with everything I had. I was convinced that the truth would not do anybody any good. The longer that the lie went on, it felt like the truth was getting further away. It felt as though I was suffering in my own, self-made, personal prison and that I was 10 years too late to speak up. For a long time, I accepted that I was going to have to continue lying about this for the rest of my life, in order to avoid anyone else getting caught up in what I saw as "my problems".

Eventually though I was forced to tell the truth. I have since come to see being forced to tell the truth as a blessing in disguise. I was summoned in front of a federal grand jury, as part of the investigation into the US Postal Team, and Lance Armstrong, to give evidence and ended up doing so over the course of 7 h. The instant relief was like removing a 100 kg weight from my back, and it was only then that I realized that I had been lugging around that burden for years, even during the best years of my career. That relief gave me the confidence I needed to continue to tell the whole truth, even if the information testified in court was sealed. So, I came out, wrote a book and started to open up. It was an incredibly difficult process. But through the pain of reliving these experiences, I felt a huge sense of catharsis, and I began to feel proud. Not of what I was admitting to, but proud of the truth-telling process. There was a lot of fallout from doing this, but I was also surprised by the amount of forgiveness. I learned that it is never too late to tell the truth. Thinking retrospectively, I regret not telling the truth earlier. Speaking out sooner would have liberated me a long time ago, and I feel sorry for those who have not shared their truths yet. For sport more widely, cycling became the example of what can happen if you are not paying attention and not governing your sport well enough. Doping is not limited to just "bad people", and it is not limited to cycling. Difficult sports and lack of governance leads to cutting corners, and initially those corners might be on the correct side of the moral line, but eventually they have the propensity to dip into the grey zone, to that dark side of sport.

Was Your Personal Life Impacted Upon by Your Doping and Subsequent Testing Positive?

I had to lie to a lot of people, including close family and friends throughout. It's not an enjoyable position to be in and leaves you feeling isolated with the stress, which takes its toll.

> "When you're living a double life, your relationships with others suffer".

In cycling, and in many other sports, you're only as good as your last result. It doesn't matter if you've had big victories if those were a year ago. This means there's always something to worry about. Doping only adds to that. With the introduction of regular anti-doping controls and unannounced doping controls, you have the extra worry that a vial of blood being taken by a stranger has the potential to change your whole life. I was surprised how little support there was from within the cycling community after my positive test. It is at that point when you quickly realize who your true friends are, because many people no longer want to be associated with you. This, in combination with being scared of the truth and not being ready for the consequences, led to periods of depression. It was only once the truth found me again that I began to feel relaxed again, and that changed me and my life forever. It's easy to forget as an athlete that there's a lot of life to live after sport. You are lucky to be competing into your 30s, and there's a lot of life to live after that. So, if you are going to live a life of doping in sport, you have to be prepared to deal with the consequences and to deal with those lies.

Several Years Have Now Passed Since This Time in Your Life. Has It Had an Impact on Your View of Professional Sports?

I look at sports from a different viewpoint these days. I still love watching sports, but I do look at sports differently now. Now I know from the inside out about the amount of pressure, how people are willing to win at all costs; it changes your perspective. We, as a society, have set up sporting competitions in a way that only values first place and doesn't truly celebrate the success of competing. In a 150-person peloton, there are 149 losers. In each Olympics competition, there is only one gold medal. How does someone stay positive, maintain a sense of achievement and feel good about their performance if the be-all and end-all is first place? Cycling specifically is all about getting a competitive edge. Shaving seconds in a wind tunnel, gaining a few watts, boosting your Functional Threshold Power. This creates a culture that fosters pushing the envelope for competitive edge, and it sets the stage for an environment where some will do whatever it takes to win. We need to think about how we, as a society, can counter that.

> "An overemphasis on winning opens the floor to a no-holds-barred approach to performance enhancement. But at what cost? Is it worth winning a race if you lose yourself in the process?"

In cycling specifically, though, I do not believe cycling is completely clean now. I do hope it is doing a lot better today because of the truth finally coming out. My hope is that younger generations of cyclists and other sport professionals will be able to learn from the past and strive to make the sport a better place for all – a place that values sportsmanship and effort rather than that first-place title. Public view of cycling was hit negatively at first by the information about doping that has come out over the last decade. But it has also made people realize how hard the sport is, and so why some of these things were happening. And it has led to a lot of changes in the sport. Anti-doping has gotten a lot better in the years since, and loopholes are getting fewer. But they are still there. My hope is that one day any existing loopholes will be gone and it will be impossible to cheat. The best thing to have come out of the exposure of doping in cycling is that it has showed us all that we need to focus more on anti-doping, across all sports. We know now what could be repeated if we do not continue that focus, and nobody wants that. Overall, I think my view, and I hope society's view of cycling, has to look at the positives that came out of this. There is a cycling boom going on right now, and I am excited to see what it is going to look like. The sport is exciting to participate in, and it is exciting to watch. The team dynamics, the strategy and the required effort. I think that excitement is only growing.

In Your Opinion, Are There Any Ways in Which These Substances Could be Better Regulated in Your Sport and in General?

It's all about education. Educating athletes from a young age. People need to be more aware of the potential impact of doping and should know that it is something that might be presented to them – that they might get that visit to the hotel room from a team doctor like I did. And they need to be ready for it. I was not. Stories from me, some of my teammates or some of my competitors who all speak out against doping have to be the best way to educate people about the risks and what your life truly becomes if you cross that line. And further than that, teaching them the *right* way to do things, the *right* ways to train and compete properly. And showing them how to reveal their natural potential, legally and safely, that can help their performance. That might be things like getting extra rest, eating more of certain food types, working with a sport psychologist. Focusing on those micro-advantages that are legal and, importantly, ethical. It's a combination of educating people on the right way to do things, and the life they will lead if they dope, whether or not they ever get caught. Because it is just not worth it. I also believe that all sports and all governing bodies should work together to tackle doping in a more professional sport-wide approach. Because it still seems as though the testers are always a step or two behind the athletes and coaches. Though the line seems to be getting ever-closer, increased funding for anti-doping agencies and research will help to close that gap so that one day, we can watch sport, whether it's basketball, baseball, cycling or anything else, and believe in it, and in the athletes, 100 percent again.

What Would Your Advice be to Individuals Considering Using Illegal Performance-Enhancement Substances?

It is never worth it. If you dope during your career, you will deal with the heavy burden of lying to people you care about, always looking over your shoulder and worrying more about getting caught than winning. That's the point I got to. You will also have a long life to live after that career is over, and you will have to sit and reflect on your choices. Always listen to the right people in your life and think about the disappointment they would feel if you were caught. The key is to remember your core values, as a person and as an athlete. That way, you can live your life with a clear conscience. You can look in the mirror and know that you are doing your best at your sport, and you are doing it the right way. And you can know that your life is going to be a lot better without it.

Do You Regret Engaging in Doping?

Yes. Sometimes it has made me wish that I had never picked up a bike in the first place. I certainly wish I had not listened to that first team doctor, swallowed that first testosterone pill and entered that dark side of sport. But I have forgiven myself for it, and I have accepted what I did and take full responsibility for it. That forgiveness from yourself is an important step. And it is what has enabled me now to be able to comfortably share my story. Maybe it is a good thing that everything happened the way it did. I hope that it has contributed a small part towards helping professional sports to get on the right path. Had I turned my back on it, said no to doping and left professional sport, I would not be here today to share my story. So maybe I am supposed to be here, and maybe it all happened for a reason, and maybe that reason is to start that process of educating through the medium of my own experiences…who knows.

Conclusion

Despite the time that has passed, Tyler Hamilton has strived for nearly a decade to shed light on the inner complexities, issues and hidden dark side of professional cycling. His account is valuable, not only due to his lived experience as an ex-professional athlete but also due to his continued tireless efforts to maintain the conversation about performance-enhancement drug use in sports. His advice is clear throughout: it is not worth it, and his story stands to testify to that. The world of professional sports is an entity like no other. From Tyler's story it has only made clearer that in order to create a positive change, we must collectively work together, as athletes, fans, governing bodies and organizations, to re-address the narrative of sport. We must now strive as Tyler has to continue the conversation and to question our processes and the things we hold valuable. We must work together, to do better.

A Hammer Thrower's Journey with Doping: Being the Phoenix of My Own Life

Quentin Bigot

Introduction

Quentin Bigot started the life of an international athlete when he was only 16 years old. Today, 12 years later, he already had several 'sport lives'. He started as a 'promising young teenage athlete', and then just 5 years later, at the age of 21, he was excluded from his discipline and all competitions as a 'doped athlete' and more recently became a 'vice world champion' in hammer throwing. In this chapter, he shares with us the journey he had to face after he was caught with anabolic steroids in his body back in 2014, following a 2-year suspension period during which he went from complete rejection of sport to rebuilding his personal entourage with people of trust, including a new personal coach, and finally being on the podium again at a major competition but this time as a 'clean athlete'. This rare testimony is filled with personal reflections on his sport life with some strong messages for younger athletes who would consider embracing a similar career of international athlete.

My Story

To imagine even for one second that the problem of doping will one day be resolved is totally unproductive. Let me explain: men and women in today's and past society have always resorted to cheating, in all areas. I would even say that things are not moving in the right direction currently, but this is my personal point of view. Based on this observation, it is more useful to envisage a realistic and attainable fight

Q. Bigot (✉)
Gandrange, France
e-mail: qbigot@gmail.com

against doping. Trying to achieve absolute zero is an illusion, no doubt an enviable goal, but it is a barbed-wire wall, enclosed by a trench and well-guarded, at that…which inevitably discourages the world of sports, a source of endless defeatism and of a mission which looks more like of a witch-hunt than the conquest of space.

The most effective and feasible lever, at an individual level, is education. For my part, when I was younger, I was never asked to attend any anti-doping meeting or symposium. I find this shocking, indeed likened to negligence committed by institutions. But then, to whom should this mission be entrusted? Sports federations? Clubs? The World Anti-Doping Agency? The impression that everyone is passing on the buck does not help advance the education of our young athletes. No awareness-raising whatsoever, a mere 'that's not good' murmured by coaches, who would rather not broach this issue let alone speak up about it freely, because according to some, this could give rise to certain intentions!

Quite the contrary, speaking up and out, untying tongues would put an end to a disastrous and equally useless taboo.

I believe that an athlete, in the course of his/her career and regardless of age or sporting level, should be made aware of these issues. One does not talk about doping to a 10-year-old in the same way as one does to a 20-year-old elite athlete. Every person in an athlete's entourage has a specific part to play at a given time, in an appropriate language, giving edifying and captivating examples. Why not include an anti-doping programme in the school curriculum on the same footing with education on information about drugs or traffic regulations? All kids take physical and sports education! The E in PSE is…education!

It always surprises me to no end that I am invited so rarely to anti-doping symposia, given that I have always desired to speak as an elite athlete and to share my experience with doping to help promote the fight against substance abuse in sports. The few times I was able to speak about my experience to youngsters, they seemed to really understand what doping is, but more than that, they could envisage the consequences of doping. Getting doctors only to speak to 12- to 17-year-olds is not necessarily the most effective strategy, given how off-putting and boring such talks can be.

So, the question is: *what does society do about athletes who have been suspended because of doping?* This is the topic I wish to discuss here.

Currently, a suspended athlete is not really monitored and vanishes for the duration of his/her suspension. When I doped, I believed that I could not succeed without a banned substance, that there was no way to achieve high performance levels without them. And did my belief change after I tested positive? No, it did not! Why would I have called myself into question, since doping helped me to achieve these results…. This is the crux of the problem!

I was extremely fortunate to be attended to in this descent into hell by people who refused to abandon me and wanted to help me. They undoubtedly saw in me, beyond the athlete who had cheated, the human being, like any other, with his background, his qualities and flaws. When I was very young, I had nothing special that predisposed me to dope myself one day! I was just an ordinary child, without any transgressions, a good student, well behaved, with loving parents. Who could swear that they would not have fallen into the trap of doping in my place? Every life, every backstory is different, and things are sometimes more complicated than they appear. Thus, I was helped by these persons, from different walks of life (family, friends, president of a club, coaches, etc.), to question myself. They suggested to me to see a psychologist, helped me to bounce back, to grow up and to change the way I saw myself and my relationship to performance. In short, they helped me become a man, the man I am today. Then, I met my current coach, who gave me self-confidence and told me that it was not doping that had made me and that I was just as able to achieve performances free of doping.

It takes a lot time to change, and above all, to believe in this change-making path. It took me several years to step back and to convince myself that I would succeed. Today, I am convinced that I am stronger than with doping. The proof? My best result dates back to 2019, in Doha, Qatar, when I became vice world champion, nearly 6 years after having doped for the last time. And do not talk to me about 'muscle memory'…after my positive doping control, I did not train for nearly 6 months, after which the result I achieved after my first throw was…55 meters! My training record whilst doping was 82 meters. As I speak, after 5 years of intensive training, with better support and more experience, ultimately, better: it is only 79 meters. So where are the 3 missing meters if not in doping?

So, supervised, supported, helped and reinstated, I pulled through. I also pulled through thanks to my current profession: train driver. Ever since I can remember, this was a dream, a passion, one I was able to turn into reality thanks to my suspension. Yes, I say 'thanks', because in the end, my positive doping test saved me and helped me fulfil my dream. My apprenticeship helped me get back on my feet: new surroundings, new colleagues, new town…new life! Only later did the desire to return to hammer throwing came, because I started missing it. Ultimately, I would say that my job helped me rebuild my life beyond sports, to relativise, to re-learn happiness and pride in myself. The return to high-level performance was a slow process, no cutting of corners. But what would have happened without this and the invaluable help from well-meaning persons? I would most likely have relapsed into doping. It is inevitable. A belief, a profound personal truth does not cease to exist just like that, without outside help or completely calling oneself into question.

Shocked to learn that athletes with a positive doping control are caught a second time? This does not surprise me!

What is undertaken to help them after their first positive doping control result and the ensuing suspension? Nothing. You cannot simply hope they will be hit by a stroke of genius in their sleep and stop believing that doping is indispensable. Look at prisoners: before they are released from prison, they pass tests, are helped to be rehabilitated in society, they are monitored regularly, get help finding a job, housing. Some bear witness to their experience, speak about it in schools…. Setting up a system, which helps suspended athletes to analyse themselves, to reinstate themselves in their sport (or not), this is what will prevent a whole slew of second-time doping offenders and consequently also first-time offenders; in fact, all these athletes will be able to speak out, help eradicate the taboo, bring down systems, become whistleblowers, cooperate in and work for the true fight against the scourge that is doping. Education and re-education are instrumental, because without such guidance, the only way to fight doping is by repression. Yet, the purpose of anti-doping controls is not to fight against doping but to catch the cheaters. At this stage, however, if an athlete is cheating, it is already too late. Everything needs to happen upstream and through education and outreach.

The second problem has to do with the athlete's entourage. Rarely does an athlete weigh the pros and cons of pills and syringes all alone. Often, third parties come into play in this decision-taking process, although I have to admit that there is a vast divide between the time an athlete envisions doping and the time the athlete actually acts on it. How many athletes have wondered about doping but ultimately did not resort to it? No doubt a vast number. And what distinguishes the athlete who acts from the one who does not? A difficult family background, some instability, a lack of self-confidence, an unhealthy entourage, an injury, etc., a string of opportunities for individual intervention, all the more so as we are all different. Many of us do not possess the wherewithal required to cope with such issues. Let us not forget that we are human beings, each one of us with our own human backstory. It is so easy to judge, without knowing all the ins and outs. It is not necessarily a question of seeking excuses, nor of forgiving outright, but it *is* a question of doing everything to understand the underlying mechanisms impelling an athlete to dope. This is how we will be able to better 'diagnose' individuals at risk and to help them. Help them not only to avoid falling into this trap but also to help them in their day-to-day life, for once the deed is done—and I know what I am talking about—the athlete will pay for it forever: image, suspension, the esteem of others, insults, even disease (e.g., cancer), etc.

Nevertheless, it is important to emphasise that doping has become less and less prevalent. Let us be gratified we are no longer back in the 1970s, 1980s and 1990s and we can assert confidently that performances are increasingly doping-free. Quite apart from the sports aspect, doping endangers the health of athletes. Is premature death or disease a worthwhile price to pay for a supposed, and above all, ephemeral, moment of glory? Athletes, please do not sacrifice your life. It is worth much more than just a medal.

Conclusion

In his narration, Quentin Bigot insists on the role of the entourage not only in the decision for an athlete to dope but also in his ability to reinvent himself as an individual and as an athlete. During his 2-year doping suspension, after being tested positive for stanozolol, Quentin rejected his passion in track and field for several months as he could not imagine competing without doping substances. He used this suspension period to pursue his passion for train driving and made of this other passion in his life his new professional career. Reinventing his personal life and meeting the right people allowed him to reinvent his approach to hammer throwing and to pursue his sport career at the highest international level. Quite interestingly, not only has Quentin reinvented his athletic passion at the highest level, but after intense training for several years, he also has reached the top level of his discipline with a better world ranking than before his suspension despite a lower performance.

This illustrates all the efforts conducted in anti-doping over the recent years, and in particular in track and field, where numerous athletes were caught for doping in various disciplines, including throwing disciplines, and either were removed from the international competitions or retired for fear of being caught for doping. Track and field is undoubtfully cleaner today than a few years ago, which permits athletes like Quentin to return to his passion for sport and to international competitions with a sense of having his true performance being appreciated at its right value. The fact that track and field was so plagued by doping in the seventies, eighties and nineties, with some world records appearing inaccessible today to clean athletes, led to the reflection a few years ago by the IAAF [International Association of Athletics Federations, now known as World Athletics as of 2019] to maintain or cancel all the old world records and start de novo with a cleaner era.

Quentin Bigot evokes in his contribution the theory of 'muscle memory'. This is a hypothesis of interest to WADA, which is currently exploring this concept through various advanced research projects. The theory would be that muscle exposed to doping, in particular to anabolic steroids, would keep the memory of such an exposure and would allow the muscle to perform better months or years after the cessation of doping. If such a theory were to be proven, it would inevitably question the duration of suspension of doped athletes which, in the current rules, might be insufficient to eliminate all benefits of doping for some doped athletes returning to competition after a 2- or 4-year period of suspension.

Athlete-centred education leading to a better prevention of doping is a notion at the heart of reflections and actions by anti-doping authorities. Different initiatives to understand the motivations to dope, to anti-doping education inserted in school curriculums, to better accompany doped athletes during their suspension periods are now appearing in various sports and countries. It took a mindset revolution for the world of sport to integrate these notions and move from completely ignoring the issue of doping, to having to face it and deal with the consequences at the athlete and sport levels. Even if much remains to be done, stories such as Quentin's personal life should give all the young athletes the incentive to continue their passion for sport and their dreams to compete at the highest level with a strong belief in a system that will protect their passion and values to compete clean.

To Take or Not to Take? Why I Chose to Stay Clean

Toby Atkins

Introduction

Toby Atkins, an ex-professional cyclist who was faced with the choice to dope, tells his story of how he became a part of elite sport and what brought him to being faced with the choice of whether or not to dope. Toby made the choice to be a clean athlete and then chose to speak out against his entourage and teammates by reporting the doping programme to the Union Cycliste Internationale (UCI). In doing so he became a whistleblower. He outlines some of the key attributes he believes made him strong enough to reject doping and speak out and also shares his thoughts on clean sport in 2021.

From Videogaming to Cycling

"You need to take these vitamins!" I never thought that just a few words could crush down the world around me. But this one did. Not only that but they also changed the trajectory of my life and my career.

My name is Toby Atkins, I'm a sport fanatic, an ex-professional cyclist and most importantly, a whistleblower. When I tell my story, I like to start at the beginning. My childhood. I get a lot of odd looks when I start here and many people ask me, why? The answer is simple. When faced with the opportunity to dope, we fall back on our morals and values. And when do we learn those? As children.

I grew up in a small town in the middle of England. A quiet place but nonetheless a fantastic town to grow up. I lived an average upbringing, my family was part of the

T. Atkins (✉)
London, UK
e-mail: tobyatkins@icloud.com

middle class, maybe on the upper edge of it? It's hard to tell as a kid! I wouldn't say I was spoilt, but my family never went without. As with a lot of families, my father was away working a lot. He ran a motorsport team (looking back this is probably where the competitive side of me came from!), which meant there was a lot of time away from home. For a lot of families, it is the norm to be closer to one parent than the other, but with my father being away a lot, it meant the time he was at home, he made count. We were always on family outings, on holidays to faraway places and generally being exposed to as much of "life" as possible. When I was 13, my family decided that it was time to push the boat out. We moved to New Zealand (NZ). For those that aren't great with geography, that's about a 24-hour flight from England. My father wanted to retire early in a relaxing place, and so we moved to a tiny town called Coromandel, population 1500 inhabitants (on a good day!). Needless to say this was a huge shock to my system. I had grown up in one of the most densely populated countries on earth, and now I was dropped into a village where the nearest supermarket was over an hour away. This kind of experience was going to go one of two ways for me. It would either be the making or the breaking of me. Thankfully, it made me. This is where my sporting story begins!

I attended a small local school that catered to ages 4–18. As you can imagine, my classes were small, but I had a great relationship with my teachers. I knew them as part of the community rather than just being my teachers. I quickly grew in confidence, and in a matter of months I had embraced the relaxed and outgoing "kiwi" lifestyle. It's about now I should point out that sport and exercise was not something that was part of my family's lifestyle. I played a bit of football and did a bit of swimming, but the extent of my family's sporting credentials were "great at watching Formula 1 on TV every second Sunday". I was the depiction of the stereotypical PlayStation kid. Slightly overweight, pale skin and a soft spot for anything containing sugar. Thankfully, that kind of lifestyle isn't very compatible with rural living in NZ, so to make friends, I started to look at sport.

I was lucky to live on top of a huge hill that overlooked the Hauraki Gulf. The views were spectacular but, as a young teenager, big hills meant one thing. Going down them, *fast*. I had learnt that I could ride my bike from home to school (about 5km) without pedalling once. My parents quickly caught on that encouraging me to ride a bike was a good thing, so I inherited my dad's mountain bike. He didn't do anything by halves, so I ended up commuting to school on a top-of-the-range trail bike, but I had no idea at the time; to me it was just a bike.

A few months passed and one scorching hot day after school I got cornered by the school Sports Coordinator, Kelvin. He had seen the bike I was using to get to school and assumed that I must be a mountain biker. He convinced me that I should be part of school relay team in an "adventure race". All I had to do was the mountain bike leg. "It's not that hard", he said. I had no idea what an Adventure Race was, but all the cool kids were doing the other legs of the race, so I cheerfully agreed and the following week turned up to the race with my bike. I probably don't need to tell you that we didn't win. It turns out, riding your bike downhill to school doesn't actually make you very fit. But that's beside the point. I was hooked. My sporting journey started here.

After that, I started riding my bike for fun. I wouldn't call it training, but I loved being out on the bike. I started exploring on two wheels and loved the freedom it gave me. A few months passed by, and I had started riding with Kelvin, the Sports Coordinator I mentioned earlier. I had not thought much of it at the time, but I had started leaving him behind on the hills. I was getting fast. I was sitting under a tree eating lunch one day and he came and sat next to me and said, "Toby, there's a race called the K1, its longer than you've ever ridden before but I think you can do it. Only thing is, it's on road bikes". I didn't have a road bike and the race was 2 weeks away. I didn't want to let him down, so I sold my first car, headed to Auckland, and bought a road bike. A week later I rode the race and was 3rd U19 having only ridden a road bike once. I guess you could say this was the start of a long ride to elite cycling!

Fast Wheel

Let's fast-forward about 4 years. I was now done with school and had started attending the University of Waikato in Hamilton, NZ. I had worked my way up to be a part of one of NZ's strongest cycling development programmes run by NZ cycling legend Gordon McCauley and was now riding elite/U23. I spent a lot of time considering my options once I had finished school. Do I move to Europe, follow the dream or do I give myself a little more time to develop? Cycling is odd like that. You get stronger the older you get, physically, mentally and emotionally. I had watched some of NZ's strongest juniors quit school and head to Europe only to be chewed up and spat out by the pressures of elite sport. I chose to give myself the time to prepare for Europe and decided to do the first few years of university before heading overseas. It was the perfect plan. I could study hard so that when my riding life was over I had something to fall back on, all whilst still being able to train close to full time. I trained hard and learnt a lot. I matured, learnt my worth and learnt about dedication and commitment. To this day I believe that it is those 2 years I waited whilst doing university that made me 'head strong' enough to deal with what was to come the following year. The end of my second year at University was drawing near which meant it was time to start searching for a contract in Europe. Any kiwi knows the hardest thing about making it to Europe is finding a contract. The euro teams don't know much about the NZ racing scene, which makes it hard for them to decide if you're worth a punt or not. Again, my choice to wait a few years paid off here as I had spent a lot of time and effort creating connections with people in sport, so that when the time came, I could make the most of my network and find a contract. Don't get me wrong. I contacted over 30 teams; 10 responded, 3 negotiated and only 1 offered me my first professional contract. I love you, cycling!

Dream Coming to Life

I signed my first contract in October. I would be heading to Italy, the home of cycling, and racing all over the continent. Six years in the making and my dream was becoming my reality. All the hours of training, the sacrifices, the injuries, it had all become worth it. The elation was incredible. After a few days of celebrating, it was time to put my head down and train like I never had before. There is no good having a contract if you can't win races. "This is where the real work starts", I told myself. "This is where you have to show them you were worth the risk".

I knew I would be flying out to the UK for Christmas and then onwards to training camp early in the New Year, so I had a few months to train. I wanted to arrive at the first team training camp ready and raring to go. I wanted to show them that even in the off season I had what it takes. The drive to succeed. In the weeks leading up towards Christmas, it all began to feel very real. I was constantly emailing back and forth organising what kit I wanted, how I wanted my bike set up, what kind of requirements I had for training camp. Every little detail was scrutinised, and I loved it. Each day I'd swing my leg over the bike with a newfound hunger to succeed. I had to. This was my chance. My chance to live my dream. The new year rolled around pretty quick. It always does when you are deep into a big training block. You lose track of time, and it feels like you are in your own "little bubble". I found myself with just 7 days left before flying to camp, and my phone started getting notifications about "not long now until your holiday in Italy". It was ironic really. It was about as far from a holiday as you can get. I would be staying in a tiny rural house in the mountains doing the most punishing training of my life! The weird thing was I was looking forward to it more than any holiday I have ever had. I suppose us athlete types are a little odd like that.

The final day rolled around, the bags were packed and I was in the form of my life. I felt incredible and I was ready to make the leap. I got on the plane in the cold early hours at London Stansted and 2 hours later stepped off in the refreshing 20-degree sunshine of Italy. "Here we go", I thought. This is what you've been dreaming of. Let's do this.

I stepped out to the arrivals hall where I was to meet the team manager and catch a ride to the team accommodation. No one was there waiting for me. "That's odd", I thought. I double-checked the times and everything lined up but no one was there. I waited for an hour and decided that something must have gotten confused in translation. I bought an Italian SIM card and set up my phone. I messaged the manager. It turned out he had completely forgotten! A little worrying considering he had just signed me up and flew me all the way from NZ. An hour later a fancy sports car sped up to me and asked, "Atkins?". "Yes, are you with the team?" I asked. To which I got a confused look and a "non capisco l'inglese". Let me translate that for you: "I don't understand English". I take a punt and assumed he was with the team as he already started to pull my bike out of its travel case and is precariously attaching it to the boot of the car.

A very quiet car ride later, I arrived at a farmhouse. No Internet. No phone. No outside world. Totally isolated in the middle of nowhere. I thought it was strange at the time. I heard the Italians were well-known for liking to keep their team training somewhat behind closed doors. Maybe that's just what it's like here, I thought. Little did I know the real reason behind the secrecy.

Over the next few days, the riders started arriving at the house. They were a great bunch of people. Only a few of them spoke English, but even the ones that couldn't made me feel welcome and helped me with my Italian. We sat down after dinner as a group, and they gave me an Italian language lesson each night. The training was hard and long, but I was prepared. I had spent months getting ready for this, and I came into it in the best form of my life. Day 3 we did a series of performance tests up a mountain. I did not look forward to mountains. I am a what they call a "rouleur" in cycling. Great at riding the front, pulling hard in the breakaway, racing over rolling terrain or setting things up for a sprint finish, but not lightweight enough to be great at climbing. That day I did beat the entire team par one. Their best climber. Things were looking good. Confidence was high. Fast forward to day 6 and I was starting to crack. If you know much about training in sport, you know that it works in cycles. Train hard, then recover to get the performance gain.

From Dream to Reality…

Day 6 was horizontal rain and horrible cold. I headed out, but turned back soon after. There was no way I should be doing that when fatigued; it was a recipe for disaster. It was at this point that I started to question the legitimacy of some of my teammates. I knew from the tests that I was strong, but these guys just never seemed to get tired. They weren't any faster than me, but they seemed indestructible. Every day they would wake up as fresh as a daisy. I went back to the team house perplexed and confused. Maybe I wasn't as good as I had thought? I must have done something wrong. Five hours later the rest of the team got home chatting to each other as if they had gone for a walk in the park. Something wasn't right.

Each morning I would sit down with the team manager at the breakfast table and talk about how I was feeling, how my legs were, how I was fitting in, how my Italian was going, discussing early season races. The idea being that they wanted me to feel included and part of the family unit. This particular morning was a little different though. This morning's talk ended with the words, "You need to take these vitamins" and a firm clasped hand sliding across the table. Today was the day I was offered performance-enhancing drugs.

It was clear I was starting to fatigue and the team manager had decided I was trusted enough to be presented with the reason why the rest of the team never seemed to tire. Testosterone. The thing that still scares me to this day was the fact he did this in front of an entire team. There was no secrecy, no shame. Just absolute certainty that this is what I needed to do. I paused and stared at him for what felt like an hour. How did this happen? How did I get here? We all heard the stories but no one expects it to happen to them. I reached out and grabbed the drugs without losing eye contact. We both knew what was expected. I hurried off to my bedroom and sat on the bed. My heart was jumping out of my chest, I couldn't think straight, and I was now facing what was and likely will be the biggest decision of my life. Do I take performance-enhancing drugs? I sat there for an hour in total panic. I'm not going to say that I didn't consider taking them, because I did. I was 5 cm from taking testosterone at one point, but I couldn't do it. I couldn't sacrifice who I am for my dreams.

I couldn't do it. I shoved the drugs in my pillowcase and went back out to the kitchen as if nothing had happened. As far as they knew, I was now one of them now.

Heartbreaking to Take the Right Decision

That day I was allowed a recovery day. I rode my bike down to the ocean. It was good for the legs but even better for the head. I knew I had to talk to someone, but I couldn't. There was no Internet or phone service at the house, so I took my phone with me and emailed the friend that helped me find my contract. He worked for a cycling organisation but is a close family friend and someone who I looked up to in all aspects of life. The email was pretty simple.

"They've offered me PEDs (Performance-Enhancing Drugs) and I don't know what to do. Help."

Thirty minutes later I was on the phone with my friend. It wasn't until that point that I appreciated the situation I was in. I was in a country where I knew no one, I had no transport, I couldn't speak the language, I had no money, there's no Internet and very limited cell phone service. It wasn't until now that I realised I was in real danger.

Later that day, I was washing my bike outside and my phone started vibrating. I answered and a female Swiss accent introduced herself as someone from the Union Cycliste Internationale (UCI). "I'm here to help you and get you out of the situation safely". I didn't realise it at the time, but because my friend worked for a cycling organisation, he had no choice but to report the incident to the UCI. Suddenly I had become one of the first whistleblowers to go through the UCI's new reformed system.

The next morning, I knew I had to make it clear where I stood. I was angry. This team had taken everything I had worked for. My dreams, the countless hours of training, the sacrifice and thrown it back in my face. I walked into the dining room and told the manager I needed to speak to him privately. We walked outside and sat in the morning sun. I reached into my pocket and placed the PEDs on the table in front of us. "I know what this is", I said. His face turned to a look of worry. "I've proven to you I'm one of the strongest people here, and you think you can do this?" I said. He started to grin, which only made me angry. He got up and ushered me to follow him. We walked through the house and into the bathroom. He closed the door behind us and my heart felt like it was coming out of my chest. He laughed, threw the PEDs in the toilet and flushed it. "You passed the test", he said. With that, he opened the door and walked off.

Cyclist Undercover

Anger was an understatement. I was livid. I rode down to the road, found cell phone service and got UCI to call me. We talked about my options. There weren't many. The best they could do was offer me a safe passage out of the country and help me walk away from the mess I was in. They couldn't do anything as it was just my word against the team. I was not very proud of it, but a lightbulb in my head came on. All I need is evidence. I asked UCI what they'd need for this to actually be followed up. The answer was proof. I agreed that I would leave the team as per her instruction, but not until I had material proof of what was going on. It was hard to arrive home and not be able to tell my friends and family the real reason why I couldn't make it as a cyclist after all the time and money they put into my dream.

The following day I sat down and told the team manager that I wanted out. I said I would leave quietly and he can tell the riders that "I didn't like the athlete life-style". Lying through my teeth was hard, but when a person puts your personal well-being at risk, it is a lot easier to live with. Later that day, I explained I had a recurring knee injury and said I couldn't ride. The stars aligned and this was my time to find proof that it wasn't "a test" and that the entire team was doping.

It took 2, maybe 3, minutes to find what I was looking for. There was no trying to hide it, no attempt to conceal, it was just sitting there in riders' bags. Vials, needles, endless pills, medical equipment. You name it, it was there. I took the photos I needed and packed everything neatly back into place. I had what I needed and now it was time to worry about myself. That day, I booked a flight back home for the following day. My flight was at 5pm. Once the team got back, I explained to the manager I was leaving and I needed someone to drop me at the airport, about a 1 hour drive. He was less than impressed by my sudden departure but surprisingly offered for me to be based out of the UK and they would fly me to and from the races. I said I would consider the offer, but for now I needed to be somewhere else. It was at this point, I think, he might have realised life was about to get very difficult for him so he decided the best he could do was have one of the staff drop me at a nearby bus stop at 6am before the riders woke up.

Home Alone

Twenty-four hours later, I arrived home, perplexed, confused, angry, upset, the list could go on. But I was safe, I spoke out and I did the right thing. I might not have been able to talk to anyone about it, but knowing that my moral values stood strong was something I was and still am very proud of to this day.

Once the UCI knew I was home safe, I didn't hear from them for over a month. I had given them damning evidence of cheating and then they dropped off the face of the planet. I felt like I had thrown my dream away. And for what? A pat on the back from the few people I could actually tell the truth to? I stopped riding my bike for 4 weeks after that. Those that know me will know that means I wasn't okay. To this day, that is the longest I haven't ridden a bike since I was 14 years old (that was 12 years ago at the time of writing this). I felt like I was at the lowest of the low. Dreams shattered and directionless.

I ended up having a conversation with my friend that even now is one of my fondest memories. He turned me around and gave me my fighting spirit back. The day after this pep talk, I got a phone call from UCI. She apologised for the radio silence and explained that because it was a criminal investigation, I could not be involved or kept updated. She explained that because of the evidence I had provided they were able to build a criminal case against the team. Riders tested positive and staff were convicted of trafficking drugs. I don't like to admit it but this reinstated my belief in the system.

So, What Happened Next?

A week after the bans and convictions were made public, I flew back to Italy to race for one of the most prestigious U23 teams in the country. I lived in northern Italy and raced all over the continent. Whilst racing, I managed to complete my studies in business management, I met some of the most incredible people in sport and am proud to say I lived out my dream after facing the biggest challenge in my life. I am also proud to say I have worked closely with UCI, the World Anti-Doping Agency and the International Testing Authority to help develop pathways for athletes in the same position as I was, as well as helping develop an educational framework to help prevent athletes from ever being put in the same position as me.

A Few Words About Clean Sport

Sport is a strange beast. It is both totally meaningless yet the most important thing on earth. It is the mortar that holds society together and the tool that humanity uses to bring cultures together. It is one of the most powerful tools we have, yet we have real issues protecting the values on which it relies. Integrity, excellence, honesty, the list of values that sport brings together is limitless. I have come to learn that people dope for a million different reasons, but I have also come to understand that no one sets out wanting to dope. We all want to live by our values and morals. Be the best we can be, but life isn't that simple. I often get asked if I hate people that dope. The answer to that is simple: No. They are exactly the same as me, but maybe their environment was different to mine. There is always a trigger that causes an athlete to step over the line and I believe the way to remove that issue is education. We cannot remove temptation from sport. It is an unfortunate trait that all humans have; we get tempted. But what we can do is educate athletes, support staff, coaches (even fans!) about anti-doping so that if they are faced with the same challenge I was, they have the tools and knowledge to say no and uphold the values of sport and humanity.

Part V
Truth in the Test Tubes?

Forensic Analysis of Seized Drugs

Emily D. Lockhart

Introduction to Novel Psychoactive Substances (NPS) and Forensic Analysis

The goal of the forensic analysis of suspected drug evidence is to identify the substance(s) present and, when applicable, determine the purity. This analysis serves several purposes: (1) scientific evidence in criminal proceedings, (2) intelligence regarding drug trafficking organizations and (3) scientific documentation that can be used to support drug scheduling actions for new drugs of abuse. Novel psychoactive substances (NPS) can fall into any number of chemical classes. Examples of these classes include synthetic cannabinoids, substituted cathinones, synthetic opioids, benzodiazepines and steroids (Figs. 1, 2, 3, 4, and 5).

This chapter will discuss matters related to the forensic analysis of seized drugs. These include topics such as (1) quality assurance practices; (2) method validation; (3) sample selection and preparation; (4) instrumental techniques; (5) structural elucidation; (6) challenges associated with seized drug analysis; and (7) reporting recommendations.

Quality Assurance Practices

Laboratories have policies in place to ensure that reports issued have a strong foundation in scientific principles. If operating within these policies, different laboratories will reach the same result and conclusions if provided with the same sample.

E. D. Lockhart (✉)
Drug Enforcement Administration (DEA), Special Testing and Research Laboratory,
Dulles, VA, USA
e-mail: Emily.D.Lockhart@dea.gov

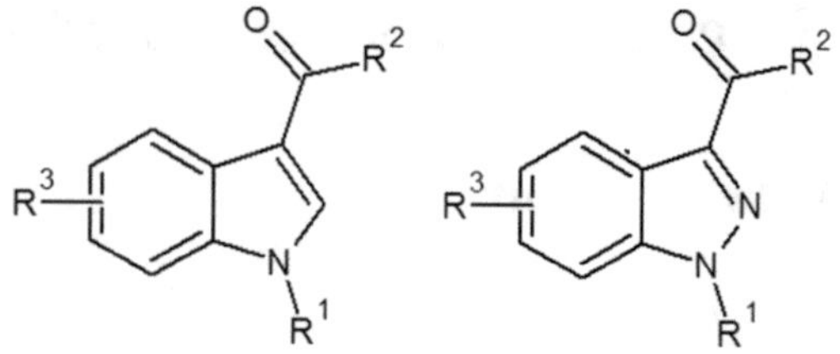

Fig. 1 Generic synthetic
cannabinoid structures

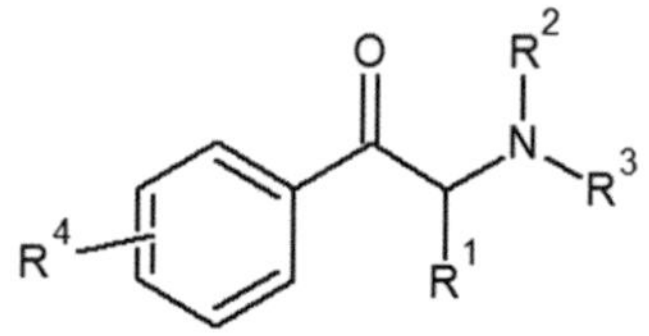

Fig. 2 Generic cathinone
structure

Quality assurance topics include (1) analyst training, (2) instrument verification and maintenance, (3) method development and validation, (4) reagent reliability, (5) positive and negative controls, (6) chain of custody, (7) sampling protocols and analytical procedures, (8) reference material verification, (9) casefile review, (10) proficiency testing and (11) accreditation and certification, among others [1]. Selected topics from this list will be discussed in further detail. Analysts must receive training in drugs of abuse and their scientific properties, proper use of instrumentation and the interpretation of data generated by laboratory equipment. Continuing education is an important aspect of maintaining expertise, particularly as new drugs of abuse continue to proliferate and new and updated instruments are developed. In addition to initial and ongoing training and education, analysts are routinely proficiency tested to ensure they have maintained competency. In these scenarios, analysts test a known prepared sample as though it were evidence. Their results are compared to the known composition. Instruments are evaluated upon installation and periodically thereafter to ensure they are performing properly. This evaluation generally consists of analysis of a test mixture and/or diagnostic testing internal to the instrument. The initial evaluation verifies that the instrument was installed properly and functions as intended, while subsequent evaluations monitor the instrument for any decline in functionality. Much like a vehicle, preventative maintenance is regularly performed to keep the instrumentation functioning properly. In addition to keeping the instruments working, the methods used on those instruments should be validated to show they work for their intended use. Method validation is discussed in more detail in a subsequent section. In regard to the analysis portion of a chemist's duties, quality policies describe appropriate sampling and analytical procedures. Acceptance criteria are outlined for each technique to determine when results are of sufficient quality for drawing scientifically valid conclusions. These policies also dictate the use of blank samples (negative controls), which are used to demonstrate that the reagents and instrument used are free from contamination. Equally important is the proper use and evaluation of positive controls

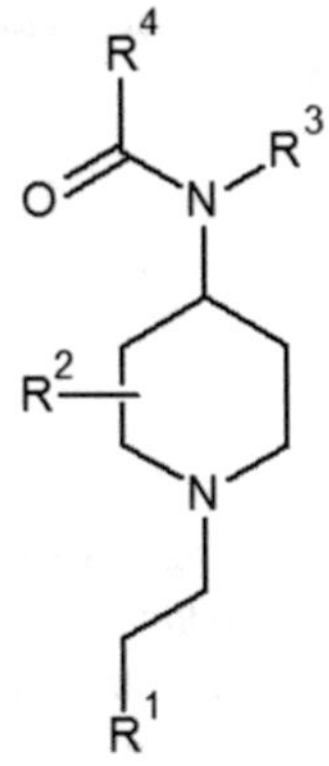

Fig. 3 Generic fentanyl structure

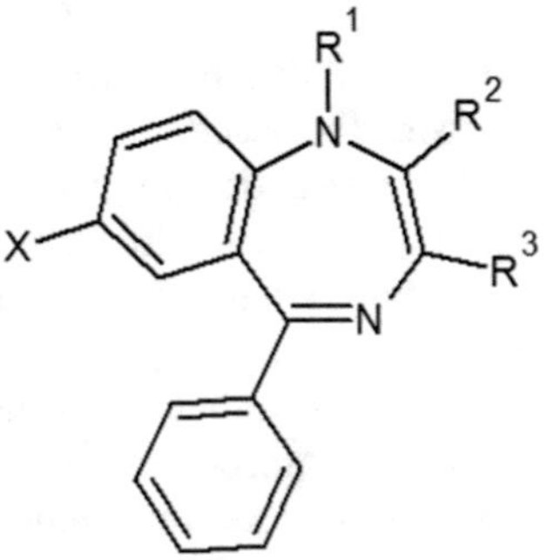

Fig. 4 Generic benzodiazepine structure

(reference materials) which are necessary for drawing conclusions by comparison to the unknown sample. All of the data generated during the analysis, along with the analyst's notes, make up the casefile. Technical review of the casefile is another aspect of quality assurance. This practice ensures analytical sufficiency has been met and quality practices were used. Many forensic laboratories seek accreditation (e.g., ISO/IEC 17025) from third-party organizations to demonstrate to their customers that their work meets a minimum standard. Additionally, individual analysts can seek certification to demonstrate their abilities in particular areas of expertise.

Uncertainty

The concept of statistical uncertainty is an important consideration in quality assurance, but it can often be confusing to a layperson. Uncertainty can apply to both qualitative and quantitative methods. It does not imply doubt but provides a range within which the true value lies. This means that it actually improves the accuracy of the reporting. Typically, uncertainty values are only applied to numbers that are critical to control status or statutory threshold; this primarily includes weight and purity. Factors involved in assessing the uncertainty associated with a weight include

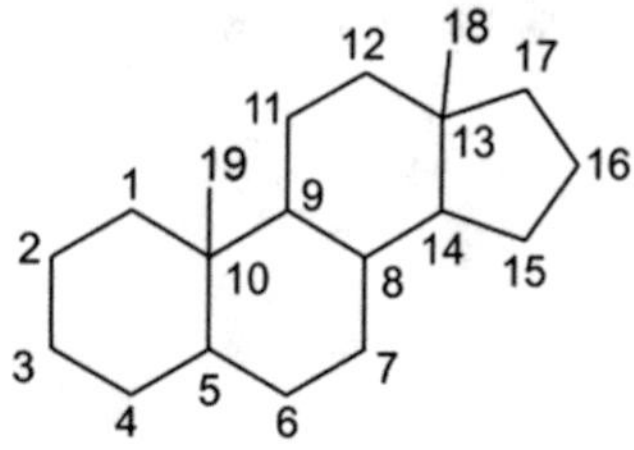

Fig. 5 Generic steroid
structure

how many weighing events occurred, the type of balance used and the operation of
the balance [1]. On a report, the uncertainty associated with a weight will appear as
a value plus or minus (±) the uncertainty. The weight and the uncertainty are reported
in the same units of measure (e.g., grams or kilograms). The uncertainty is calculated at a predefined degree of statistical confidence (e.g., a weight reported as
1.7845 g ± 0.0007 g at 95% confidence indicates that the true weight value has a
95% probability of being between 1.7838 g and 1.7852 g). Factors involved in
assessing the uncertainty associated with quantitation include sample homogeneity,
sample preparation and the equipment used [1]. The statistical principles used for
reporting the uncertainty associated with a purity is the same as with weights (e.g.,
on a report, a purity will appear as 85% ± 4% indicating that the true purity value
has a 95% probability of being between 81% and 89%). When it comes to qualitative methods, individual techniques have limitations; therefore, they have uncertainty. The uncertainty for qualitative methods is generally not represented
numerically. This uncertainty can be minimized by using multiple instrumental
techniques on multiple portions of the sample [1].

Method Validation

Method validation is another important aspect of a laboratory's quality assurance
practices. Having strong methodological foundations for the formation of scientific
opinions is critical and will therefore be discussed in further detail. Method validation demonstrates that "the performance limitations of the method are understood
and quantifiable criteria for its satisfactory performance exist" [2]. In other words,
method validation shows that the method is fit for its intended purpose.

Considerations for Qualitative Methods

A qualitative method validation provides evidence that a particular method can
identify a specific drug while minimizing the chances of false positives and/or false
negatives. The documentation produced during the validation notifies the analyst of
method limitations. Qualitative method validation occurs over the lifetime of the

instrument so, as new drugs emerge and are evaluated, they are added to the validation [3]. For separatory methods (such as chromatography methods), it is strongly encouraged that at a minimum the following parameters be investigated: *selectivity* (the ability of the method to isolate the drug and assessing interference of other components commonly seen in drug mixtures), *repeatability* (short-term precision) and *reproducibility* (long-term precision). Evaluation of the data includes, but is not limited to, the assessment of peak shape, intensity and precise results for both short- and long-term studies [1, 3]. For confirmatory methods (such as mass spectrometry), it is recommended that at a minimum *accuracy* is investigated. The spectrum generated by the instrument must match the spectrum generated by a reliable source using verified reference materials. Specific criteria of what constitutes a "matching" spectrum may vary from laboratory to laboratory, but generally, the two spectra should have the same overall pattern [1, 3]. Other parameters that may be considered include the *limit of detection* (lowest amount of analyte that can be detected and identified), *robustness* (altering method parameters to determine any changes to accuracy) and *ruggedness* (assessing factors external to the method such as the analyst and instrument) [1, 3].

Considerations for Quantitative Methods

For the purpose of quantitative methods, the validation must show that the technique accurately determines the amount of drug present. For quantitative methods, it is strongly encouraged that at a minimum the following parameters be evaluated: *selectivity* (defined above), *linearity* (the mathematical relationship between concentration and response), repeatability (defined above), *accuracy* (achieving the correct value) and *ruggedness* (defined above). Evaluation of the data includes, but is not limited to, the assessment of peak shape, intensity, precise results for short-term studies and an accurate quantitative result when compared to the known prepared purity [3]. Another parameter to be considered, especially in the case of complex matrices such as food products or plant material, is *recovery*. The efficiency with which the drug can be extracted from the matrix is critical to accurately determining purity [3].

Sample Selection and Preparation

Sample Selection

Statistical and non-statistical sample selection can be appropriate depending on the customer's needs. In order to make an inference about the whole population (e.g., 500 vials of unknown liquid), a statistical sampling would be required. If it is sufficient to simply state whether there is a drug present in any items of the population, a non-statistical sampling may be appropriate. Once sampled, each selected unit must be analysed to meet minimum analytical sufficiency as outlined by quality assurance policies [1]. The most common form of statistical sampling used in forensic drug laboratories is hypergeometric sampling. There are a number of resources available detailing its use in this setting [1–5]. Statistical sampling allows the analyst to assign a probability that a certain percentage of the population (meaning a certain percentage of the samples) contains a particular drug [1]. Non-statistical sampling only allows the analyst to make a statement about the samples which were tested, without making a conclusion about the entire population. An example of a non-statistical method is the "square root" method. Many laboratories also have policies in place that allow them to only test one unit of a population [1]. Regardless of which sampling technique is used, the procedure must be clearly outlined in the resulting report so that the reader can understand how many units were tested and whether that testing allows a statement regarding the qualitative results of the entire population. For example, samples analysed after statistical sampling may have a reporting statement such as "[Substance Identified] confirmed in [#] units tested of [#] units received indicating, to at least a 95% level of confidence, that at least 90% of the units in the population contain the substance" [3]. Using a non-statistical sampling technique will result in a statement such as "[Substance Identified] confirmed in [#] unit(s) tested" appearing on the report [3]. When using non-statistical sampling, the weight of both the tested and untested portions is reported for clarity and transparency.

Powders, Tablets and Capsules

Sample preparation varies depending on the instrumental techniques selected for the analytical scheme. For most routine instrumentation, powders (Fig. 6) are ground to improve homogeneity and diluted to an appropriate concentration (based on the method validation results) using a solvent in which the target analyte is known to be soluble. Tablets are ground and capsules are opened and subsequently treated the same as a powder. It is not uncommon for forensic laboratories to encounter counterfeit pharmaceutical tablets that may or may not contain the proper active ingredient (Fig. 7). As such, it is critical that samples be properly tested rather than using tablet imprints to determine the contents of the tablets.

Liquids and Suspensions

A liquid is a homogenous solution containing a solvent and drug (Fig. 8). Alternatively, a suspension is a liquid containing solid particles of material that do not dissolve. During the first step of analysis, liquids and suspensions are tested to

Fig. 6 Heroin powder.
Courtesy: DEA

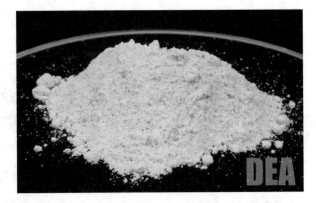

Fig. 7 Counterfeit
oxycodone tablets
containing fentanyl.
Courtesy: DEA

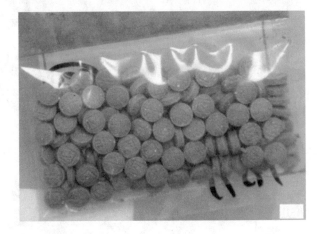

determine if they are composed of aqueous or organic solvent. If possible, the liquid
is directly diluted to an appropriate concentration using a solvent in which the target
analyte is known to be soluble. If the sample is aqueous, liquid-liquid extractions
may be performed to transfer the drug into a solvent appropriate for analysis, or a
technique that is appropriate for aqueous samples will be selected for the analysis.
Suspensions are generally separated into the solid and liquid portions and prepared
separately as described for the powder and liquid samples above.

Plant Material

Plant material samples (Fig. 9) are extracted using a solvent in which the target
analyte is known to be soluble and diluted to an appropriate concentration. Matrices
such as plant material often have a large number of natural components that may
also extract with the target analyte. Careful consideration should be given to choose
an appropriate extraction solvent.

Fig. 8 Testosterone
cypionate liquid.
Courtesy: DEA

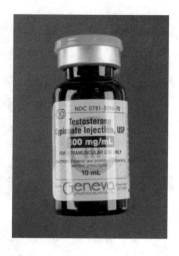

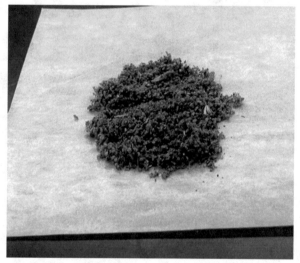

Fig. 9 Plant material dosed with a synthetic cannabinoid (Spice). Courtesy: DEA

Other Matrices

It is not uncommon to see drugs of abuse in other forms, such as food products—
like gummies, chocolates or baked goods—or beauty products, such as lotions.
Smuggling techniques are ever-evolving and becoming more scientifically advanced.
Chemical concealment techniques include complexing drugs with metals or paint
and the addition of "protecting groups". These techniques make field detection
more difficult. It can often prove challenging to liberate the target analyte from
these complex matrices.

Instrumental Techniques

General

Within the forensic drug analysis community, it is generally accepted—and recommended—that each unit to be tested is subjected to a minimum of both a separatory and a confirmatory test on separate portions of the sample [1]. This assures that the results are representative of the entire sample and that no inconsistent results are observed. Not all techniques are appropriate for all drugs. It is important for the analyst to understand the limitations of different instrumental techniques so that a proper analytical scheme is built for each sample. An analytical scheme can be defined as "a combination of selected techniques used to reach a scientifically supported conclusion" [1]. In order to assist in selecting appropriate techniques, analysts often use presumptive tests to assist in guiding their analysis. Presumptive tests provide general information on what drug classes may be present [2]. Alone, they do not provide sufficient data to form a reportable conclusion. Alternatively, confirmatory tests provide specific information about a substance's chemical structure and may provide sufficient data to form a reportable conclusion. As part of quality assurance policies, a negative control and a positive control should be tested for all techniques.

Colour Tests

Colour, or spot, tests are very quick and easy presumptive tests commonly performed in forensic drug laboratories. A small amount of sample is tested using a reagent. If a particular functional group, or portion of a molecule, is present, a colour change will occur [2] (Fig. 10). While this test alone is insufficient to identify a specific drug, it can give the analyst an idea of whether the substance is an opium derivative, an amphetamine, a natural cannabinoid, etc.

Thin Layer Chromatography (TLC)

Thin layer chromatography (TLC) is a presumptive test that uses a piece of glass, called a plate, which is covered in a thin film with which the sample interacts. The sample is applied to the bottom of the plate and placed in a chamber containing a solvent or solvent mixture. As the solvent is absorbed and moves up the plate via capillary action, the components of the sample mixture separate. The final locations of the spots on the plates are visualized using UV light or developing reagents [2]. The analyst compares the retention factor of the sample to that of a reference

Fig. 10 Sodium
nitroprusside colour test
turns blue in the presence
of secondary amines such
as 4-methylmethcathinone
(4-MMC) Test kit:
NarcoPouch Test 923.
Courtesy: DEA

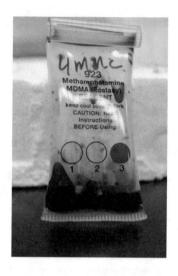

material. Both the retention factor and spot colour, if using a developing reagent,
should match.

Gas Chromatography (GC)

Gas chromatography (GC) is a separatory technique that uses gas and heat to separate the components of a mixture. First, the sample is volatilized. Then, it passes
through a heated hollow column. The change in temperature and interaction of the
volatilized sample with the interior of the column allows different compounds to
reach the detector at different times. Evaluation of the data includes, but is not limited to, the assessment of peak shape, intensity and comparison of the retention time
of the sample to that of the reference material [3]. These characteristics can be
observed in Fig. 11. When GC is used in this manner, it is typically equipped with a
flame ionization detector (FID). With this type of detector, the sample is burned
when it exits the column and the change in voltage is detected [6]. In addition to
presumptive testing, this detector is commonly used for quantitation. This detector
works well for compounds containing C-H bonds (very common in drugs of abuse)
[2]. Other types of detectors that may be useful in forensic drug analysis include, but
are not limited to, a nitrogen phosphorous detector (NPD), an electron capture
detector (ECD), a thermal conductivity detector (TCD) and a mass spectrometer
(MS, which will be discussed in a later section) [2, 6].

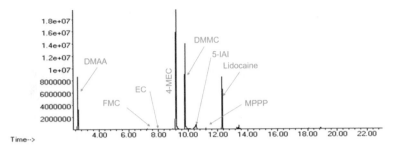

Fig. 11 GC-FID of a mixture of cathinones from a seized product. Courtesy: DEA

Liquid Chromatography (LC)

Liquid chromatography (LC) is a separatory technique that functions similarly to GC. Instead of using gas to push the sample through the column, LC uses liquid buffer, such as water or acetonitrile. Interaction of the sample with the column makes some substances move through the column faster than others, separating the components of the mixture. Similar to GC, evaluation of the data includes, but is not limited to, the assessment of peak shape, intensity and comparison of the migration time of the sample to that of a reference material [3]. One benefit of LC is that it is a non-heated technique, meaning it can be used to analyse thermally labile compounds. LC also works well for substances that do not volatilize easily such as large molecules [6]. It also has a lower limit of detection than its gas counterpart, so it can be used to detect trace components in a drug mixture [6]. Common LC detectors include a diode array detector (DAD) which collects the UV/Vis spectrum of the components in the mixture and mass spectrometric detectors (of which there are many types). Other types of LC detectors include but are not limited to a refractive index detector and a fluorescence detector [6].

Infrared Techniques (IR)

Infrared spectroscopy (IR) is a confirmatory technique that measures the interaction of the test sample with infrared light. The spectrum of the sample should match the overall pattern of the reference material taking into consideration the defined resolution of the method used [3]. For pure substances, no sample preparation is needed, which makes IR a quick and easy technique. Unfortunately, many drug samples are adulterated and contain more than one substance. This is a consideration the analyst must make prior to developing the analytical scheme. It may be possible to do a series of solvent washes or a liquid-liquid extraction to isolate the different substances for collection of IR spectra. Infrared spectroscopy does not work well for samples containing a lot of water. The –OH absorption band in water or other solvents can obscure a large portion of the spectrum. The broad nature of the –OH band

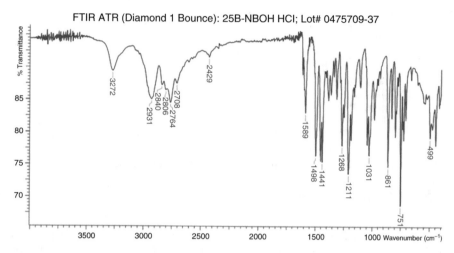

Fig. 12 Infrared spectrum of 25B-NBOH (a phenethylamine hallucinogen)

can be observed in between 2000 cm^{-1} and 3500^{-1} cm in Fig. 12. Typically, IR instruments are coupled with an attenuated total reflectance (ATR) accessory. This accessory is ideal for the analysis of solid samples. IR instruments can also be combined with GC to allow the separation of a mixture via GC followed by the detection of the separated analytes via IR. This detection can be done in both the vapour and condensed phase.

Mass Spectrometry (MS)

Mass spectrometry (MS) is perhaps the most frequently used confirmatory technique in forensic drug laboratories. There are two primary types of ionization that occur in MS detectors used for forensic drug analysis. Electron ionization substantially fragments the molecule providing some detail about the chemical structure. Alternatively, chemical ionization results in less fragmentation. This technique is particularly useful when determining the molecular weight of an analyte [6]. There are a number of mass spectrometers available. Quadrupole MS detectors use a voltage to allow ions of a specific mass to travel to the detector [6]. In time of flight MS detectors, the size of the fragments is determined by measuring the speed of the ion [6]. Ion trap MS detectors use an electric field to trap molecules and subject them to ionization. Then the voltage is increased to allow ions of a specific mass to travel to the detector [6]. The overall fragmentation spectrum of the sample is compared to that of a standard. Evaluation of the data includes checking the relative ion abundances and molecular ion [3]. These characteristics can be observed in Fig. 13. Distinguishing between isomers—substances with identical molecular

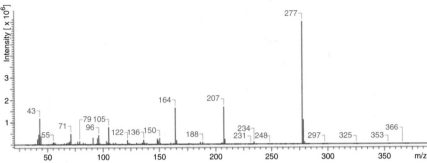

Fig. 13 Mass spectrum of meta-fluoroisobutyryl fentanyl (a fentanyl-related compound)

formulas—using MS requires a thorough evaluation of the data as the data is often similar. Other techniques, such as IR, LC and nuclear magnetic resonance (NMR), may be more appropriate for differentiating isomers.

Nuclear Magnetic Resonance (NMR)

Nuclear magnetic resonance (NMR) is a confirmatory technique that can provide both qualitative and quantitative data. While not a separatory technique, it can be used to analyse simple mixtures. NMR uses a magnetic field to determine the chemical structure of a molecule. Proton NMR is the most common form used in forensic laboratories. Carbon NMR or fluorine NMR may also be useful in forensic applications. Similar to MS and IR, the spectrum of the sample is compared to that of the reference material. This includes the evaluation of multiplicity, relative signal intensity and chemical shifts [3] (Fig. 14). It should be noted that proton NMR is not ideal for use with aqueous samples. NMR requires the use of deuterated solvents (hydrogen atoms are replaced with deuterium) so that protons from the solvents do not obscure the sample spectrum.

Other Instrumentation

The techniques mentioned above are the workhorses of a forensic drug analysis laboratory. There are a number of other instruments that may be used to analyse drugs of abuse such as NPS. For example, X-ray crystallography can be used to determine the structure of a crystal or particle of powder [2]. Inductively coupled plasma (ICP) mass spectrometry can be used to detect different elements [2]. Isotope-ratio mass spectrometry (IRMS) can measure the relative abundance of

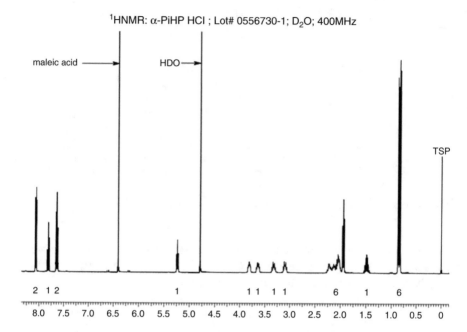

Fig. 14 Proton NMR spectrum of α-PiHP (a substituted cathinone)

different isotopes in a sample. This particular technique can aid in determination of geographic origin or synthetic route [2]. In recent years, large strides have been made in the area of portable instrumentation. Raman spectroscopy is one of the most common techniques used for field applications. This technique measures the light scattered when a laser is pointed at the sample [2]. In addition to Raman and IR instruments, which have been around for some time, portable MS and bench-top NMRs have become available. Ion mobility spectrometry (IMS) is another common technique used for the detection of drugs in the field. This technique measures how quickly the ionized material moves through an electrical field [2]. The demand for reliable instrumentation that can provide quick results in the field is ever increasing.

Structural Elucidation

With the continued evolution of NPS, a new challenge has presented itself: what happens when no reference material is available for comparison? Structural elucidation is the process of determining the chemical structure of a compound. There is a significant amount of expertise required to truly elucidate a chemical structure. This can be a time- and labour-intensive process. Commonly, this process includes the use of NMR and MS. It is first necessary to determine the exact mass of the substance. This can be done using direct analysis in real time (DART)-MS or another soft ionization technique. Knowing how much the molecule weighs allows analysts to determine possible molecular formulas. Several one-dimensional (1D) and two-dimensional (2D) NMR experiments are routinely used for determining chemical structure. These include proton, carbon, fluorine, correlation spectroscopy (COSY), nuclear Overhauser effect spectroscopy (NOSEY), total correlation spectroscopy (TOCSY), heteronuclear multiple bond correlation spectroscopy (HMBC) and heteronuclear single-quantum correlation spectroscopy (HSQC). These experiments provide information on how the individual atoms interact with carbons and protons up to 3–4 bonds away. Predictive software is available to aid in interpreting this vast amount of data, but review by an expert is necessary to verify the proposed structure. Fragmentation patterns from the MS data provide additional information on the chemical structure and can support or negate a structure proposed using NMR. Because many drug structures are so similar—particularly in the realm of NPS—it is common to see the same fragments in different compounds. Critical evaluation of all data generated is important, especially when interpreting data from an unknown substance. This thorough analysis allows for the identification of very similar substances, such as isomers. The identification of new substances prompts the purchase or synthesis of reference materials so that the substance may be identified more easily in the future.

Challenges Associated with Seized Drug Analysis

The forensic analysis of seized drugs brings with it a slew of challenges to include (1) complex matrices, (2) limited sample size, (3) thermal lability and (4) structural similarity. As discussed previously these substances may be present in complex matrices, such as on plant material, or in combination with other similar substances. This can complicate sample preparation—when the analyst is trying to extract any substances of interest from the matrix—and analysis, where there may be a number of additional compounds interfering with the target analyte.

Sample size may be limited. It is not uncommon for forensic drug laboratories to receive paraphernalia—such as pipes, spoons, digital scales and needles—that contain only a very small amount of drug material (Fig. 15). The analyst may only get one opportunity to produce quality data that can be used for reporting.

Some drugs of abuse are thermally labile, meaning they degrade when analysed using a technique that applies heat. A relevant example of this phenomenon in the area of sport is mebolazine (dimethazine) (Fig. 16). Not only is this molecule so large (633 g/mol) that it may not be detected using standard GC-MS parameters, but it is a dimer of another steroid called methasterone. When heated, mebolazine breaks along the N—N bond to form methasterone. This exemplifies the importance of testing materials with both heated and non-heated techniques.

Many NPS are structurally similar. This further emphasizes the importance of selecting appropriate analytical techniques to differentiate these substances.

Fig. 15 Blotter paper is
typically dosed with small
amounts of potent drugs.
This seizure was found to
contain 25H-NBOMe,
25C-NBOMe,
25I-NBOMe, fenproporex
and caffeine.
Courtesy: DEA

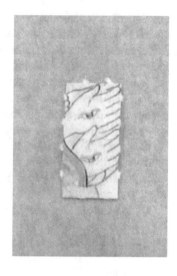

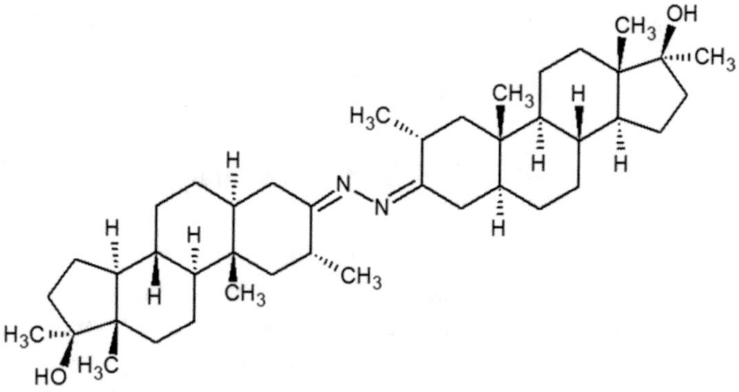

Fig. 16 Mebolazine (dimethazine)

Switching out a carbon for a nitrogen in a chemical formula produces small, but meaningful, differences in the data (Fig. 17).

Reporting Recommendations

The Scientific Working Group for the Analysis of Seized Drugs (SWGDRUG) is an international committee that puts forward internationally accepted minimum recommendations and best practices for the forensic drug analysis community. Several of these recommendations have been submitted to and accepted by the American Society for Testing and Materials (ASTM) International, a standard developing organization. SWGDRUG also works closely with and endorses several European

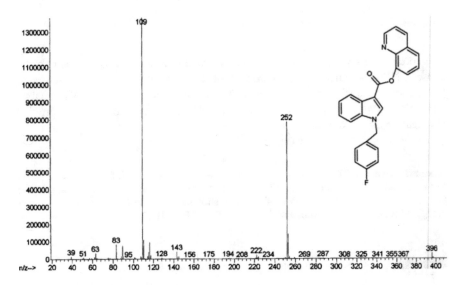

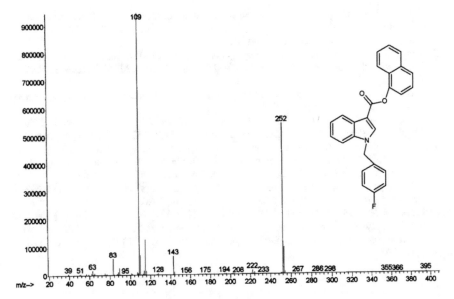

Fig. 17 MS spectrum of FUB-PB-22 (top) and FDU-PB-22 (bottom). Courtesy: DEA

Network of Forensic Science Institutes (ENFSI) documents. All of these organizations have recommended standards for reporting [7, 8]. A substance is typically only reported after data generated by the sample is compared to authenticated reference material or characterized via structural elucidation. The report should provide clear conclusions and explain how the sample was treated to reach these conclusions.

Conclusion

The forensic analysis of seized drugs is a critical component to combatting the abuse of NPS and other emerging drugs. From the moment a sample is submitted to the laboratory, quality practices guide its journey to identification. The analyst applies thoughtful analytical schemes to elicit the necessary information to provide a scientifically valid conclusion. These conclusions are essential to support law enforcement and drug policy efforts.

Acknowledgements Thank you to the members of the DEA Special Testing and Research Laboratory's Emerging Trends Program—past and present. It has been an inspiration to see your unwavering perseverance in the face of the NPS phenomenon. I am forever grateful for your thoughtful counsel and friendship over the years. DEA PRB 10-15-20-34

References

1. Scientific Working Group on the Analysis of Seized Drugs (2019) SWGDRUG recommendations edition 8.0. https://www.swgdrug.org/approved.htm. Accessed 31 Aug 2020
2. Bell, S (2006) Forensic chemistry. Pearson Education
3. Drug Enforcement Administration Office of Forensic Science (2019) Analysis of drugs manual. https://www.dea.gov/sites/default/files/2019-10/Forensics/ADM%20R4%202019_Public%20 Posting_Final2.pdf. Accessed 31 Aug 2020
4. Bates JW, Lambert JA (1991) Use of the hypergeometric distribution for sampling in forensic glass comparison. J For Sci Soc 31:449
5. European Network of Forensic Science Institutes (2017) Guidelines on sampling of illicit drugs for qualitative analysis. https://enfsi.eu/wp-content/uploads/2017/05/guidelines_on_sampling_ of_illicit_ drugs_for_qualitative_analysis_enfsi_dwg_2nd_edition.pdf. Accessed 31 Aug 2020
6. Harris DC (2007) Quantitative chemical analysis, 7th edn WH Freeman and Company
7. Scientific Working Group for the Analysis of Seized Drugs (2017) Supplemental document SD-5 for part IVA reporting examples. https://www.swgdrug.org/Documents/SWGDRUG%20 Reporting%20 example%207-11-12.pdf. Accessed 31 Aug 2020
8. European Network of Forensic Science Institutes (2017) Minimum reporting requirements for the analysis of controlled drugs https://enfsi.eu/wp-content/uploads/2017/05/minimum_ reporting_requirements_for_the_analysis_of_controlled_drugs_2013-09-25.pdf. Accessed 31 Aug 2020

Analysis of New Chemical Entities in a Sport Context

Mario Thevis and Tiia Kuuranne

Introduction

Methods and substances in anti-doping partly overlap with those of toxicological and forensic interest. However, the objective of doping practises is performance enhancement in sport context, which often involves chemical entities emerging in the market from the drug development programmes of the pharmaceutical industry, aiming at medical treatment of clinical patients for indications requiring improved oxygen transfer (e.g., erythropoietin (EPO) receptor agonists and hypoxia-inducible factor (HIF) activating agents) and increase of lean muscle mass (e.g., selective androgen receptor modulators (SARMs)).

Approximately 30 laboratories are accredited globally by the World Anti-Doping Agency (WADA) for the analysis of anti-doping samples collected within the test missions of anti-doping organizations (ADOs). For an efficient and updated anti-doping analysis, sensitive and cost-effective initial testing procedures (ITP, "screening") are needed, with the possibility of smooth integration of representative target substances within already-established analytical pipelines.

The objective of an ITP is to target characteristic metabolites or markers in the biological matrix and via method of choice, at adequate analytical sensitivity and reasonable sample volume, in order to discover from the large sample population

M. Thevis
Center for Preventive Doping Research – Institute of Biochemistry, German Sport University Cologne, Cologne, Germany

European Monitoring Center for Emerging Doping Agents, Cologne, Germany

T. Kuuranne (✉)
Swiss Laboratory for Doping Analyses, University Center of Legal Medicine, Genève and Lausanne, Centre Hospitalier Universitaire Vaudois and University of Lausanne, Epalinges, Switzerland
e-mail: tiia.kuuranne@chuv.ch

© The Author(s), under exclusive license to Springer Nature Switzerland AG 2022
O. Rabin, O. Corazza (eds.), *Emerging Drugs in Sport*,
https://doi.org/10.1007/978-3-030-79293-0_17

those suspicious ones that require more specific confirmation procedures (CP) before completing the full test menu. The procedures shall be validated and included within the scope of the mandatory ISO 17025 accreditation for the reporting of an adverse analytical finding (AAF, "positive result"), which requires, e.g. availability of characterized reference material, good comprehension of the method specificity as well as the exclusion of any other explanation (clinical, pathological or non-prohibited substance) as source of the analytical finding.

According to the strict liability principle of the World Anti-Doping Code, it is not necessary for the anti-doping organization (ADO) to demonstrate the intent, fault, negligence or knowing use of the athlete to establish an anti-doping rule violation [1]. However, for the fair process, the ADO with responsibility for result management shall provide the athlete with an impartial hearing panel, as well as with the opportunity to provide an explanation to the analytical finding. More and more often, the efforts are made to clarify the origin of the finding, namely, references to unintentional administration or inadvertent exposure to a prohibited substance, as well as the time, the dose and the route of administration. The anti-doping laboratories are often consulted during the result management or the disciplinary procedure in order to receive an unambiguous statement to support the result management. For science-based expertise, the pharmacokinetic characteristics of the drugs should be well known and studied in humans. For new chemical entities, especially for those emerging outside the *bona fide* industry, the details are scarcely or not at all available. The aim of this discourse is to present the analytical context, processes and regulatory requirements of the WADA-accredited anti-doping laboratory with regard to discovery of new chemical entities and their incorporation to routine analysis.

Prohibited Substances in Sport

Regarding the analytical capabilities and test menus, the anti-doping laboratories shall comply with the list of substances prohibited in sport as established under the World Anti-Doping Program [2]. The list is updated annually, drafted by the WADA Prohibited List Expert Group and consulted among the stakeholders before being approved and coming into force. The division of the substances to ten (10) classes of the list (Table 1) is based on the pharmacological properties of the substances, and, except for the fixed classes S4.5 (metabolic modulators) and S7. (narcotics), these classes are open for flexibility to include other substances with similar chemical structure or similar biological effect(s) in addition to those examples named on the list.

From the laboratory perspective, the categorization is not exactly identical with the analytical pipelines, i.e., all the substances of a given class are not analysed in the same analytical procedure, as the division between the analysis processes is based on the chemical, physical and metabolic properties instead [3]. An example could be given on the group of anabolic androgenic steroids (AAS), for which an

Table 1 Classes of substances prohibited in sport [2]

Event	#	Class	Examples
At all times	S0.	Non-approved substances	S48168 (ARM210, Rycal®)
	S1.	Anabolic agents	
		S1.1 Anabolic androgenic steroids	Boldenone Stanozolol
		S1.2 Other anabolic agents	Enobosarm (ostarine, S-22) LGD-4033 (ligandrol)
	S2.	Peptide hormones, growth factors, related substances and mimetics	Erythropoietin (EPO) GHRP-2 (pralmorelin)
	S3.	Beta-2-agonists	Higenamine Terbutaline
	S4.	Hormone and metabolic modulators	GW501516 (GW1516, endurobol) Tamoxifen
	S5.	Diuretics and masking agents	Furosemide Hydrochlorothiazide
In competition	S6.	Stimulants	
		a: Non-specified stimulants	Amphetamine Cocaine
		b: Non-specified stimulants	Cathinone analogues (e.g. mephedrone) Methylphenidate
	S7.	Narcotics	Oxycodone Morphine
	S8.	Cannabinoids	Marijuana JWH-018
	S9.	Glucocorticosteroids	Prednisolone Triamcinolone acetonide
[1]	P1.	Beta-blockers	Bisoprolol Propranolol

[1]Beta-blockers are prohibited in particular sports, e.g. archery and shooting

extensive set of sample preparation procedures (with and without hydrolysis or derivatization) and gas chromatographic (GC) and liquid chromatographic (LC) separation techniques are interfaced with multi-stage mass spectrometric (MS^n) analysis to cover the full pattern of target metabolites. Furthermore, for the exogenous substances, the scope of the analysis is qualitative, whereas the analysis of endogenous AAS for athlete biological passport purposes requires a quantitative approach.

As discussed earlier in this book, specific criteria are established for characteristics of a substance to be considered as prohibited in sport; most importantly it has the potential to enhance or it enhances sport performance. Even if the definition may appear clear and undisputable, enhanced sport performance is not always easy to demonstrate unequivocally. The experimental setup for a descriptive population with an adequate reference group regarding, e.g., exercise, stress, recovery, sleep and nutrition is not easy to arrange, in addition to inter-individual variation in compliance, physiological characteristic and response.

According to the anticipated duration of the performance-enhancing effect, the classes of substances are prohibited either at all times (classes S0–S5) or only in competition (classes S6–S9). For example, the administration of AAS (S1) or EPO (S2) has the potential to provide long-term advantage, whereas the impact of administration of ephedrine (S6) is temporary. A particular position of class S0 should be also emphasized, as it was established as a tool to control new emerging substances without marketing approval. With this amendment any pharmacological substance, which is or has been under drug development, potentially fulfils the criteria for being prohibited in sports but is not yet included in the list, is prohibited at all times. The same class includes also designer drugs and drugs aimed at veterinary use, if not covered already by another existing class on the prohibited list.

In forensic and toxicological context, the most interesting types of compounds emerging in the market are novel psychoactive substances stimulants (NPS), which are often linked to criminal acts and/or intoxications. According to the categorization by the United Nations Office on Drugs and Crime (UNODC), NPS include both natural and synthetic compounds (Table 2) [4]. Information on the availability and entrance of the NPS in the market is certainly interesting also in the sport context as the athletes, nevertheless, are not a group isolated from the rest of the society.

Table 2 Categorization of new psychoactive substances (NPS) by United Nations Office on Drugs and Crime (UNODC) [4]

Group	Examples[1]
Aminoindanes	5,6-Methylenedioxy-2-aminoindane (MDAI) N-Methyl-2-aminoindane (NM-2AI)
Phencyclidine-type substances	Phencyclidine (PCP) Ketamine
Phenylethylamines[1]	1-(2,5-Dimethoxy-4-ethylphenyl)-2-aminoethane (2C-E) p-Methoxymethamphetamine (PMMA)
Piperazines	1-Benzylpiperazine (BZP) 1-(3-Chlorophenyl)piperazine (mCPP)
Plant-based substances	Khat (*Catha edulis*)[2] Kratom (*Mitragyna speciosa*)
Synthetic cannabinoids[1]	HU-210 JWH-018
Synthetic cathinones	Mephedrone[1] Pyrovalerone
Tryptamines	5-Methoxy-N,N-dimethyltryptamine (5-MeO-DMT) 5-Methoxy-N,N-dipropyltryptamine (5-MeO-DPT)
Other substances	1,3-Dimethylamylamine (DMAA) Flualprazolam

[1]Groups/substances indicated by name on the WADA Prohibited List of Substances
[2]Khat contains cathinone and cathine which belong to the class S6 substances of the WADA list. Cathine is a threshold substance and prohibited when the urinary concentration exceeds 5μg/mL

From the sports perspective, these substances belong mainly to those classes of substances, which are prohibited only in competition, and the theoretical doping scenario, though very different from the hallucinogenic or psychedelic goals of drug-of-abuse scene, could be related rather to the attempts to improve attention span or alertness, tolerance to pain as well as increased aggressivity or combativeness. And, inversely, many of the performance-enhancing drugs (PEDs) are neither psychoactive nor otherwise interesting for sensation-seeking or intoxication purposes, and a wider source of information is needed to target the emerge of new substances with doping potential.

Origin of New Performance-Enhancing Drugs

The lead molecules of the pharmaceutical, especially biopharmaceutical industry, both for human and animal medication, are an interesting source of emerging compounds for doping use—much more often than in the scene of drug abuse. The most attractive properties of the substance for doping use are those with features to enhance oxygen transfer to muscle tissue (e.g., HIF activators) or to increase the lean muscle mass and/or performance (e.g., SARMs).

Pharmaceutical companies dedicate significant scientific, administrative and financial resources in the drug discovery processes when new molecular entities are involved, with the aim of returning the investment from clinical indications and not from doping practises, which could be a non-desired "by-product" of the marketing approval instead. The development processes are long in comparison with the patent protection term, and it is clear that sharing the sensitive information on the lead molecule before marketing approval could be considered as a risk for a maximized product lifecycle. In order to match the analytical method capability with the increased risk of doping practises with the new molecules, timely information on the drugs in development pipelines and their metabolic and pharmacokinetic (DMPK) profiles are valuable assets to the anti-doping laboratories but require trustworthy partnering and memorandums of understanding regarding the limited use of material provided for method development purposes.

In the doping context, it is important to emphasize the approved preparations for animal use, even those having entered the market already years ago, as an important source of products for human doping purposes. For example, anabolic steroids, e.g., boldenone and trenbolone, are available only for veterinary practises; nevertheless, they represent a significant number of reported AAFs of this category of substances. According to the annual laboratory testing figures of 2018, the WADA-accredited anti-doping laboratories reported 34 cases associated with boldenone and 79 with trenbolone, corresponding to approximately 2 % and 6 % of all findings of anabolic androgenic steroids (AAS), which comprised 44% of all the AAFs of that year [5].

New chemical entities originating from illicit or black markets pose a completely different and less controlled problem for the method development. The merge in the market can be very local and short term, depending often on the reactivity of the national drug legislation to regulate the new chemical entity according to the drug schedules. The marketing sector of these products is not necessarily the elite athlete population, as most of the performance-enhancing drugs can be estimated to be used by recreational athletes or other individuals who are outside of the anti-doping programmes and testing [6].

It therefore can be estimated that the first observations on these products are made by the customs, police and healthcare professionals. Regarding more analytical aspects, very little if anything is known about the DMPK profile of the designer drugs, which are also prone to high inter-batch variation regarding quantity and purity of the active molecule and additives. No pharmacokinetic nor metabolic data are available, which will require different approaches, e.g. in vitro assays, to estimate the correct target compound, intact substance or metabolite(s) in urine. Taking into consideration a fast turnover of the illicit products in the market and management of the Prohibited List, one mechanism for the inclusion of a substance to the list is the Monitoring Program [7], which is established by WADA to study the patterns or trends of misuse in sports. These selected substances are not prohibited, but associated with doping potential, and followed up on anonymous basis in the routine samples by anti-doping laboratories in order to obtain statistical information on the prevalence.

An example of the entrance via monitoring programme is pseudoephedrine, specified stimulant and class S6b substance from which the prohibition status was removed in 2004 and which was transferred then to the Monitoring Program. Pseudoephedrine was incorporated again in 2010 in the Prohibited List with the threshold of 150 µg/mL due to observed patterns of prevalence and evidence of high risk of misuse in sports. Designer compounds most often encountered for are amphetamine, cathinone and hallucinogenic compounds, but not very often for solely performance-enhancing effects. However, some examples in sport context could be given, such as desoxymethyltestosterone [8, 9] (DMT) and tetrahydrogestrinone (THG) [10]. The necessity of the complementary analytical approach was demonstrated in early 2000s in the "BALCO case", where a designer steroid THG was synthesized by Bay-Area Laboratory Co-Operative specifically for doping purposes. THG possesses an extensively conjugated π-electron system, which was tailored to remain non-detected by the prevailing GC-MS^n-based routine analysis, e.g. due to the low volatility. The target compound was identified in the syringe provided to the UCLA laboratory and concluded to exhibit anabolic effects [8]. In this case, an LC-MS^n approach to the routine analysis was the method of choice as the conjugated structure is capable of stabilizing well the electronic charge and high proton affinity allows for high sensitivity via electrospray ionization (Fig. 1). Whichever is the source of information regarding new PEDs, sharing of knowledge among anti-doping laboratories and with ADOs plays an essential role in method implementation to maintain the harmonized analytical testing at global level.

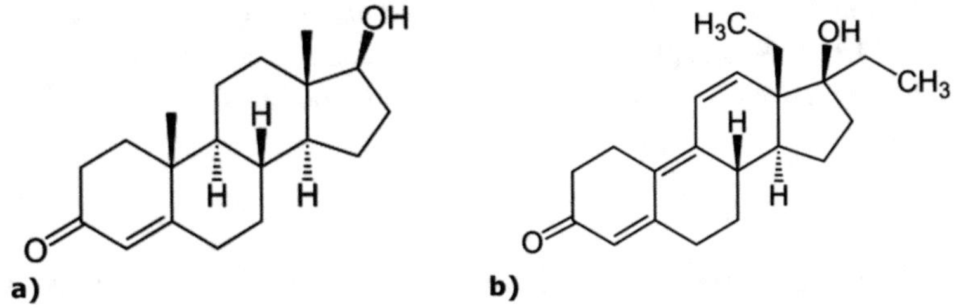

Fig. 1 Testosterone (**a**), model compound of the anabolic androgenic steroids (class S1.1), is amenable to GC-MS analyses with electron impact ionization, whereas for conjugated structure of THG (**b**), the method of choice is based on LC-MS techniques interfaced with ambient ionization techniques, such as electrospray (ESI)

Target Compounds and Biological Matrix of Choice

Xenobiotics are transformed in the body most often by the liver and excreted in water-soluble form in urine. Metabolic reactions are categorized roughly into two main groups, phase I (functionalization) and phase II (conjugation), and they are catalysed by multiple overlapping and potentially polymorphic enzymes, e.g., by members of cytochrome-P-450 or UDP-glucuronosyltransferase families. Additionally, there are various other confounding factors, such as age, gender, dosing regimen, physical stress and medication, which may create a very individual pattern for the spectrum of metabolites present in the biological matrices.

For successful targeting, sophisticated compromises should be made between method sensitivity and number of target analytes to establish an ITP that covers all the potential stages of the excretion profile. In case the production is not made according to good manufacturing practises and/or it is designed for doping use, the anti-doping laboratory faces an additional task in suggesting the metabolic fate and the suitable sample matrix of an unknown chemical entity. The selection has a crucial impact on the analysis strategy as it defines the sample preparation and chromatographic conditions chosen for the ITP. Very often, the urine analysis focuses on the metabolized species of the intact compound with a prolonged detection window after the administration, whereas the blood sample could serve the purpose of identification of the parent compound, although within a shorter time-frame from the administration, especially for those chemical entities which are too large to pass through the renal filtering system. A blood sample, if deemed necessary, has also the benefit of providing better quantitative information on the identified substance, owing thanks to the more stable consistence than urine, which is impacted by the hydration status of the body.

According to the WADA rules, any biological matrix can be collected within the anti-doping programme. Similar to clinical and forensic chemistry and along improved analytical performance regarding sensitivity of the LC-MS-based technologies, various approaches have been studied and presented in hair and saliva testing, as well as in dried blood spot (DBS) [11–13]. Nevertheless, low concentrations (lower than in urine) and limited sample volume still restrict these approaches from being applied to the full menu of analytical screening and the routine anti-doping samples being mainly urine and blood (serum and whole blood) specimens.

From Discovery and Method Development to Routine Analysis

Although during the previous years method development in anti-doping laboratories has shifted towards high-resolution (HR)-based MS applications and non-scanning analysers, many ITPs, especially GC-MS/MS-methods, are based on selective sample preparation (e.g., enzymatic hydrolysis, liquid-liquid extraction and derivatization), combined with targeted and filtered data acquisition of pre-defined precursor ion-product ion transitions.

Consequently, the recorded data is obtained at highest possible sensitivity, but it is limited only to already known compounds, and, although providing with a straightforward data evaluation for the presence/absence or targeted species and relatively compressed data file size, these applications are bound to the knowledge and settings prevailing at the time of sample preparation and analysis. Implementation of non-scanning analysers, such as time-of-flight or Orbitrap, has enabled non-targeted and non-restricted acquisition of the HRMS data.

The increased selectivity of the HRMS often allows for reducing the sample preparation event to a minimum of "dilute-and-inject" –type of a process where the urine sample is only diluted with a relatively high proportion of aqueous buffer prior to chromatographic separation, electrospray ionization and MS analysis of the intact population of soluble compounds in urine. The number of analytes to be recorded is thus significantly higher than in targeted analysis and practically limited only by their mass-to-charge ratio (m/z), selected mode of ionization polarity (positive or negative), ionization and matrix suppression. Efficient data processing methods are required to extract the relevant information from the extensive set of raw data ("digital matrix") [14], and the great benefit of this approach is the possibility to access the non-filtered primary data in a retrospective manner, in case more information is gained from the emergence of new chemical entities, in order to study its prevalence without the need of re-extracting the biological sample again.

The great challenge with this approach is the digital space required for the data storage, as the file sizes could be at high megabyte to gigabyte level per one injection. Retrospective as well, but bearing an effect of deterrence, the testing authority may apply the strategy to place an anti-doping sample for long-term storage up to 10 years from the sample collection day, to request further analyses at any given moment within the storage period and to proceed to pursue an anti-doping rule violation. The trigger for the further analysis may arise from the implementation of new methods or instruments, which allow for discovering new substances or more representative metabolites, from improved sensitivity of the most recent

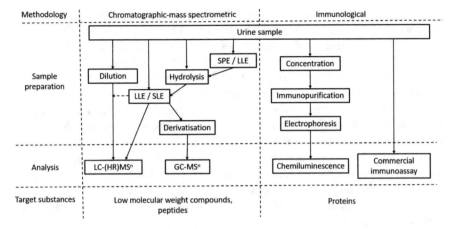

Fig. 2 Schematic illustration of an analytical strategy for routine anti-doping urine analysis. Abbreviations: *GC* gas chromatography, *HR* high resolution, *LC* liquid chromatography, *LLE* liquid–liquid extraction, *MS* mass spectrometry, *SLE* supported liquid extraction, *SPE* solid phase extraction

technological implementations as well as from the investigational and intelligence tools which may refer to misuse of new chemical entities emerging in the market at that time.

In order to carry out the routine analyses of wide coverage of analytes, within the expected turnaround time, with fit-for-purpose sensitivity and reasonable sample consumption, the anti-doping laboratories apply typically two to four different chromatographic-mass spectrometric procedures to the analysis of the urine samples, which offer a versatile platform for low molecular mass molecules and peptide analysis (Fig. 2). Specific immunological methods are also adapted from biochemistry, clinical chemistry and protein analysis to complete the toolbox for the detection of proteins, such as EPO, which not only are large in size but also present endogenously in urine at low concentrations and which often require specific analytical techniques or sample preparation procedures capable of distinguishing between endogenous and exogenous origin of the target substances.

Today, one initial testing procedure may typically incorporate the monitoring of 200–300 substances, which each require characterization and validation. It is therefore quite obvious that the aim of the strategic planning is to develop an ITP that is a well-considered compromise between the number of target substance and analytical sensitivity. Facing the challenge of the extensive list of prohibited substances with a wide spectrum of chemical properties and size, the ITP methods should be general enough to provide the flexibility to additions of new compounds without changes in critical conditions. The anti-doping laboratory may choose their own approach for the tailoring of their own ITP structure, as long as the methods meet the minimum required performance levels and the identification criteria established by WADA [15]. These limits define the highest acceptable concentration levels of substances, which the developed method shall routinely be capable of detecting.

The criteria are established by categories of substances (e.g., 100 ng/mL for most substances of class S6, stimulants) with the aim of harmonizing the analytical sensitivity among the anti-doping laboratories. For the method development and identification purposes, representative (preferably certified) reference material should be available. Considering the occasionally short lifecycle of the NPS, the commercial production of the material is slow, especially for the metabolites, whereas the excretion studies in human subjects may be hampered due to illicit source of the drug and due to lack of pharmaceutical preparation and ethical approvals required for human administration. In vitro and in silico predictions can be made to estimate the metabolic fate of the substances for the preliminary method settings (i.e., estimations on chromatographic retention time and mass spectrometric ion transitions). For confirmation procedure and reporting, however, positive control sample (spiked urine sample or characterized excretion urine sample) is needed to ensure identification of the target analyte [16].

Result Management

The analytical method is validated for performance characteristics to meet the needs of the given application (e.g., for selectivity) according to the quality procedures of the anti-doing laboratory.

However, prior to reporting, the anti-doping laboratory should assess the analytical finding for any prevailing scientific knowledge regarding, e.g., analytical artefacts, microbial or chemical degradation, endogenous origin or possibility of non-prohibited substances as the source of analytical finding that could cast a doubt on the doping scenario and on the validity of the result. In the routine analysis of tens of thousands of routine samples, originating from athletes who often use multiple prescribed drugs and over-the-counter products, additional information to method validation can be obtained. Illustrative example for accumulated information is S1.2 compound andarine (SARM S-4), which is targeted in the ITP by its O-dephenylated metabolite in urine (Fig. 3). The same metabolite may also result from the administration of anti-androgen flutamide, which is not a prohibited substance.

Consequently, the anti-doping laboratory should take additional measures, i.e., monitoring for the presence/absence of specific flutamide metabolite 2-hydroxyflutamide in the CP, to accurately identify the original source of O-dephenylandarine [17]. After the laboratory reporting, there are also other result management steps which will have an impact on the result interpretation and pursuing an anti-doping rule violation (ADRV). For instance, the athlete may have illnesses or pathological conditions that require administration of certain medication. Therapeutic use exemption (TUE) could be granted, the substances are already known, and the obstacles encountered in result interpretation (if any) are linked to the permitted dosing route or regimen. The question regarding intentional use versus inadvertent exposure to a prohibited substance is significant for the result

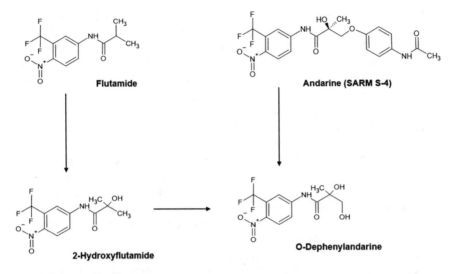

Fig. 3 Overlapping metabolism of non-prohibited flutamide and class S1.2 substance andarine

management and disciplinary process, however, not always unequivocal to define based on the analytical observation.

Regarding new chemical entities, especially those originating from illegal and non-controlled sources, very little is often known about the expected target concentrations in urine samples or about the elimination profile for those cases where the substance is categorized as prohibited only in competition. In general, threshold substances excluded, the laboratory analysis is aimed at qualitative purposes, and consequently, the analytical report does not include quantitative details on the result. A urine sample is not the matrix of choice to estimate the dose nor time of exposure, as the apparent estimated concentration of the substance in the urine sample is impacted by the hydration and urinary flux at the time of sample collection. Some support can be obtained from the specific gravity measurement of the sample, but ideally, these measurements should be done in a blood matrix, in which the composition is much more stable than urine due to rigorous physiological control mechanisms.

Conclusion

New chemical entities of pharmaceutical drug development and products from illicit sources feed the market with new substances of doping potential. For efficient anti-doping analysis and result management, the accredited laboratories and other anti-doping operators should be ready to adapt the prevailing processes for these needs and before reporting a new chemical entity as an AAF, many analytical and regulatory details should be clear.

First of all, the substance should comply with the prohibited criteria and be categorized for the aspects related to prohibition at all times or only in competition. At the laboratory level, a fit for purpose routine ITP shall be selected in order to target the new compound and/or its representative metabolites in the correct sample matrix. Adequate reference material shall be available for the unambiguous identification of the substance, and the method shall be validated and introduced within the scope of ISO 17025 accreditation of the laboratory prior to reporting.

The laboratory should have excluded any other source that doping practises for the AAF, including pathological and clinical conditions (endogenous production) and non-prohibited medication that could result in the finding via metabolism. Some alarms of the presence of new chemical entities could be suspected in conjunction with the routine analysis and by the unusual data or exceptional behaviour of an anti-doping sample. Still quite often the methods are targeted to the monitoring of pre-defined compounds in order to obtain high sensitivity and smooth processing of the acquired data.

The most efficient sources of information, however, are the continuous exchange of experiences with other anti-doping laboratories, knowledge of the sport and investigational tools from the ADOs, active monitoring of other overlapping branches of analytical sciences (clinical, forensic and toxicology), as well as WADA monitoring programmes and collaboration with pharmaceutical industry, and early-warning systems and statistics of the customs, police and other authorities (e.g. UNODC). This information, combined with efficient long-term sample storage programmes and direct dialog with the ADOs, could be used for further analysis of the samples within 10 years from the sample collection and as a deterrence tool to tackle the emergence of the new chemical entities.

References

1. World Anti-Doping Agency (2015) Anti-Doing Code. https://www.wada-ama.org/sites/default/files/resources/files/wada_anti-doping_code_2019_english_final_revised_v1_linked.pdf. Accessed 28 Oct 2020
2. World Anti-Doping Agency (2020) International Standard, Prohibited List 2020. https://www.wada-ama.org/sites/default/files/wada_2020_english_prohibited_list_0.pdf. Accessed 28 Oct 2020
3. Schänzer W, Thevis M (2017) Human sports drug testing by mass spectrometry. Mass Spectrom Rev 36:16–46
4. United Nations Office on Drugs and Crime (UNODC) (2020) Early warning advisory on new psychoactive substances. https://www.unodc.org/LSS/SubstanceGroup/GroupsDashboard?TestType=NPS. Accessed 30 Sept 2020
5. World Anti-Doping Agency (2018) Anti-doping testing figures. https://www.wada-ama.org/sites/default/files/resources/files/2018_testing_figures_report.pdf. Accessed 30.09.2020
6. Sagoe D, Molde H, Andreassen CS et al (2014) The global epidemiology of anabolic-androgenic steroid use: a meta-analysis and meta-regression analysis. Ann Epidemiol 24:383–398
7. World Anti-Doping Agency (2020) The 2020 Monitoring Program. https://www.wada-ama.org/sites/default/files/resources/files/wada_2020_english_monitoring_program.pdf. Accessed 30 Sept 2020

8. Sekera MH, Ahrens BD, Chang YC et al (2005) Another designer steroid: discovery, synthesis, and detection of 'madol' in urine. Rapid Commun Mass Spectrom 19:781–784
9. Gauthier J, Poirier D, Ayotte C (2012) Characterization of desoxymethyltestosterone main urinary metabolite produced from cultures of human fresh hepatocytes. Steroids 77:635–643
10. Catlin DH, Sekera MH, Ahrens BD et al (2004) Tetrahydrogestrinone: discovery, synthesis, and detection in urine. Rapid Comm Mass Spectrom 18:1245–1249
11. Thomas A, Geyer H, Schänzer W et al (2012) Sensitive determination of prohibited drugs in dried blood spots (DBS) for doping controls by means of a benchtop quadrupole/Orbitrap mass spectrometer. Anal Bioanal Chem 403:1279–1289
12. Holly D, Cox HD, Miller GD, Lai A et al (2017) Detection of autologous blood transfusions using a novel dried blood spot method. Drug Test Anal 9:1713–1720
13. Reverter-Branchat G, Bosch J, Vall J, Farré M et al (2016) Determination of recent growth hormone abuse using a single dried blood spot. J Clin Chem 62:1353–1360
14. Thevis M, Walpurgis K, Thomas A (2020) Analytical approaches in human sports drug testing – recent advances, challenges, and solutions. Anal Chem 92:506–523
15. World Anti-Doping Agency (2019) Minimum required performance levels for detection and identification of non-threshold substances. https://www.wada-ama.org/sites/default/files/resources/files/td2019mrpl_eng.pdf. Accessed 30 Sept 2020
16. World Anti-Doping Agency (2015) Minimum criteria for chromatographic-mass spectrometric confirmation of the identity of analytes for doping control purposes. https://www.wada-ama.org/sites/default/files/resources/files/td2015idcr_-_eng.pdf. Accessed 30 Sept 2020
17. Perrenoud L, Schweizer Grundisch C, Baume N et al (2016) Risk of false positive results to SARM S-4 in case of therapeutic use of antineoplastic/antiandrogen drug containing flutamide: a case study. Drug Test Anal 8:1109–1113

Hair Testing of Doping Agents: Potential and Limitations

Detlef Thieme and Patricia Anielski

Diagnostic Value of Blood, Urine and Hair

The main purpose of blood is transportation of substances—including drugs—to remove metabolic waste products away from cells. It is undisputed that blood concentrations of compounds represent the most universal monitor for current endogenous processes or exogenous manipulation. Acute drug influences, e.g., impairment, amnesia, hallucination or psycho-stimulations, cannot be properly evaluated based on urinary or hair concentrations. Urinary or hair concentrations are both totally redundant for any biological processes. Renal excretion and hair incorporation represent both passive processes which are not regulated to maintain normal values and undergo huge biological variations. Substance levels in these matrices characterize concentrations which are *typically* averaged over hours to days (urine) or weeks to months (hair). Urine is very often unrivalled, in particular if the respective substance is prohibited at all times. Any qualitative verification of steroid abuse, e.g., the detections of urinary long-term metabolites, does not require the proof of a recent administration and relevant biological effects. Respective findings (long-term metabolites of dehydrochloromethyltestosterone or methandienone) can often be detected for several months, which seems clearly superior to blood or hair testing.

D. Thieme (✉) · P. Anielski
Institute of Doping Analysis Dresden, Kreischa, Germany
e-mail: Detlef.Thieme@idas-kreischa.de

© The Author(s), under exclusive license to Springer Nature Switzerland AG 2022
O. Rabin, O. Corazza (eds.), *Emerging Drugs in Sport*,
https://doi.org/10.1007/978-3-030-79293-0_18

Renal Excretion vs. Hair Incorporation

Renal filtration and urinary excretion represent the predominant pathway to eliminate pharmaceutical compounds from the organism. High lipophilicity appears to
be a pre-requisite for most biological activities of pharmaceutical compounds to be
able to pass membranes and attach respective receptors. This holds for all psychoactive compounds (drugs) but is also essential for any androgenic-anabolic compound.
These substance classes are logically not markedly excreted as unchanged drug and
need to undergo bioconversion (metabolism) prior to urinary elimination. This typically includes hydroxylation of a molecule and/or conjugation with glucuronic or
sulphuric acid. Resulting metabolites are significantly more polar and often more
acidic than corresponding parent compounds, are rapidly removed from the blood-
stream by renal filtration but are in return no longer eligible for efficient hair incorporation. The according approach, i.e., parent compounds, are preferential
candidates for hair incorporation (and potential analysis), whereas urine testing
needs to identify suitable metabolites which are unequivocally diagnostic for the
incorporation of a corresponding parent compound and provide sufficient temporal
detection windows. Long-term metabolites of certain anabolic steroids are ideal
examples of legally defensible detection of steroid incorporation over weeks or
months. The situation in hair testing is similarly complex. To illustrate a different
situation, the so-called incorporation rate, i.e., the ratio of hair incorporation over
blood level (AUC), was defined by Nakahara [1] to illustrate concentration ratios
between circulating blood and hair. This parameter was found to vary between ~1
(basic compounds, e.g., cocaine) and 3600 (neutral acidic, THC-COOH), indicating
that identical blood level may result in 3600 times higher hair concentrations if the
chemical structure provides so (e.g., cocaine vs. cannabis). Moreover, protein binding, e.g., the complexation of anabolic steroids to its binding proteins, can markedly
reduce biological effect and hair incorporation. Respective data (i.e., hair incorporation rates) require controlled administration studies and are hence not available for
the doping substances (except few stimulants). Empirical case data (see Fig. 4) provide a qualitative insight into hair incorporation but typically lack reliable data on
substance intake. However, the reduced incorporation rate can well be compensated
by higher blood levels and longer circulation times. THC-COOH and the highly
polar ethanol marker ethyl glucuronide represent two polar drug markers for a successful application of hair testing. Conversely to the low incorporation rate into hair,
there is an elevated risk of washout of respective acidic or polar drugs from hair. In
conclusion there is a consensus that only proximal segments (typically 0–3 cm
strands) are suitable for hair testing, whereas older (terminal) segments bear the risk
of false-negative results. Long-term detection in hair is critically dependent on the
stability of xenobiotics in hair (vs. washout). External contaminations need to be
taken into consideration in hair testing of social drugs which can be easily spread
via air or contact to drug users (in particular when applied by smoking or sniffing,
e.g., cocaine or in animal testing (potential spreading via urine or saliva).
Contamination of hair by doping agents (mostly steroids) was recurrently observed
in forensic cases of its manufacturing in underground laboratories.

Quantitative Interpretations of Hair Concentration

Generally, the potential to explore typical doping scenarios depends on multiple biochemical, pharmaceutical, pharmacokinetic and administrative aspects, i.e., dosage, repetition frequency or risk of unannounced out-of-competition doping controls. Hair concentration represents the temporal average over the collection time. The hair concentration in a typical 3 cm segment signifies the total drug intake in the last 3-month period (Fig. 1), irrespective of individual doses and frequency of intake. Interpretation of most hair tests is focused on drug abuse and restricted to semi-quantitative evaluations, based on empirical forensic databases to discriminate between abuse categories, e.g., abstinence, single use, recurrent use and heavy use of cocaine. Hair that is unprotected is exposed to environmental impact, and hair concentrations can be affected by external factors. In particular, contamination of hairs with smoked (or sniffed) drugs—in particular cannabis and cocaine—is crucial in drug abstinence control but should be less important in doping cases. Transdermal administrations (testosterone cream) could well result in false-positive contamination if contacts between a patient and an athlete cannot be excluded. Contamination via urine or saliva needs to be considered in animal testing. Although there are precautions to identify external contamination of hairs—i.e., pre-washing procedures—it is common consensus that these indicators cannot reliably differentiate incorporation from contamination. Moreover, the gradual reduction of hair concentration following cosmetic treatment is well-approved. Several studies have tested the impact of hair washing, bleaching, colorizing or perming certain drugs [2]. Besides specific chemical degradation of special compounds (cocaine, cannabis), there is a general effect of the deterioration of the hair surface structure leading to enhanced washout of (any) xenobiotic compound from (any) hair. This general

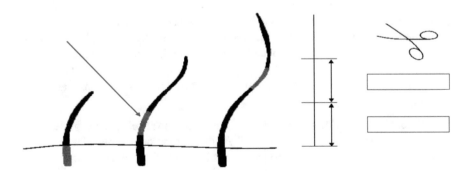

Fig. 1 Time course of hair formation and potential incorporation of drugs. The estimated time span between administration and initial hair detection in humans is 1–2 weeks. Owing to the average growth rate of 1 cm/month, the compound could be detected over 2 months in the proximal segment. Subsequently, the affected hair segment will continuously migrate into corresponding distal segments

effect is least crucial for basic drugs which are tightly bound to the natural hair pigment melanin, e.g. clenbuterol or cocaine. Hair concentrations were found to be rather constant over months [3] giving access to serious long-term profiles by hair segmentation. Logically, hair concentrations of these drugs depend significantly on the amount of melanin, and hence on hair colour, which is far less important for neutral drugs like most steroids. Practically, dark hair incorporates higher concentrations of these substances than similarly exposed blond or white hair.

Hair Testing and Anti-doping Testing

There have been many approaches to use hair as complementary testing in doping control. A general limitation is due to the fact that prohibition of substance use in sport is partially limited to certain times (e.g., *prohibition* of stimulants, or opiates *in-competition*), dosages and/or administration pathways (e.g., permitted therapeutic inhalation of certain dosages of beta2 agonists). These acute effects cannot be properly addressed by hair testing, which provides information on average dosages administered over the collection time, i.e., typically several weeks to months. In contrast, substances *prohibited at all times* and irrespective of its administration pathways were traditional targets of hair testing of doping agents. Numerous attempts have demonstrated the potential of hair analyses to identify synthetic steroids and other anabolic agents, either as target analysis or screening procedures [4–13]. The quantitative discrimination power of hair concentrations of endogenous steroids is too low to identify, e.g., testosterone abuse. Endogenous variations and external effects (washout) are rather high, and only administrations in large doses of testosterone are reliably detected, in particular following transdermal administrations or injections of free testosterone. Additionally, other substance classes were found to be suitable targets for anti-doping hair testing, e.g., S1.2, other anabolic agents, or S4, hormone and metabolic modulators. Interestingly, even testing for polar acidic diuretics was reported to be rewarding because their relative high dosages appear to counterbalance the poor incorporation. As an example, hydrochlorothiazide was found to be reproducibly detectable in hair following multiple doses [14].

Suitability of hair testing of upcoming substance classes is not yet completely investigated:

- Efficient incorporation and detection of growth hormone-releasing peptides, hormones or secretagogues is highly unlikely due to their large molecular masses.
- Incorporation of selective androgen receptor modulators (SARMs, see Example 3) seems to be comparable to steroids. However, due to their relatively high potency (low dosage and serum concentrations), a sensitive detection in hair appears rather critical.
- In contrast, HIF-1a stabilizers, taken orally at rather high dosages, represent a promising interesting target for future investigations.

The advantage of hair testing to complement adverse analytical findings in urine is therefore dependent on the specific constellation:

- Any temporal differentiation of substances prohibited in-competition only deems to be condemned to failure.
- Certain substances—typically small basic molecules—which are well- and stably incorporated into hair can be reliably confirmed in hair. In return, its absence in hair provides valid indications against relevant (i.e., biologically active) administration in the respective timeframe.
- Testing of neutral compounds in hair, in particular steroids or SARMs, is much less sensitive and sustainable, i.e., requiring careful consideration of potential washout. In particular synthetic steroid esters (e.g., nandrolone decanoate) or long-term metabolites of steroids (e.g., dehydrochloromethyltestosterone [15], stanozolol [16]) were found to persist in urine at low concentrations over months. Respective urinary findings at late stage of excretion can hardly be confirmed (or excluded) by hair tests for sensitivity reasons.

Example 1: Basic Compounds, e.g., Clenbuterol
The chemical properties of clenbuterol are almost ideal for hair testing. The molecule is rather stable, slightly polar and rather basic. It is predominantly excreted unchanged in urine; 40% of the administered dose was detected in 48 h [17]. According to the poor metabolism and rather slow elimination of clenbuterol, its blood, urine and hair concentrations are well correlated. Typical urinary concentrations are detected in presumptive doping cases, ranging from 0.02 to 20 ng/mL; hair concentrations between 0.2 and 60 pg/mg were reported [18]. Comparison of absolute substance amounts in a urine (2 mL volume) vs. hair (default weight ca. 20 mg) demonstrates that the total amount of clenbuterol available for detection is 0.04–40 ng in urine vs. 0.004–1.2 ng which differ by a factor of ca. 10. Hair testing of clenbuterol is therefore an efficient testing method, as clenbuterol is rapidly eliminated by renal filtration, but efficiently and stably immobilized into hair. Negative findings or hair concentrations below 5pg/mg were detected in presumptive contamination cases (Fig. 2), whereas clenbuterol abuse is typically accompanied by levels higher than 15 pg/mg [19]. Moreover, valid concentration profiles can contribute to case interpretation. Constant levels were detected in cases of long-term food contaminations. In contrast, the reduction of clenbuterol concentration in hair from 4.5 pg/mg (distal segment 3–6 cm) to zero (proximal segment 0–3 cm) was observed in another follow-up case. This suggested a significant reduction of clenbuterol intake—either by changing diet or stopping intake—in a presumptive doping case.

Example 2: Neutral Compounds, e.g., Steroids
Incorporation of neutral steroids into hair seems much less efficient and less reproducible. It appears likely that the external infiltration via sweat and sebum is more relevant than incorporation from blood. This is supported by the observations that hair colour does not significantly influence hair concentration [20–21], and gradual washout of steroids (e.g., reduction of cortisone by half in 3–4 months [22]) is

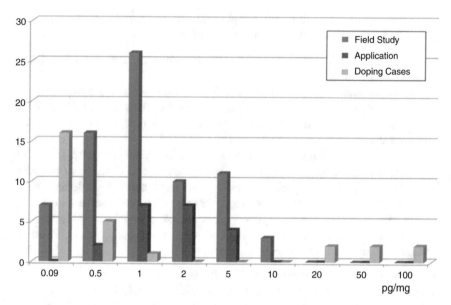

Fig. 2 Hair concentrations of clenbuterol were found to be clearly dose dependent and rather stable. The category 'Field Study' refers to presumed contamination cases, while 'Application' signifies concentrations resulting from controlled oral administration at low levels [18]. This seems to permit a semi-quantitative differentiation between potential contaminations resulting in negative or low hair concentrations from highly suspicious levels (i.e. > 5 pg/mg)

pervasive. Due to insufficient controlled administration studies dealing with hair incorporation of exogenous steroids, the concentration distribution of the endogenous testosterone might be insightful to estimate potential hair concentrations. Testosterone is produced in healthy male adults at daily rates of 6–8 mg. Logically, replacement therapy applies similar dosages, whereas abuse dosages in bodybuilding or powerlifting—focused on significant muscle gain—are starting at ~30 mg/ day. The endogenous production corresponds to typical blood concentration levels between 2 and 10 ng/mL (Table 1). Urinary concentrations of testosterone (excreted as glucuronide) undergo large inter- and intra-individual variations which are due to physiological, pathological or genetic influences. 'Normal' unsuspicious values may range until 200 ng/mL, i.e., the warning level for follow-up analyses. Extra to this, urinary metabolites like androsterone or etiocholanolone are excreted in urine at 'normal' concentrations up to 10,000 ng/mL and are analytically available for subsequent confirmation analyses. In contrast, testosterone hair concentrations of normal untreated males are typically below 5 pg/mg (representing an internal threshold for further follow-up analyses).

This example demonstrates that normal values are monitored best in blood samples, whereas individual variations of renal filtration or hair incorporation hugely reduce the benefit of quantitative interpretations. Moreover, the example shows clearly that substance amounts available in a routine test sample—and hence the sensitivity of testing procedures based on comparable technology—differ

Table 1 Comparison of endogenous concentrations of testosterone, detection limits and resulting total substance amounts in typical control samples to compare potential method sensitivity in blood, urine and hair

Testosterone	Concentration range	LOD	Max amount in a control sample
Blood	2–10 ng/mL	0.2 ng/mL	20 ng (in 2 mL)
Urine	0–200 ng/mL	1 ng/mL	4000 ng (in 20 mL)
Hair	0–5 pg/mg	1 pg/mg	250 pg (in 50 mg)

dramatically, i.e., the absolute amount of testosterone in a urine test exceeds the hair level by a factor of ca. 10.000, which is in line with the aforementioned variations in hair incorporation efficacy.

Example 3: Administration Study of a Selective Androgen Receptor Modulator (GSK 2881078)

All SARMs need to exhibit comparable physicochemical properties—i.e., mainly high lipophilicity—to be able to migrate to the location of intended biological effects, i.e., androgen receptors within the cytoplasm. Moreover, a high stability of respective drugs seems to be desirable to facilitate a long duration of biological effectiveness—and hence long detection windows in doping control. Recent reports on ligandrol indicated detection windows of 22 days in urine following a single oral administration of 10 mg, without testing hair samples. Trace amounts of ligandrol and its hydroxy metabolite were detected in horse hair following oral administration [23]. Owing to the structural diversity of SARMs and very limited amount of reference data, an oral administration study of GSK 2881078 was conducted to estimate its metabolism and incorporation rate into hair. To compare preferential suitability of hair or urine, a single dose of 1.5 mg GSK2881078 was orally taken, followed by a second administration of a single 0.76 mg dose after an 8-week washout period [24]. Interestingly, the half-life of the drug (as well as its hydroxy metabolites) was observed to be higher than 4 days, resulting in the detection window of a single therapeutic administration of 42 days (parent compound) and 38 days (longest excreted hydroxy metabolite), respectively (Fig. 3). Corresponding hair samples, investigated with identical instrumental technique, permitted detection of low amounts in a short time window, followed by traces detectable up to 9 weeks (Fig. 3). This substance category of chemically stable, lipophilic neutral compounds, which is slowly excreted in urine and detectable for a very long time, but not well incorporated into hair, seems preferentially detectable in urine.

Review of Empirical Forensic Data

Empirical case data are—next to administration studies—valuable sources of forensic interpretation. Systematic high-dose administration studies of steroids are—as well as controlled administration of drugs of abuse—ethically unacceptable, and case reference data are therefore widely accepted in forensic hair testing. We have

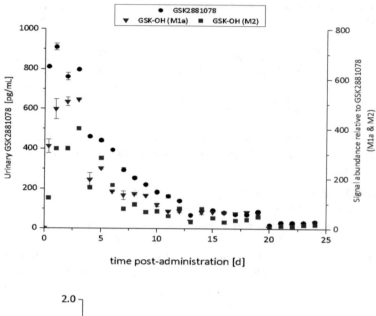

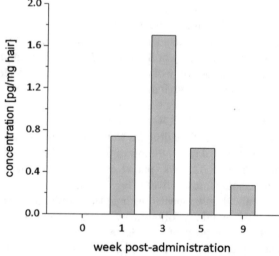

Fig. 3 Concentration profiles of GSK2881078 (and its metabolites) in urine (top) and hair (bottom). Adapted from Rading A, Anielski P, Thieme D, Keiler AM (2021) Detection of the selective androgen receptor modulator GSK2881078 and metabolites in urine and hair after single oral administration. Drug Test Anal 13 [1]:217–222, Figures 3, 4. https://doi.org/10.1002/dta.2943, licensed under the terms of the Creative Commons Attribution License (https://creativecommons.org/licenses/by/4.0/)

received related urine and hair specimens in 145 forensic cases between 2012 and 2019. The suspects were typically accused of possession or trafficking of doping agents, i.e., 82% being males who typically pretended self-consumption and often provided information on recent steroid intake. However, these data were often biased, as self-consumption is less prosecutable than dealing with steroids. Moreover, the reliability of the mostly black-market steroids was far too poor to draw any quantitative conclusion. However, these empirical 'snapshots'—in particular the correspondence between simultaneous hair and urine testing—provide some interesting insight.

Most of the doping relevant findings were coincidentally identified in both matrices in the majority of cases (282 of 554 findings, Table 2, Fig. 4) using comparable analytical screening methods, in particular identical instrumentation. The overall sensitivity (i.e., true positives over total cases) of both approaches seems to be very similar. Hair testing appears to be superior to urine in cases of basic compounds (e.g., clomifene, Table 2) or when identifying testosterone. This needs to be differentiated from endogenous testosterone in urine testing but can be detected as its intact exogenous esters in hair, which is apparently more specific (Table 2). The detection in urine is apparently more efficient in cases of injectable depot preparations (e.g., nandrolone) or wherever specific urinary long-term metabolites are monitored. Maximum detection times in those cases are difficult to estimate, and reference data from respective long-term studies are not available. Anecdotal reports suggest that respective detection windows of long-term metabolites or depot injections are often underrated (Fig. 5).

Table 2 Contingency table describing association between the detection of any doping agent (top), clomifene, testosterone and nandrolone, respectively, in hair and urine

Total $n = 554$		Hair	
		Positive	Negative
Urine	Positive	50.9%	22.9%
	Negative	26.2%	
Clomifene $n = 20$		Hair	
		Positive	Negative
Urine	Positive	20.0%	5.0%
	Negative	75.0%	
Testosterone $n = 75$		Hair	
		Positive	Negative
Urine	Positive	65.3%	6.7%
	Negative	28.0%	
Nandrolone $n = 38$		Hair	
		Positive	Negative
Urine	Positive	55.3%	28.9%
	Negative	15.8%	

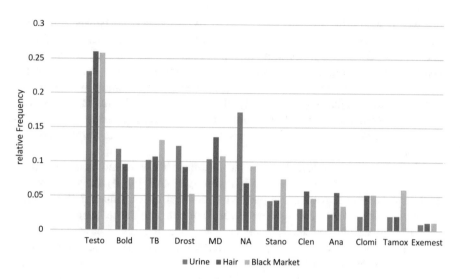

Fig. 4 Comparison of prevalence (i.e., its occurrence in confiscation statistics of doping agents testosterone, boldenone, trenbolone, drostanolone, metandienone, nandrolone, stanozolol, clenbuterol, anastrozole, clomifene, tamoxifen, exemestane) and its detection frequency in blood and urine

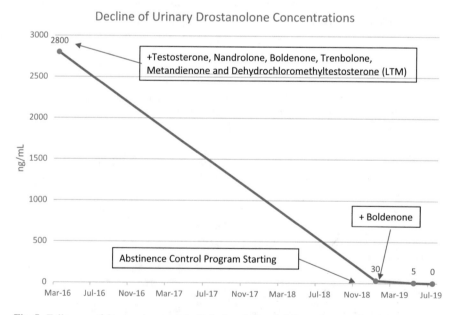

Fig. 5 Follow-up of drostanolone metabolite's (i.e., 2α-methyl-5α-androstane-3α-ol-17-one) concentrations in urine within an abstinence control programme. The absence of most steroids—which were initially detected at the beginning of abstinence control—suggests a compliance of the accused female powerlifter. This very slow urinary concentration decline—accompanied by negative hair tests—seems to be indicative for certain steroid esters

Conclusion

Hair and urine tests are never equivalent but often complement each other:

- Urine exhibits unique detection potential whenever long-term metabolites are available, e.g., in cases of dehydrochlormethyltestosterone, metandienone or stanozolol. Respective markers are detectable for several seems or even months following abuse. Similar detection potential in hair deems impossible due to limitations in sensitivity, hair length and washout.
- A similar situation appears likely for SARMs, which are slowly excreted and sensitively detected in urine, resulting in very long detection windows in conventional urine testing.
- Hair tests are extremely valuable in cases of basic anabolic agents (clenbuterol) or anti-estrogens (tamoxifen, anastrozole, exemestane), which are well-incorporated into hair and easily detected. Stability in hair, in particular concerning degradation and/or washout, appears to be good.
- The potential detection of intact testosterone esters, which are not excreted into urine, in hair constitutes a significant benefit. Confirmation of synthetic testosterone esters could prove its abuse in 28% of testosterone cases exhibiting unsuspicious urinary steroid levels.
- Owing to different temporal biochemical excretion and incorporation mechanisms, only half of the doping relevant findings were found to be coherent between urine and hair testing. Proven urinary findings remaining unconfirmed in hair (22.9%) and positive hair tests corresponding to blank urine findings (26.2%) similarly contributed to the case statistics. It is, therefore, important to clarify that hair analysis is not prohibited in anti-doping practice, but it was acknowledged by the Society of Hair Testing [25] as well as WADA [26] that it cannot be used to override the validity of a doping test. Hair analysis is occasionally used to collect additional information on doping practice or chronicity of exposure.

References

1. Nakahara Y, Kikura R (1996) Hair analysis for drugs of abuse. XIII. Effect of structural factors on incorporation of drugs into hair: the incorporation rates of amphetamine analogs. Arch Toxicol 70:841–849
2. Cooper GA et al (2012) Society of Hair Testing guidelines for drug testing in hair. Forensic Sci Int 218:20–24
3. Schlupp A et al (2004) The beta-agonist clenbuterol in mane and tail hair of horses. Equine Vet J 36:118–122
4. Auer MK et al (2020) Steroid 17-hydroxyprogesterone in hair is a potential long-term biomarker of androgen control in congenital adrenal hyperplasia due to 21-hydroxylase deficiency. Neuroendocrinology 110:938–949
5. Devi JL et al (2018) Determination of testosterone esters in the hair of male greyhound dogs using liquid chromatography-high resolution mass spectrometry. Drug Test Anal 10:460–473

6. Choi TLS et al (2018) Detection of seventy-two anabolic and androgenic steroids and/or their esters in horse hair using ultra-high performance liquid chromatography-high resolution mass spectrometry in multiplexed targeted MS(2) mode and gas chromatography-tandem mass spectrometry. J Chromatogr A 1566:51–63

7. Kwok KY et al (2017) Detection of anabolic and androgenic steroids and/or their esters in horse hair using ultra-high performance liquid chromatography-high resolution mass spectrometry. J Chromatogr A 1493:76–86

8. Shah I et al (2014) Hair-based rapid analyses for multiple drugs in forensics and doping: application of dynamic multiple reaction monitoring with LC-MS/MS. Chem Cent J 8:73

9. Strano-Rossi S et al (2013) Screening for exogenous androgen anabolic steroids in human hair by liquid chromatography/orbitrap-high resolution mass spectrometry. Anal Chim Acta 793:61–71

10. Deshmukh NI et al (2012) Determination of stanozolol and 3'-hydroxystanozolol in rat hair, urine and serum using liquid chromatography tandem mass spectrometry. Chem Cent J 6:162

11. Deshmukh N et al (2010) Analysis of anabolic steroids in human hair using LC-MS/MS. Steroids 75:710–714

12. Bresson M et al (2006) Doping control for metandienone using hair analyzed by gas chromatography-tandem mass spectrometry. J Chromatogr B Analyt Technol Biomed Life Sci 836:124–128

13. Anielski P et al (2005) Detection of testosterone, nandrolone and precursors in horse hair. Anal Bioanal Chem 383:903–908

14. Gheddar L, Raul JS, Kintz P (2019) First identification of a diuretic, hydrochlorothiazide, in hair: Application to a doping case and interpretation of the results. Drug Test Anal 11:157–161

15. Sobolevsky T, Rodchenkov G (2012) Detection and mass spectrometric characterization of novel long-term dehydrochloromethyltestosterone metabolites in human urine. J Steroid Biochem Mol Biol 128:121–127

16. Schanzer W et al (2013) Expanding analytical possibilities concerning the detection of stanozolol misuse by means of high resolution/high accuracy mass spectrometric detection of stanozolol glucuronides in human sports drug testing. Drug Test Anal 5:810–818

17. Baselt R (2020) Disposition of toxic drugs and chemicals in man. Ed Biomed Pubn:12

18. Krumbholz A et al (2014) Statistical significance of hair analysis of clenbuterol to discriminate therapeutic use from contamination. Drug Test Anal 6:1108–1116

19. Dumestre-Toulet V et al (2002) Hair analysis of seven bodybuilders for anabolic steroids, ephedrine, and clenbuterol. J Forensic Sci 47:211–214

20. Anielski P (2008) Hair analysis of anabolic steroids in connection with doping control-results from horse samples. J Mass Spectrom 43:1001–1008

21. Calamari CV et al (2020) Hair as an alternative noninvasive matrix: sources of variation in testosterone levels. Domest Anim Endocrinol 72:106477

22. Krumbholz A et al (2013) Diagnostic value of concentration profiles of glucocorticosteroids and endocannabinoids in hair. Ther Drug Monit 35:600–607

23. Cutler C et al (2020) Investigation of the metabolism of the selective androgen receptor modulator LGD-4033 in equine urine, plasma and hair following oral administration. Drug Test Anal 12:247–260

24. Rading A et al (2021) Detection of the selective androgen receptor modulator GSK2881078 and metabolites in urine and hair after single oral administration. Drug Test Anal 13:217–222

25. Society_of_Hair_Testing. Consensus of the Society of Hair Testing on hair testing for doping agents. 1999 [cited 2020 11. Dec]; Available from: www.soht.org/consensus/9-nicht-kategorisiert/88-consensus-on-doping-agents

26. WADA. International Standard for Laboratories (ISL), 5.3.4.5.6 Alternative Biological Matrices. 2020 [cited 2020 12. Dec]; Available from: www.wada-ama.org/en/resources/laboratories/international-standard-for-laboratories-isl

Part VI
The Next Challenge

What Will the Next Challenges Be?

Audrey Kinahan and Mark Stuart

Keeping ahead of doping in sport requires a sustained and innovative approach to assess what new substances are being used by athletes and to determine those that have the potential to be abused in the future. Such work involves a comprehensive and ever-changing assessment of new and historical science, global and government regulations, cultural and recreational practices and popular opinion supported by a multi-faceted strategic methodology, which seeks to both uncover what substances are actually being used by athletes and then assess whether they really do improve performance. As highlighted in previous chapters, the World Anti-Doping Code ("the Code") outlines the framework used to decide whether a substance is banned in sport. Specifically, article 4.3 of the Code outlines the principle that to be considered for inclusion a substance is either a masking agent or meets at least two of three equally weighted criteria. These criteria are: have proven or potential performance-enhancement abilities, actual or potential health risk, or its use is a violation of the "spirit of sport". New drugs that are approved for human use invariably come with a wealth of data about their risks to health which can often be used to reasonably determine whether such risk would apply in the doping context. The concept of "spirit of sport" is also well-defined by the Code and is most likely to be met if a clear *intention* to cheat with the substance can be determined.

A. Kinahan (✉)
Eirpharm, Ennis, Co. Clare, Ireland

Prohibited List Expert Advisory Group, World Anti-Doping Agency (WADA),
Montreal, QC, Canada
e-mail: pharmacy@eirpharm.com

M. Stuart
Centre for Metabolism and Inflammation, Division of Medicine, University College London,
London, UK

International Testing Agency, Lausanne, Switzerland

© The Author(s), under exclusive license to Springer Nature Switzerland AG 2022   243
O. Rabin, O. Corazza (eds.), *Emerging Drugs in Sport*,
https://doi.org/10.1007/978-3-030-79293-0_19

Striving for an Evidence-Based Approach

When assessing a substance for the Prohibited List, the most challenging criteria to determine with any robust evidence-based approach is whether a substance actually improves performance. Unfortunately, performance-enhancing effects of emerging substances or novel psychoactive substances (NPS) are rarely demonstrated in double-blind, peer-reviewed, randomised clinical trials using performance-enhancing doses in elite athletes. Conducting any human studies using illegal, unapproved or designer drugs for the purpose of demonstrating performance enhancement would normally not be permitted for safety and ethical reasons as very little supporting preclinical information is usually available. Even when sufficient preclinical data is available to allow these types of studies to be conducted, there can be limitations with respect to using sufficiently high doses to demonstrate performance enhancement. As these challenges become more apparent with emerging doping substances, it is evident that a combination of different types of clinical and preclinical studies, including animal and in vitro research, will need to be used to determine performance-enhancing potential. As modern society demands alternatives to animal testing, the development of appropriate in vitro models to evaluate potential doping effects of a substance is a further challenge. In vitro tissue-engineered models of human skeletal muscle are currently being used to model diseases such as muscular dystrophy, with a view to assessing treatments for muscle injury and disease with some success [1–3]. Currently bio-engineering approaches are in development to predict clinically relevant drug responses, and these may have a future role in predicting a substance's performance-enhancement potential.

Key Partnerships with the Biopharmaceutical Industry

For legitimate medicines in clinical development, the World Anti-Doping Agency (WADA) has formal arrangements with the International Federation of Pharmaceutical Manufacturers and Associations (IFPMA) [4] and several leading international pharmaceutical companies involving the early stage sharing of information and expertise with respect to investigational substances, particularly to establish detection methods prior to marketing of those substances identified as having a potential for doping. Pharmaceutical industry analysts regard the development of a new drug through the regulatory process to cost from 985 million USD [5] to 2.6 billion USD [6] and to take 10–15 years. The approval rate for drugs entering clinical development is reckoned to be less than 12% [6]. The challenge from an anti-doping aspect is to encourage more pharmaceutical companies, who range from multinational conglomerates to niche single-drug start-up companies, to include doping potential in their clinical development programme. While some regulatory authorities may include anti-doping in their pre- and post-approval risk management plans, the challenge is to extend this knowledge to all companies and regulatory agencies.

The Challenge of Global Harmonisation

In accordance with the Code, a key principle of the Prohibited List is that it harmonises the substances and methods that are prohibited in the majority of countries and thus by definition it is a global document. The implementation of the List affects every elite sports person irrespective of the country they reside or train in; the List's application should therefore be consistent. While there is a move to develop international Standards of Care [such as with the GINA (Global Initiative for Asthma) guidelines [7]], countries differ in access to medicines, medical practice and the regulatory status of medicines. These differences, in turn, can be a barrier to the uniform application of the List. Regulatory status with regard to the sale and supply of pseudoephedrine is one area where inconsistency is noticeable between different counties. This substance is included in products to treat nasal congestion and symptoms of cold and flu. As pseudoephedrine can be used to synthesise methamfetamine in underground laboratories, there are restrictions on its availability, with tighter restrictions in those countries where methamfetamine has a significant abuse problem. In Ireland and the UK, for example, there is a limit on the amount that can be purchased over the counter, and it is sold under the supervision of the pharmacist. In the USA, there is a limit on the monthly purchase per person, and photo identification is required to make a purchase, while in Australia these products are available with a prescription only. Inter-country differences in the regulatory status of the currently permitted substance tramadol may also pose dilemmas regarding treatment options for sports physicians. The legal status of this synthetic narcotic varies throughout the world. There is a Scheduled Controlled Drug in almost all countries, but there are differences in how it is scheduled. In Europe, North America, Australia and New Zealand, it is available on prescription, while in Egypt, tramadol is scheduled as an illegal substance, as it is regarded that there is a significant abuse issue with Egypt [8, 9]. The use of and access to a range of pain medications has been widely debated in the sports medicine community [10], and while tramadol is not prohibited for use in sport, this substance has been associated with abuse and addiction worldwide. A third example of a challenge to the implementation of the List is the brand names used in medicines. While substances are regarded as permitted or prohibited in sport based on the List, this is generally translated in each country as associated with a specific product being allowed or banned for use in sport. The Vicks nasal inhaler product range available in the United Kingdom contain substances that are permitted for use in sport, while in the USA the same brand name Vicks inhaler has also been used to market a nasal product which contained the prohibited stimulant l-methamfetamine [11]. One unfortunate British Olympian [12] learned, at his expense, when he purchased the inhaler in the USA in the belief it was the same one as in the UK and subsequently tested positive for methamfetamine at the 2002 Winter Olympics. At that time, the International Olympic Committee (IOC) List did not distinguish between the d- and l-isomers, of which the former is a stimulant, but the issue was addressed in the first WADA List by nuancing that the nature of fault is dependent on the methamfetamine isomer found in the athlete's sample. From this example, the challenge for the List is with respect to the inconsistencies in branding of medicinal products. The marketing of the same brand name for a medicine which contains different substances depending on the country of sale is outside of the control of WADA and thus could be a potential barrier to the uniform implementation of the List. When considering a harmonised application of the Prohibited List, there are cultural aspects that need to be considered, particularly in the way products are consumed as foods in different parts of the world. The Prohibited List already contains examples of substances that are available in foodstuffs in one part of the world but also marketed in commercially produced supplement products in other parts of the world. An example of such a substance is the alkaloid higenamine, which is included in section S3 of the Prohibited List as a prohibited beta-2 agonist and found naturally in a variety of plants such as *Nelumbo nucifera* (lotus seeds), *Nandina domestica* (fruit) and *Aconitum carmichaelii* (root). The laboratory reporting level for higenamine is 10 ng/mL (i.e., 50% of the MRPL for beta-2 agonists). A lotus seed powder extract, containing higenamine, when dosed at 679.6 µg of higenamine three times daily for 3 consecutive days resulted in urinary higenamine concentrations above this level [13]. In contrast, higenamine contained in a traditional Chinese medicine of a throat lozenge containing *Nandina domestica* fruit yielded urinary results below the level [14]. It should be noted that there are always significant variabilities in the actual doses obtained from natural products due to differences in cultivation, harvesting and extraction processes. Irrespective of origin, as naturally or commercially available, the advice given to athletes is to avoid higenamine-containing supplements [15] and extracts to eliminate any risk of testing positive for this substance. Exposure in foodstuffs is not a new phenomenon, and the case of poppy seeds is one that has been in the spotlight in the anti-doping community in the past. Poppy seeds naturally contain small amounts of the prohibited opioid morphine and are actually the source of pharmaceutical-grade morphine products globally. They are also commonly used in baking, such as on bagels which are popularly consumed in North America and in Europe. For morphine, the level of detection in a doping control test has been set to a threshold of 1.0 µg/mL, with a decision limit of 1.3 µg/mL. While it is still possible to have a positive test [16], the introduction of a urinary threshold is necessary to implement into the testing process to reduce the risk of an athlete testing positive for morphine with normal consumption of common food products. Setting reasonable detection thresholds for new substances is one way to maintain harmonisation of the Prohibited List while accommodating global differences in areas such as product regulation or dietary customs in different countries. However, as with higenamine, the advice given to athletes is to avoid poppy seed-containing foods before competition. While the WADA principle of global harmonisation may be an obstacle for the Prohibited List, it is not one that cannot be overcome. It is crucial that whenever a new substance or method is added to the List, that WADA conducts an impact assessment which includes an evaluation from a global and local aspect on the specific impact of any changes. If a specific local issue is identified, WADA often coincides the addition of the substance to the list with a targeted education initiative in that country or particular population at greater risk of inadvertent doping with the substance.

Monitoring New Use of Old Drugs

Keeping ahead of doping practices not only involves assessing new drugs that come onto the market but also constantly reviewing emerging patterns of drug abuse of substances that were developed decades ago, but which are only now being uncovered as potential doping agents. In this sense, the WADA Monitoring Program is an important and strategic tool to initiate further investigation into whether a drug is being widely used in sport, and the investigation of many substances that have been on the market for some time starts with the data obtained through the Monitoring Program. Substances are often placed on the Monitoring Program after anecdotal reports of abuse or after scientific research suggests a performance-enhancing effect might be conceivable. By being on the Monitoring Program, a substance is subject to testing by laboratories, and the reports are analysed by WADA to determine the prevalence of use of the substance in athletes. It is helpful to determine the extent of use, rather than to establish whether the drug works to improve performance, and can be the catalyst to initiate further research if evidence of intention to improve performance is detected. Meldonium is one particular substance developed almost 50 years ago that has come under recent scrutiny through the WADA Monitoring Program process. This drug was invented in the 1970s in Latvia, which was part of the Soviet Republic at the time, and has since been used to treat patients with heart conditions, with claims that it has cardioprotective and anti-ischaemic effects and increases work capacity [17]. It was used in the 1980s to boost the stamina of troops fighting at high altitudes in Afghanistan [18]. However, the suspected abuse of the drug by athletes was only uncovered by WADA as late as 2014 after reports of its use at the London 2012 Olympic Games, and at that point, it was added to the WADA Monitoring Program to further understand the prevalence of use by athletes. In 2015, the widespread use of the drug was also uncovered at the Baku European Games where 66 athletes (8.7%) competing in 15 of the 21 sports at the Games tested positive for the drug under the WADA Monitoring Program, including 13 medallists [19]. WADA subsequently added meldonium to the Prohibited List in January 2016, a move which resulted in many positive drug tests in athletes around the world. The uncovering of the abuse of meldonium prompted WADA to further investigate other Soviet-era substances that could potentially be performance enhancing but have gone under the WADA radar until now. One such drug that has since surfaced is bemitil, which again was developed in the 1970s and reported to have been used by Soviet troops in Afghanistan to increase endurance and increase work capacity. It was also reported that the substance was used to prepare the athletes of the USSR team for the Moscow 1980 Olympic Games [20]. The drug came under investigation by WADA as a potential performance-enhancing drug and was placed on the WADA Monitoring Program in 2019. This constant retrospective monitoring is key to systematically reviewing old science in order to keep abreast of new science and doping trends. Another more recent consideration raised by WADA stakeholders was to include the strong pain-relieving ketobemidone as an example of a prohibited narcotic drug. This drug was developed in 1942 and is currently only available in Denmark, Norway and Sweden [21]. Conceivably this is comparable to other narcotic drugs on the Prohibited List, although whether there is any real evidence to indicate the drug is actually being abused in sport seems less clear.

Keeping up with the Supplements Industry

As highlighted in previous chapters, the rapidly expanding, evolving and largely unregulated dietary sports supplements industry is an increasing challenge for maintaining the integrity of the List as many emerging substances are contained in dietary supplements. With such high profits to be made, the sports supplement industry invests huge resources into the scientific development of new substances and health products targeted at both athletes and the wider population. Market analysts predict that the fast-growing sports supplements sector is expected to be valued at about 350 billion USD by 2023 [22]. Of this, the global sports nutrition segment market size is predicted to be worth 31 billion USD by 2027 [23]. The use of such supplements is increasing, particularly in the largest market, the USA, where a US 2011 government health study [24] reported that more than half of US adults used a dietary supplement between 2003 and 2006, compared to 40% of adults between 1988 and 1994. The advertising media spend in the USA is 640 million USD for nutritional supplements [25]. Similarly, the market in Europe is currently valued at nearly 15 billion USD (2019) and increasing at a compound annual growth rate (CAGR) of 9.3% per annum [26]. Online sales are increasing, particularly in emerging economies such as India, China and Brazil. According to data published by the Ministry of Food Processing Industries, Government of India, in 2017, online retail has grown significantly in India, at a CAGR of 50–55% from 2009 to 2013 [23]. A small section of this industry has been shown to be aggressively promoting sports supplements some of which are found to contain prohibited substances such as anabolic steroids, growth promoters, stimulants and beta-2 agonists. It is recognised that athletes have had positive anti-doping tests as a result of both the deliberate and accidental presence of prohibited substances in supplements [27]. Risk mitigation services, such as NSF Certified for Sport and Informed Sport which audit manufacturing sites of supplement manufacturers, certify raw materials and final products as suitable for those subject to anti-doping rules and may reduce the potential exposure of an athlete to the better known prohibited substances, but ultimately athletes are subject to "strict liability", which means they are responsible for the presence of a prohibited substance in their bodies irrespective of whatever risk minimisation process applied. Some supplement manufacturers are also misleading athletes by taking either older previously marketed medical substances and repurposing them or using newly extracted botanicals and including them in sports supplements because they may not be specifically named on the Prohibited List. The undiscerning athlete could be deceived by these unscrupulous marketing tactics. In one example, the amfetamine-like stimulant, methylhexaneamine, which is known by numerous names including DMAA (1,3-dimethylamylamine), and was previously sold as a medicine for nasal congestion in the 1970s [28], emerged as an ingredient in sports supplements in 2009. It was heavily marketed as a "natural" stimulant as it was purported to be extracted from geranium oil; however, regulatory authorities do not have any evidence to substantiate this claim. DMAA was regarded as unsafe [29], and regulatory authorities proceeded to remove them from the market from 2012 onwards [30–33]. For a stimulant such as methylhexaneamine, even though not specifically named in the 2009 List, it was regarded as prohibited as it has similar chemical structure and biological effects to amfetamine and other substances in Section S6 of the List. Methylhexaneamine was first named on the List as a non-specified stimulant for the 2010 List. It was reclassified in the following year as a specified stimulant in recognition of its deliberate inclusion in some nutritional supplements and confusion associated with the various names used for this substance. As substances are specifically named on the List, they become routinely known in doping control testing. Regulatory authorities and public health conduct follow-ups and act to reduce or remove the supply from the market [29–32]. However, as each substance is prohibited, another supplement comes to be used in its place, and a similar pathway is followed. For example, over the past number of years, similar patterns have occurred for higenamine, octopamine, synephrine and octodrine (dimethylhexylamine, DMHA) and potentially the new names go on. The challenge to the integrity of the List is that these supplements are not regulated to the same standards as medicines in most jurisdictions around the world. This anomaly is recognised by sport's governing bodies such as the IOC [27].

The largest sports supplement market is the USA, whereby once on the market, the burden is on the regulatory authority, the Food and Drug Administration (FDA), to prove that the product is unsafe or illegal. Steven Tave, who has overseen the FDA's Office of Dietary Supplement Programs, has acknowledged that there are "regulatory gaps" and "that at a minimum that the dietary supplement market isn't perfectly regulated" [34]. Within the European Union, while there are some inter-country variations, sports supplements are in general regulated as foods, with greater regulation for certain substances and when therapeutic claims are made. The current situation is under review by the European Committee for Standardisations [35].

In Australia, the lightweight regulation is recognised as a consumer health issue and unsatisfactory, and so this is currently being redressed. From 30 November 2020, in order for sports supplements with therapeutic claims, containing higher-risk ingredients, to be advertised and supplied, they must be included in the Australian Register of Therapeutic Goods (ARTG). Such supplements will be obliged to meet the same legal requirements that ensure the quality, safety and efficacy as for medicines, including advertising standards [36]. This will include products that are marketed for enhancing muscle, mental focus, metabolism, stamina or testosterone levels or as weight reduction, pre-workout or post-workout supplements. This has also happened in Canada, where supplements are now required to meet quality, safety and efficacy standards to be registered as a Natural Health Product [37]. Some governments are recognising that this is a challenge for public health and also for the integrity of sport practice. It is welcome that governments now are starting to enhance the regulatory requirements for sports supplements in the context of public health. However, until this issue is resolved globally, the challenge to the List of unregulated sports supplements remains.

Misinformation and Popular Misconceptions

Very few supplements that are not already on the Prohibited List have been shown to directly improve performance. The International Olympic Committee published a consensus statement in 2018 stating that only a few known performance-enhancing supplements might be considered to have an adequate level of support to suggest that marginal performance gains may be possible. These supplements include caffeine, creatine, nitrate, sodium bicarbonate and possibly also beta-alanine [27]. Despite this extensive review of the supplements used by athletes, companies continue to make unsubstantiated claims about the performance-enhancing effects of their products. Ecdysteroids are one such class of drug that are widely and heavily marketed to athletes as dietary supplement, with claims to increase strength and muscle mass during resistance training, to reduce fatigue and to ease recovery [20] and being advertised as a permitted and natural alternative to anabolic agents that athletes could use without testing positive for a drug test. Whether or not they are scientifically accurate, such claims are taken seriously by WADA, and often these supplement marketing campaigns prompt a full investigation of the substance. Although there is yet to be a robust scientific study demonstrating any actual performance-enhancing characteristics of these commonly available supplements, WADA proactively supported research projects that led to putting ecdysterone on the monitoring programme, to gather information about the prevalence of the use of this substance in the athlete population. The use of thyroid hormones by athletes is another example of the perpetuation of misguided beliefs regarding the actions of these drugs in the athlete community. Circumstantial evidence indicates that thyroid hormone preparations are being abused by some athletes with the misconception that these drugs can reduce body weight. However, a number of studies [38, 39] have shown that thyroid hormones are actually not effective for weight loss. The use of low doses of thyroid hormones will ultimately not alter the circulating level of thyroid hormones and will have no impact on performance, and the use of high doses will induce toxic side effects, potentially life threatening, which would counter any possible improvement in performance.

Evolving the Prohibited List in Response
to Current Challenges

The Prohibited List is a constantly evolving document, and maintaining it is an ongoing process. New scientific literature and prevalence data is constantly monitored by WADA as it is published. An example of the ever-changing review of prohibited substances can be seen with the glucocorticoid category which have been prohibited during competition by oral, intravenous, intramuscular and rectal routes since 1985 when they were prohibited by the IOC and since 2004 by WADA under the World Anti-Doping Code. At the time of initial prohibition, their use by local injection into the joints (intra-articular) was not considered to result in systemic levels of the drugs that could be performance enhancing compared to the other prohibited routes of administration. One of the biggest challenges for laboratory analysis and results management over the years that followed was being able to differentiate the route of administration using the urine testing. Given these drugs are only banned during the in-competition period, a further challenge was to determine whether the drugs were administered inside or outside of the competition period. To address these challenges, WADA sponsored a number of scientific studies [40–42] with the aim of improving the accuracy of distinguishing systemic routes from other local routes of administration. These initial studies led to the finding that administration of permitted local injections of glucocorticoids resulted in urine levels similar to the existing prohibited routes, which presented the possibility of an Adverse Analytical Finding after permitted use, and a potential to achieve a performance-enhancing effect after a permitted local administration. This prompted WADA to convene a number of independent expert working groups to evaluate all the known evidence in the area, who confirmed that in fact local administration of glucocorticoids could lead to potentially performance-enhancing levels. This led to the decision in 2020 to ban all local injections of this class of drugs to be introduced in the January 2022 edition of the Prohibited List. Given the widespread use of these drugs as medical treatments, a 1-year delay was implemented so to allow time for appropriate education on the change to both athletes and the medical community and to develop guidelines on the use of glucocorticoids medically to avoid risk of a positive doping test through legitimate medical use. Occasionally, as new scientific evidence emerges, drugs are taken off the Prohibited List. An example of this is with the substance argon. In 2014, both xenon and argon were added to the List following evidence of abuse of xenon by Russian athletes [43, 44], and studies indicated that xenon increases erythropoietin (EPO) which encourages formation of red blood cells which can lead to performance enhancement. It was postulated that abuse of argon could have similar effects. However, argon was subsequently removed from the list in 2020 following re-evaluation by WADA who determined that it no longer met the criteria for inclusion, on the basis that it was unlikely to have any performance-enhancing properties similar to xenon and, in fact, the scientific opinion suggested that it could even be detrimental to performance.

Intelligence and Investigations to Uncover New Doping Substances

The work to gather new global intelligence on doping is ongoing and ever-evolving. In 2015, new provisions were included in the World Anti-Doping Code which provided WADA with the authority to initiate and undertake its own investigations, leading to the formation of the Pound Independent Commission and the McLaren Independent Investigation, which exposed widespread and systemic doping activities among Russian athletes. These changes to the Code were shortly followed by the launch of the WADA *Speak Up!* programme in 2017, providing a confidential route of communication to the WADA Intelligence and Investigations team to report concerns about potential anti-doping rule violations or misconduct. In conjunction with analytical and scientific activities, it now plays a critical role in gathering new insights into drug use and trafficking worldwide and actively initiates investigative approaches in response to allegations raised by informants and whistleblowers. Such information is closely followed by the WADA Prohibited List Expert Group to often determine the emergence of new doping substances. Keeping ahead of novel psychoactive substances specifically requires a truly global effort, and many collaborations with international drug and law enforcement agencies are in place to provide the greatest access and sharing of intelligence between organisations. One such collaboration is that of WADA and the United Nations Office on Drugs and Crime (UNODC). UNODC actively monitors emerging trends on new psychoactive substances, which are defined as substances of abuse that have become recently available and pose a potential public health threat, but are not currently controlled by international drug conventions. Such substances are often marketed as "legal highs", "research chemicals" or "herbal highs". In recent years, substances which have been identified through this partnership, and subsequently assessed by the WADA Prohibited List Expert Group for their abuse in sport, have included synthetic cannabinoids and novel hallucinogens and stimulants including synthetic cathinones, phencyclidine-type substances and phenethylamine derivatives. Through the UNODC Early Warning Advisory (EWA) on new psychoactive substances, WADA has access to a wealth of global prevalence data, chemical details and laboratory analytical methods which are used to proactively assess novel psychoactive substances in the doping context as soon as they are identified [45]. WADA also initiated a programme to monitor the appearance and distribution of new substances and products of concern on the Internet as illustrated in the operation Energia jointly conducted with Interpol and the École des Sciences Criminelles of the University of Lausanne, Switzerland.

Global Collaboration to Address the Challenges

The decision to ban a substance is complex and requires a matrix of data that collectively show the potential to enhance performance or harm to health. To keep ahead of the cheats, the approach to discovering new substances being abused in sport requires a sustained systematic approach at every step of the way. This is integral to how WADA undertakes the decision-making process for prohibiting drugs in sport, employing a multitude of investigative techniques to address the issues presented in an informed and evidence-based way. The mechanisms for determining the status of a drug involves comprehensive investigation of existing research to establish the known scientific facts about a substance, which could range from a simple literature search to requesting detailed unpublished clinical trial data from drug companies. If this does not yield the evidence required to understand how a substance works, WADA regularly initiates and funds further scientific research to fully understand the substance in question. Determining whether a substance is actually problematic as a doping agent in sport is also a key piece of the assessment for any new drug. WADA has a number of mechanisms to achieve this, from the global surveillance achieved through the Monitoring Program through to analysing drug information and prevalence data of actual use at major sporting events, to proactively acquire such substances and develop its assessment and analytical capabilities. An annual consultation process for the Prohibited List ensures that global stakeholders including national anti-doping organisations and government agencies around the world are actively engaged in the decision-making process for determining new doping substances. Once a substance is banned by WADA or an important change is made to the List, a strong and targeted communication and education campaign is essential to alert and inform the sporting community of the new status of the substance to ensure athletes and their support personnel can change their practices to ensure they do not fall foul of a doping offence. This is particularly well-illustrated with the significant change to the injectable glucocorticoid rules coming into force as of 1 January 2022 with an information campaign organised, which includes publication at the scientific and medical level, a communication campaign and educational tools to inform the athletes and their medical entourage. Strong alliances between the sports and anti-doping communities, science and research and the food and pharmaceutical industries, with the key support of public authorities, are essential to uncover and address the new challenges in doping worldwide. Global collaboration and the ability to achieve consensus decisions applicable worldwide are the most effective ways to overcome the biggest challenges faced in the fight against doping.

References

1. Broer T, Khodabukus A, Bursac N (2020) Can we mimic skeletal muscles for novel drug discovery? Expert Opin Drug Discov 15:643–645
2. Smith AST, Davis J, Lee G, Mack DL, Kim DH (2016) Muscular dystrophy in a dish: engineered human skeletal muscle mimetics for disease modeling and drug discovery. Drug Discov Today 21:1387–1398
3. Khodabukus A, Prabhu N, Wang J, Bursac N (2018) In vitro tissue-engineered skeletal muscle models for studying muscle physiology and disease. Adv Healthc Mater 7:e1701498
4. WADA and IFPMA strengthen collaboration in the protection of clean sport (2020). https://www.wada-ama.org/en/media/news/2020-07/wada-and-ifpma-strengthen-collaboration-in-the-protection-of-clean-sport
5. Wouters OJ, McKee M, Luyten J (2020) Estimated research and development investment needed to bring a new medicine to market, 2009–2018. JAMA 323:844–853
6. A tough road: cost to develop one new drug is $2.6 billion; approval rate for drugs entering clinical development is less than 12%. https://www.policymed.com/2014/12/a-tough-road-cost-to-develop-one-new-drug-is-26-billion-approval-rate-for-drugs-entering-clinical-de.html
7. Global Initiative for Asthma – GINA. https://ginasthma.org/
8. Bassiony MM et al (2015) Adolescent tramadol use and abuse in Egypt. Am J Drug Alcohol Abuse 41:206–211
9. Fawzi MM (2011) Some medicolegal aspects concerning tramadol abuse: the new Middle East youth plague 2010. An Egyptian overview. Egypt J Forensic Sci 1:99–102
10. Vernec A, Pipe A, Slack AA (2017) Painful dilemma? Analgesic use in sport and the role of anti-doping. Br J Sports Med 51:1243–1244
11. Mendelson JE et al (2008) The clinical pharmacology of intranasal l-methamphetamine. BMC Clin Pharmacol 8:4
12. Wilson E (2002) The Guardian. Speed freak
13. Yen CC et al (2020) Potential risk of higenamine misuse in sports: evaluation of lotus plumule extract products and a human study. Nutrients 12:285
14. Okano M, Sato M, Kageyama S (2017) Determination of higenamine and coclaurine levels in human urine after the administration of a throat lozenge containing Nandina domestica fruit. Drug Test Anal 9:1788–1793
15. UKAD. Issues warning regarding higenamine to athletes. https://www.ukad.org.uk/news/article/ukad-issues-warning-regarding-higenamine-to-athletes
16. Thevis M, Opfermann G, Schänzer W Urinary concentrations of morphine and codeine after consumption of poppy seeds. J Anal Toxicol 27(1):53–56. https://doi.org/10.1093/jat/27.1.53
17. Schobersberger W, Dünnwald T, Gmeiner G, Blank C (2017) Story behind meldonium-from pharmacology to performance enhancement: a narrative review. Br J Sports Med 51:22–25
18. Reuters Staff (2018) Factbox: five facts about meldonium. Reuters. https://www.reuters.com/article/us-olympics-2018-doping-fivefacts-factbo-idUSKCN1G20IT
19. Stuart M, Schneider C, Steinbach K (2016) Meldonium use by athletes at the Baku 2015 European games. Br J Sports Med 50:694–698
20. Oliynyk S, Oh S (2012) The pharmacology of actoprotectors: practical application for improvement of mental and physical performance. Biomol Ther 20(5):446–456. https://doi.org/10.4062/biomolther.2012.20.5.446
21. Ketobemidone (2006) Contributors to Wikimedia projects. https://en.wikipedia.org/wiki/Ketobemidone
22. Prescient & Strategic (P&S) Intelligence Private Limited, Global Sports Nutrition Market Size, Share, Development, Growth and Demand Forecast to 2022 - Industry Insights by Type (Sports Food, Sports Drinks, Sports Supplements), by Distribution Channel (Supermarkets and Hypermarkets, Convenience Stores, Drug Stores, Others). https://www.psmarketresearch.com/market-analysis/sports-nutrition-market

23. Sports nutrition market size, share & trends analysis report by product, by distribution channel, by region and segment forecasts, 2020–2027. https://www.reportlinker.com/p05741317/Sports-Nutrition-Market-Size-Share-Trends-Analysis-Report-By-Product-By-Distribution-Channel-By-Region-And-Segment-Forecasts.html?utm_source=GNW

24. National Center for Health Statistics (US) (2012) Health, United States, 2011: with special feature on socioeconomic status and health. National Center for Health Statistics (US)

25. 25 Days of Data – Day 18 – healthcare trends. http://www.kantar.media/QQqFaDF

26. Europe dietary supplements market size, trends. https://www.fortunebusinessinsights.com/industry-reports/europe-dietary-supplements-market-101918

27. Maughan RJ et al (2018) IOC Consensus Statement: Dietary Supplements and the High-Performance Athlete. Int J Sport Nutr Exerc Metab 28:104–125

28. Use of recreational drug 1,3-dimethylethylamine (DMAA) associated with cerebral hemorrhage (2012) https://doi.org/10.1016/j.annemergmed.2012.04.008

29. DMAA in products marketed as dietary supplements, FDA, August 2018 https://www.fda.gov/food/dietary-supplement-products-ingredients/dmaa-products-marketed-dietary-supplements

30. MHRA https://assets.publishing.service.gov.uk/government/uploads/system/uploads/attachment_data/file/404785/Final-determinations-Vol4_1_pdf

31. The TGA decision to ban DMAA. TGA, August, 2012 https://www.tga.gov.au/behind-news/tga-decision-ban-dmaa

32. Anvisa alert to risk of consumption of food supplement. July 2012 https://www.jurisway.org.br/en/article.asp?id_dh=8233

33. Stimulant Potentially Dangerous to Health, FDA Warns. FDA https://www.fda.gov/consumers/consumer-updates/stimulant-potentially-dangerous-health-fda-warns

34. Long J (2020) FDA supplements chief identifies 'regulatory gap'. Natural Products Insider. https://www.naturalproductsinsider.com/regulatory/fda-supplements-chief-identifies-regulatory-gap

35. FprEN 17444. https://standards.iteh.ai/catalog/standards/cen/d101ae80-5ba4-45cd-aa43-5971cb1cf1ee/fpren-17444

36. Therapeutic Goods Administration Press Release 24 September 2020 https://www.tga.gov.au/media-release/declaration-certain-sports-supplements-are-therapeutic-goods

37. Health Canada (2010) About natural health products. https://www.canada.ca/en/health-canada/services/drugs-health-products/natural-non-prescription/regulation/about-products.html#a2

38. Dubois S et al (2008) Thyroxine therapy in euthyroid patients does not affect body composition or muscular function. Thyroid 18:13–19

39. Roef G et al (2012) Body composition and metabolic parameters are associated with variation in thyroid hormone levels among euthyroid young men. Eur J Endocrinol 167:719–726

40. Criteria setting for the misuse of glucocorticosteroids (2020) Study LSDD-Lausanne. https://www.wada-ama.org/en/resources/research/criteria-setting-for-the-misuse-of-glucocorticosteroids-study-lsdd-lausanne

41. Improved methodology for detecting and confirming the abuse of glucocorticosteroids. (2014) https://www.wada-ama.org/en/resources/science-medicine/improved-methodology-for-detecting-and-confirming-the-abuse-of

42. Criteria setting for the misuse of glucocorticosteroids (2014) Study LNDD-Paris. https://www.wada-ama.org/en/resources/science-medicine/criteria-setting-for-the-misuse-of-glucocorticosteroids-study-lndd-paris

43. McGrath M (2014) Wada brings in ban on xenon and argon, but has no test. BBC News. https://www.bbc.com/news/science-environment-28970855

44. The Economist (2014) Breathe it in. https://www.economist.com/science-and-technology/2014/02/08/breathe-it-in

45. International monitoring of New Psychoactive Substances – The UNODC Early Warning Advisory on NPS. https://www.wada-ama.org/sites/default/files/resources/files/wada-levissianos-unodc.pdf. Accessed 21 Jan 2021

Epilogue

In writing this book on emerging drugs and novel psychoactive substances, we aimed at focusing on the perspective of sport, which, despite its unique specificities, represents only a microcosm of our global society. However, considering the dynamic and multifaceted nature of the subject, we feel that most of the considerations being made will find an appeal to a wider societal context beyond sport.

The athletic population is a fascinating subset of society to monitor, often heralding new trends to enhance human performance. Athletes are constantly looking for new methods to achieve higher scores, and they are very demanding on themselves and on their entourage. This obsession for constant improvement might lead to incorporate cutting-edge technologies or preparatory methods in their daily routines which might reach a culmination during high-level competitions, where years of dedication and sacrifices are played in one event, often on a few seconds of a lifetime. Deviations can inevitably accompany this desire to perform at the highest level of human abilities, despite the risks and damaging consequences that these might have at both the health and professional level.

The deliberate choice of this manuscript was to explore the various angles of the relationship between sport and drugs by inviting high-level contributors from various sectors of interest with the intention to generate as much resonance as possible and inform a diverse audience on the ever-changing threat posed by emerging drugs on "clean sport" and values.

From a purely technical standpoint, analytical science in the field of sport is not very different than in other cutting-edge analytical sectors. Similar principles of quality and rigor apply to the selected methods and ultimately to the interpretation of the results. Even if anti-doping requires a higher level of proof and certainty than in some other sectors of forensic or criminal science, the methods applied have to remain versatile to accommodate not only the variety of substances faced but also the novelty and the high level of specificity and sensitivity required. In other terms, the level of precautions and the mandatory standard of proof differ in the case of

O. Rabin, O. Corazza (eds.), *Emerging Drugs in Sport*, https://doi.org/10.1007/978-3-030-79293-0

sport making it often more challenging to sanction an athlete for doping than to condemn an individual for years in prison before a criminal court.

In this book, the latest analytical methods applied in the field of drug control in sport to unmask emerging drugs were covered from the perspective of anti-doping and forensic laboratories, also discussing how the use of alternative matrices to the traditional urine or blood fluids, such as hair analysis, can be incorporated to strengthen case adjudication but not without taking into account their limitations and the risk of misinterpretation of scientific information when presented before a court such as the Court of Arbitration for Sport.

Modern challenges in doping can take the form of innovative and promising therapeutic methods, such as gene and cell therapies deviated from their medical intent to become new doping methods. This challenge has been identified by anti-doping authorities almost 20 years ago and evolved from simply tracking a transgene to the more subtle DNA modifications recently generated by gene editing. Even if initially considered impossible by many, intense research in this field yielded some direct and indirect detection tools to reveal gene doping. While gene manipulation remains a preoccupation for anti-doping authorities, no serious indication of abuse in sport exist yet.

The court challenges, when science and law come into play to adjudicate doping cases, is an essential dynamic to the anti-doping system. Both fields nurture one another to bring the quintessence of facts and context before a case is adjudicated by a legal panel. This symbiosis between legal evidence and science is also well covered in the book with its strength in the current system but also some weaknesses that do represent opportunities for improvement in a system that constantly evolves. Integration of forensic logic or use of artificial intelligence, for example, will require intellectual agility from the non-scientists when such tools are more frequently used to resolve doping cases. It is essential to position the fight against doping in sport in a more global effort of curving down the current trend of increased consumption of illegal drug in our societies.

The authors strongly believe that consumption of natural or synthetic drugs without a proven medical need is not a recommendable path to a better and healthier society. Quite the contrary, their consumption should be seen as our societies falling short of providing satisfactory physical and mental environments to its individuals providing them with suitable environments to develop and grow harmoniously under their auspices. Various philosophical opinions stating that drugs enhance performance or make athletes feel better or that they should be made available freely to all-level athletes ignore the health risks and the loss of human lives due to drug use in sport or in other sectors of society. Just looking at the opioid crisis around the world gives us a scale of where inappropriate use of some pain medicines or of illegal opioids can take us. This book offered the floor to renown philosophers and allowed them to engage in an open discussion on the moral and ethical dimensions and consequences of drug use in sports.

Jointly, we feel it should be a collective endeavour to provide valuable alternatives that are compatible with moral and health rules collectively adopted and enforced. In essence, this is not a moral judgement but a call for giving more attention to the cause rather than the symptoms while identifying and providing more support to the most fragile individuals in our societies, and some athletes happen to be among them. Sport should be a conduct to a healthier lifestyle, not the opposite, and high-level athletes should continue to act as role models to fully deserve the iconic role that some are given today in our modern societies. Athletes cannot escape their societal responsibility.

As this book is written during the COVID-19 pandemic, the role played by each individual not to harm others should allow us to reflect in further depth on the impact of individualistic and selfish behaviours on our collective health. In the context of sport, where values and rules are inherent to the practice and also part of what makes the essence of sport practice with the purpose of enhancing human capabilities and skills to their best, it was of paramount importance for us to include in this book the experiences of athletes who were confronted with doping. It is rare to hear the reflections on doping directly from the athletes themselves and, despite the difficulty in collecting such direct and sincere testimonies, we were pleased that some of those contacted agreed to share their stories and provided their intimate convictions in an insightful way. Unfortunately, too few athletes agree to speak out and deny the benefit for themselves and for the athlete community to openly share their views.

Our system tends too often to ostracize doped athletes, when in reality we have to learn from them. Each doping story is different even if the fundamental context remains common. Yuliya Stepanova was trapped in a nationwide institutionalized doping system and could not escape this collective system until she turned into a whistleblower when meeting her future husband. She decided to sacrifice her Olympic dreams to tell the truth about being embedded into a doping programme as a female track and field athlete in Russia. Her dreams turned into an exile from her motherland. With Tyler Hamilton's testimony, we shift gears from nationwide doping to team doping. He was a prominent cyclist, a lieutenant of the infamous Lance Armstrong, and conquered an Olympic gold medal before seeing his dreams vanishing before his eyes when caught for blood transfusion a few days after receiving the Olympic laurels. He reflected on his years as a professional cyclist and took us deeper into the mindset from being a clean athlete to a doped athlete and how this decision accompanied him for years since such a decision was made in a few minutes in a hotel room. Quentin Bigot shared with us his experience on his years as a doped hammer thrower and how, after he was caught and sanctioned, he reinvented his approach to his sport and today competes clean at the highest international level.

This is an experience of doping taking us through the meanders of what an individual doping experience is and how you can come out of doping being stronger not only as an individual but also as an international athlete. All these experiences from collective doping to individual doping are a unique set of stories pointing at the imperative need to better inform and educate the athletes on the risks of doping, to better provide them with the tools to guide their choices when confronted with a doping situation. We heard from them that doping is not a fatality and doping takes its toll in mental and physical well-being shaping their lives in ways they did not intend. In this context, it was important to include the insights of an elite athlete who rejected doping when confronted with it. This was the case of Toby Atkins who agreed to share his experience and reflections on how his personal ethos led him to refuse performance-enhancing drugs when he was confronted with it as a professional cyclist. All these testimonies conclude unambiguously that you live better without doping than with doping as an athlete or as a human being during and after a sport career, because there is necessarily a life after sport.

Extreme behaviours vis-à-vis sport and association with drugs are well-illustrated by a selection of clinical cases encountered at the "Clinica Parco dei Tigli" in Padua (Italy), where behavioural disorders were treated for individuals whose insatiable passion for sport took them beyond the limits of physical and mental tolerance. The antipodes of sport values are reached when extreme self-perception leads to the negation of the health and sport benefits. Rules in sport are also, and often primarily, established to protect the health and well-being of the participants. Anti-doping rules are no exceptions.

A sector that benefited from a certain immunity vis-à-vis proper quality control remains the sector of dietary/nutritional supplements. The weak legislations in various countries permit the distribution of dietary supplements containing active principles that can create a significant health risk to unaware consumers. Analysis conducted in the anti-doping context constantly reveal the undisclosed presence of synthetic drugs in products advertised for various health reasons. In some cases, they even contain non-approved chemicals or legal medicines at therapeutic or even supra-therapeutic doses exposing the consumers to significant risks.

Some athletes have experienced positive doping tests because of the consumption of such contaminated or adulterated dietary supplements. Beyond sport, it should be considered as a serious public health issue that some highly unscrupulous manufacturers expose populations to pharmacologically active drugs, some of which are not even approved by regulatory drug agencies. About 15 years after WADA started to address this issue, it seems that some manufacturers have taken strong steps to ensure quality and traceability of their dietary supplements; unfortunately, in the context of weak legislations or easy access on the Internet, some manufacturers continue to supply risky products to the athletic population and to the general public. Facing such a large-scale issue, we start seeing countries such as Australia and some European countries taking the matter seriously and recently raising legislative and administrative barriers to the importation and distribution of such products. As advocated by WADA many years ago, one can come out of the current preoccupying situation only by combining strong legislation, adequate quality controls of the end products and serious sanctions for the manufacturers or distributors that do not rigorously ensure that their products are absolutely safe for human consumption.

Analytical science applied to anti-doping have made great progress over the past few years. Judging by the number of cases reported after the Olympic Games during re-analysis campaign notably conducted by the International Olympic Committee, tens of doping cases were reported long after the Olympic medals were distributed on the podiums and the fireworks ceased above the Olympic stadiums. Strong integration of investigation capacity and science knowledge in the anti-doping field only starts to reveal its potential and will likely grow in the coming years. Various initiatives are currently being developed to strengthen these joint activities, and the book lifted the veil on some of the most recent operations. This illustrates how the anti-doping system evolved from a passive mode to a more *proactive* role. This book incorporates such a shift by offering a unique set of testimonies from people who are in the first line of law enforcement operations aiming to disrupt illegal drug manufacturing and distribution around the world. Operations have multiplied over recent years at the national level, and we can read about the situation in Italy, which is often perceived as an entry door of drugs into Europe, to a more international level involving Europol and Interpol to dismantle large crime organizations operating on a worldwide scale. It is reassuring to note that such broad operations against PEDs or other counterfeit drugs are gaining interest in many countries as use or trafficking of such drugs is taken more seriously and sometimes criminalized by some countries. It is a trend that is likely to increase in the coming years as cooperation of international police and custom forces becomes more efficient and rewarding in terms of concrete results of dismantling trafficking networks around the world.

Use and abuse of drugs in society existed for decades and will certainly continue to permeate in our societies for many years. Time is now that we collaborate more to inform, educate and protect population at risk. Facing the scale of this issue, no organization has sufficient resources or competence to address the issue in its complex globality. Beyond intersectorial collaborations, partnerships between international organizations with a vested interest in better controlling drugs of abuse are mandatory when facing organized crime activities which have long bypassed border controls. It is by combining the efforts and knowledge of strong official actors in the field and in the mutualization of their respective resources that we will be able to provide the level of scientific knowledge and scale of field operations that will create an efficient level of disruption to organized crime around the world. However, combining our efforts to a multiple angle approach and combining our efforts and resources whenever possible should allow us to collectively limit progression of those drugs and hopefully regain a form of control in the protection of the most vulnerable individuals.

WADA has established this activity within its walls, and it now relies upon partners such as UNODC, WHO, Europol, World Customs Organization and others to exchange information and develop our knowledge and capacity while mapping out networks of illegal activities to disrupt criminal organizations and strike at the heart of their systems in both sport and societal environments. Scientists also intensify their collaborations and sharing of knowledge as exemplified by the annual Conference on Novel Psychoactive Substances and the recently created International Society for the Study of Emerging Drugs (ISSED). Multilevel collaborations supported by a strong network of expertise will certainly lead to more efficient operations in the field with more disruptive effects on illegal drug manufacturing and distribution.

This book presents a snapshot of the situation as we observe and analyse it at the beginning of this new decade. It was not structured with the intention to be an exhaustive overview of the phenomenon but rather to share selected insights on the complexities and practicalities of doping in sport with ramifications on drug use in society. Written by high-level contributors who act daily at the heart of the system, it is aimed at being an invitation for readers to discover more on the various subjects covered in an engaging way. It includes views, daily challenges and strategies and anticipates trends for the future as foreseen by leaders in the field. Numerous challenges do exist and will continue to exist for some time. But knowing the level of commitment by some actors in the regulation and the law enforcement sides, these factors act more as strong stimulators and ultimately as drivers for collective progress than anything else. By intelligently addressing our individual and collective shortfalls, remaining critical on our failures and successes and aiming at developing novel creative solutions, in a few years from now, we will generate that change in the playing field that athletes and sport fans will be able to appreciate across different sports and countries. We will carry on working with and convincing public and sport authorities that doping and the protection of the health of athletes deserve full consideration. We have already made significant progress over the past two decades or so, and without claiming that doping can be forever eradicated, we can now set a more reasonable goal that doping can be reduced to a level having limited or no significant impact in sport and that those who decide to dope, whatever their motivation may be, are unlikely to continue unpunished and will have, one day or another, to face sport and human justice.

For those of us who wish to preserve the values embedded in sports, the dreams of children who want to become athletes, like their favourite heroes on television or in gaming, and ultimately the health of those practising sport at all levels, we have a collective duty to educate and to preserve some societal ideals in a world where the temptation to cheat is constant and the moral values of some public figures are often doubtful. Sport is a wonderful school not only for children to develop and learn but also for adults in their personal and collective accomplishments. This is certainly why some unique set of rules were created specifically for drugs in sports and have to be adhered to by all. Let us ensure that we collectively preserve those values that have been fundamental in the perdurance and the development of our societies.

Index

Printed in the United States
by Baker & Taylor Publisher Services